Addiction Medicine

Addiction Medicine

Editor: James Burke

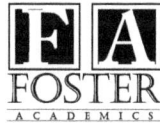

FOSTER
ACADEMICS

www.fosteracademics.com

www.fosteracademics.com

FA
FOSTER
ACADEMICS

Cataloging-in-Publication Data

Addiction medicine / edited by James Burke.
     p. cm.
Includes bibliographical references and index.
ISBN 978-1-63242-793-9
     1. Drug abuse--Treatment. 2. Substance abuse--Treatment. 3. Drug addiction.
4. Addicts--Medical care. I. Burke, James.
RC564 .A23 2019
616.86--dc23

Foster Academics,
118-35 Queens Blvd., Suite 400,
Forest Hills, NY 11375, USA

ISBN 978-1-63242-793-9 (Hardback)

Contents

Preface

The medical specialty which deals with the treatment of addiction is known as addiction medicine. It often overlaps with other areas, like mental health counseling, public health, psychiatry, psychology, internal medicine, etc. Acute intervention, detoxification, abstinence-based treatment, rehabilitation, harm reduction and individual and group therapies, are some of the common therapies that fall under addiction medicine. Relapse prevention is an important aspect in the treatment of substance abuse, especially alcoholism. Supportive psychotherapy and interpersonal therapy are extremely effective treatments for substance abuse. This book unravels the recent studies in the field of addiction medicine. It includes some of the vital pieces of work being conducted across the world, on various topics related to addiction medicine. Doctors, researchers and students actively engaged in this field will find this book full of crucial and unexplored concepts.

After months of intensive research and writing, this book is the end result of all who devoted their time and efforts in the initiation and progress of this book. It will surely be a source of reference in enhancing the required knowledge of the new developments in the area. During the course of developing this book, certain measures such as accuracy, authenticity and research focused analytical studies were given preference in order to produce a comprehensive book in the area of study.

This book would not have been possible without the efforts of the authors and the publisher. I extend my sincere thanks to them. Secondly, I express my gratitude to my family and well-wishers. And most importantly, I thank my students for constantly expressing their willingness and curiosity in enhancing their knowledge in the field, which encourages me to take up further research projects for the advancement of the area.

Editor

Substance use disorder treatment retention and completion: a prospective study of horse-assisted therapy (HAT) for young adults

Ann Kern-Godal[1*], Espen Ajo Arnevik[1,2], Espen Walderhaug[1] and Edle Ravndal[3]

Abstract

Background: Keeping substance use disorder patients actively engaged in treatment is a challenge. Horse-assisted therapy (HAT) is increasingly used as a complementary therapy, with claimed motivational and other benefits to physical and psychological health. This naturalistic study aimed to assess HAT's impact on the duration and completion of treatment for young substance users at Oslo University Hospital.

Methods: Discharge and other data were derived from the Youth Addiction Treatment Evaluation Project (YATEP) database for patients (n = 108) admitted during an 18-month period. An intention-to-treat design, and univariate and multivariate analyses were used to compare those receiving treatment as usual (n = 43) with those who received treatment as usual plus HAT (n = 65).

Results: Despite a lack of randomization, the baseline characteristics of the two groups were similar. However, more HAT participants completed treatment (56.9 vs 14 %, p < 0.001), remained in treatment for longer (mean 141 vs 70 days, p < 0.001) and had a significantly higher chance of completing their treatment than those not given the HAT program. Excluding time in treatment, and after controlling for the potentially confounding influence of age, sex, education, number and severity of substances used, psychological distress and number of temporary exits, the adjusted odds ratio for treatment completion was 8.4 in the HAT group compared with those not participating in HAT (95 % CI 2.7–26.4, p < 0.001).

Conclusion: The study found a statistically significant association between HAT participation and time in treatment, and between HAT participation and completion of treatment. This association does not infer causality. However, it adds supporting evidence for the development of an innovative therapy, and warrants investment in further research in relation to its inclusion in substance use disorder treatment.

Keywords: Addiction, Substance use, Treatment completion, Duration of treatment, Dropout, Horse-assisted therapy (HAT), Equine-assisted psychotherapy (EAP), Alternative/complementary treatment

Background

Retention in treatment improves the prognosis for substance use disorder patients [1–3]. Early dropouts are reported to have the same outcome as untreated patients [3]. There have been four major reviews of dropout from addiction and substance use disorder treatment [3–6], and these involve more than 500 studies undertaken over almost 40 years. They report that despite wide diversity in treatment methods [7], patient failure to complete therapy (usually referred to as dropout) often exceeds 50 %. Completion of treatment is associated with successful outcomes [3, 4, 8, 9]. The optimal duration of treatment is debatable and may depend upon the treatment method [10], but 90 days is often identified as the minimum time period for effective treatment [2, 3, 11–13]. In addition, many substance use patients exit treatment for various reasons and then re-enter treatment after varying periods of absence [3, 4, 13]. There is a continuous struggle to find

*Correspondence: ann@godal.com
[1] Department of Addiction Treatment, Oslo University Hospital, Sognsvannsveien 21, Building 22, 0424 Oslo, Norway
Full list of author information is available at the end of the article

treatment modalities that motivate patients to remain for sufficient time to enable beneficial change in morbidity [10]. Treatment factors such as method, staff–patient alliance and interaction, and satisfaction, although less frequently studied, have been found to be among the best predictors of outcome [6]. Reported studies of alternative or complementary treatment methods are rare [14], including those for substance use disorders.

Horse (or equine)-assisted/facilitated therapy is an innovative complementary approach to psychotherapy that actively involves horses or other equines in the therapeutic process. Challenges in this rapidly developing field of experimental therapy include increasing the provision of a high-cost therapy, which is often of unknown quality, to vulnerable population groups with little substantiating evidence of associated benefits [15].

Since the 1990s, there has been a dramatic increase in the number of equine programs that claim to provide psychotherapy and/or education and development. However, equine-assisted/facilitated psychotherapy is still very much in an evolutionary phase, lacking a generally accepted theoretical framework. There is a variety of emerging schools of thought, approaches and terminology [16–18]. The term horse-assisted therapy (HAT) is used in this paper.

A review of the literature and media relating to psychotherapy involving horses has revealed a growing number of studies and "opinion-based" material in the psychosocial area with a variety of factors at play, including motivation. These include claims that the size, strength, warmth, body language and herd behavior of horses can be used with therapeutic benefit when working with clients who are mistrusting, depressed and anxious [16, 18–21], or who lack the boundary setting or other skills needed to deal with everyday living [22, 23] or who have issues related to self-esteem, self-efficacy or resilience [24, 25]. In addition, there are claims that the horse "mirrors" the patient and provides immediate, honest feedback, untainted by the usual human and social constraints [16, 21], and that the horse can promote trust in vulnerable clients, particularly those with traumatic backgrounds [20, 26]. Dell and colleagues refer to the importance of the horse's consistency, and nonverbal and nonjudgmental relationship with Inuit youth undergoing substance abuse treatment [27]. In general, the horse is reported to be a motivational force for treatment [28–30].

However, the studies are usually small and rarely documented in an adequate or systematic format. There have been two published systematic reviews of peer-reviewed literature of psychotherapeutic programs involving horses [15, 31]. The first reviewed material in 16 databases, identifying 103 studies, of which 14 met the selection criteria. Only two of these were rated as having evidence of (moderate) effectiveness [31]. The second, in mid-2014, reviewed 14 studies identified from a more restricted search and found that all 14 were compromised by threats to validity. The authors concluded that psychotherapy involving equines should not be marketed but that research should continue with improved methodology [15]. Since then, findings from a randomized controlled study have been published. The study found that long-term psychiatric patients at risk of violence responded positively to a program of equine-assisted psychotherapy [32].

Many horse centers offer therapy for substance use, or addiction programs [33], but few studies are reported. We found nine specific HAT and substance use disorder-related papers or theses, only one of which was in a peer-reviewed journal [27]. None of them met the inclusion criteria for the two systematic reviews.

Most reported studies of HAT, including those relating to substance use and addiction, conclude with a recommendation for further research. However, few HAT programs have the resources, patient numbers, diagnostic homogeneity, or the research capacity and skills required.

In 2010, Oslo University Hospital's Department of Addiction Treatment—Youth provided a unique research opportunity to study HAT. It had approximately 100 new patients per year with a primary diagnosis of substance use and/or addiction. In addition, it had 37 years' experience of HAT in a residential psychiatric setting [22]. Since 2010, the hospital's resident herd of five specially selected and trained horses has worked exclusively with the department's young patients in a structured, substance use disorder-relevant program of HAT.

As far as we are aware, this is the first peer-reviewed quantitative study of the inclusion of HAT in a substance use disorder treatment program. Our objective was to assess whether HAT patients remained in treatment longer and were more likely to complete their agreed program of treatment. We hypothesized that HAT participation was associated with both longer time in treatment and completion of treatment.

Methods

The study covered an 18-month treatment period from January 1, 2011. It was part of a larger, ongoing, mixed-methods project to investigate the impact of HAT on substance use disorder treatment outcomes.

Patient participation was voluntary. All necessary patient consent and data inspection authority approvals were obtained as part of the Youth Addiction Treatment Evaluation Project (YATEP). The study was reviewed and approved by the Norwegian Regional Committee for Medical Research Ethics, and performed according to their guidelines and the Helsinki Declaration.

Patients

The study sample comprised inpatients and day patients admitted between January 1, 2011 and June 30, 2012 to the Department of Addiction Treatment—Youth at Oslo University Hospital. The department treats men and women aged 16–26 years (but patients up to 35 years of age may be accepted) who have a primary diagnosis of mental and behavioral disorders due to psychoactive substance use (ICD 10). One hundred eleven patients entered treatment during the 18-month period. Three patients were discharged to other institutions for ongoing treatment, leaving 108 patients in the study.

Study design

At entry to treatment, all participating patients who had provided written informed consent were registered in the YATEP database. Recording usually started in the first week. The database comprises basic patient information, psychological tests, discharge status, and HAT participation data. Additional patient demographic, morbidity and treatment information, plus the dates of any temporary exit from treatment, can be drawn from the hospital's electronic patient journal when required and matched anonymously to the YATEP database records. All individuals were followed from treatment entry to discharge.

Measures

The study outcomes were: (1) completion of treatment (primary outcome), (2) time in treatment (measured using number of treatment days), and (3) completion of 90 days of treatment or more (included because it is often identified as a critical period for effective treatment [2, 3, 11–13]).

Discharge status was categorized as (1) treatment completed, or (2) dropout. Treatment completed was defined as staying in treatment for the duration of the recommended treatment plan. This was determined by examining the YATEP discharge report and the clinician's journal record. Those who left the program but returned within a 30 day period to continue with the remainder of the treatment course were considered to have completed treatment. Leaving the program but returning within a 30 day period was termed "temporary exit." The number of days of temporary exit was excluded from the total treatment days at discharge. Dropout was defined as patient initiated treatment termination, or expulsion for rule violation prior to completing the agreed treatment period.

Psychological distress was measured using the Hopkins Symptom Check List 25 (HSCL-25), which is one of the assessment items in the YATEP. It consists of 25 questions that map respondents' anxiety and depression [34]. It is scored on a scale from 1 (not bothered) to 4 (extremely bothered). The form is frequently used in Norwegian research projects with 1.75 as the risk cutoff in normal Norwegian populations [35]. In the analysis for this study, HSCL-25 was used as an indicator of psychological distress.

Severity of substances used was categorized as more severe [heroin, amphetamine, benzodiazepine, gamma hydroxybutyrate (or GHB) and cocaine] or less severe (cannabis and alcohol).

Treatment as usual (TAU)

The treatment site is part of the specialist health care system in Norway. Patients are referred by general practitioners and specialists or from other hospital departments. They must have a primary diagnosis of mental and behavioral disorders due to psychoactive substance use (ICD 10). The social services authority has oversight of this process. The treatment is a person-centered program which comprises individual and group therapy based on a biopsychosocial model with emphasis on mentalization-based theory and practice [36]. An individual treatment plan, which includes treatment goals, is prepared in cooperation with each patient. Medical treatment is offered, as well as assistance/counselling for accommodation, education, employment, living, adjustment and support. Psychological treatment is tailored to the individual's specific problems and treatment goals. The likely duration of treatment is decided with the patient as part of the treatment plan, in accordance with their needs. It can include movement between units, such as from inpatient to day patient. In the day unit, as patients become more established in school, work or a domestic situation, the therapist gradually reduces contact until discharge.

The HAT intervention

HAT is an integral part of the department's program of addiction treatment [37]. It comprises $12 \times$ 90-min sessions of body-orientated psychotherapy with horses. The animals have been selected and trained for this work to be strong, secure, responsive and interactive. Patients and staff are insured against injury by the hospital. Serious incidents and injuries must be recorded.

All patients are eligible to participate in HAT, but must be referred by their treating clinician. The referral can be requested by the patient or suggested by the clinician. A final decision on suitability and the treatment objectives of the individual's HAT participation (for example, to strengthen boundary setting, or reduce anxiety, depression or aggression, etc.) are agreed at a preparatory meeting between the HAT therapist, the patient and the clinician. Patients have the opportunity to meet the horses and become involved in care activities (such as feeding) from their first day in treatment. They normally start the HAT program within 2–3 weeks. HAT therapists become part of the patient's clinical team, with full access to the patient's clinical record. Patients are encouraged to attend and participate fully but can choose not to undertake an activity, such as mounted work. Specific activities, level of participation and response at each HAT session are recorded by the HAT therapists in the patient's electronic hospital journal.

The sessions are planned and provided by two qualified therapists who are also Norwegian Level 1 Riding Instructors. The program design is structured for small groups (maximum four participants per session), but includes provision for individual work on specific needs if required. It involves a three-way interactive (positive triangulated) process in which the patient works in emotional safety with the horse on activities selected with his/her therapist to address agreed goals. During sessions, the horse will respond naturally to environmental factors (for example, the proximity of other horses, or a sudden loud noise). Similarly, it will react to the physical and emotional state of the patient (for example, a request lacking focus or clarity is unlikely to produce the desired movement from the horse, and an aggressive request may be met with resistance). The therapist, in leading the process, can both read and influence the horse, and provide reflective feedback to the patient on the relationship, reactions and responses between the horse and patient.

Activities can involve any combination of herd behavior observation, stable duties, and ground, mounted and/or driving work with the horses. Observation of the herd can promote discussion of social interaction and relationships and stable duties promote responsibility, routine and reliability. Groundwork is used to address issues relating to boundaries/contact, anxiety/trust, communication/connection, mastery (of new skills, the horse and self), body awareness and focus. Mounted work addresses posture, balance/centering, coordination, rhythm/regulation, mastering of anxiety and focus. Carriage driving can be used to promote forward thinking and outlook, and, with other passengers, it can engender a sense of empowerment, group responsibility and care. These activities involve good healthy exercise, having fun, and learning new skills. However, while physical exercise, fun and skill acquisition are important, the prime purpose of this program is therapy and contribution to successful treatment.

The focus of the first four sessions is on getting to know about horses, herd behavior, basic handling and safety. The following eight sessions are tailored to meet the individual's therapy objectives using a range of group and individual ground-based, mounted or driving exercises as outlined in the stable manual (unpublished).

The HAT program has been developed at Oslo University Hospital over time, largely by Lysell [22], a qualified and experienced body-oriented psychotherapist. It also draws on theoretical and practice material from a number of relevant equine-assisted therapy schools [16, 20, 38–42]. It uses many of the usual equine-assisted/facilitated therapy exercises but places stronger emphasis on those relevant to substance use disorders, such as boundary setting, development of trust and control of emotional affect. It differs from most other horse therapy programs in two aspects. First, the patients have responsibility for the horses after hours, giving greater emphasis on care, routine, reliability and responsibility (all relevant to substance use recovery). Second, after the four introductory sessions, the HAT program does not follow a sequenced routine. Rather, specific activities and therapeutic processing are targeted at individual patient needs and are sequenced at appropriate points throughout the patient's HAT program.

HAT treatment outcome is not assessed per se. It is included as part of the patient's overall treatment outcome assessment, as measured by change in the YATEP psychological instruments and, in particular, by whether individuals complete their agreed substance use treatment program.

Statistical analysis

In this naturalistic, intention-to-treat study, univariate and multivariate analyses were used to assess the relationship between treatment completion and HAT plus a range of patient factors (gender, age, education, number and severity of substances used, psychological distress and number of temporary exits). We included time in treatment as an additional outcome measure. It is assessed using univariate analysis of both the mean (113 days) and the reported critical minimum period for effective treatment (90 days). However, we excluded time in treatment from the logistic regression because of the obvious relationship between longer time in treatment and treatment completion.

Pearson Chi squared and independent-samples t test were used to test the relationship between discharge status and HAT. Odds ratio (OR) was used to test the strength of the relationship. Potential confounding variables relating to the patient (age, sex, education, number and severity of substances used, and psychological distress), time in treatment (mean time and temporary exits) and HAT participation were controlled for using logistic regression analysis. Linear and other interactive associations were checked. SPSS Version 21 (IBM Corp., Armonk, NY, USA) was used.

Results

Study participants' characteristics

The study involved 108 individuals: 78 males and 30 females (27.8 %). At the time of entry to treatment, 14 (13.0 %) were aged less than 20 years, 74 (68.5 %) were 20–26 years and 20 (18.5 %) were aged 27 years or older (Table 1). The mean age (results not shown) was 23.1 years (range 17–33 years, SD = 3.4). Females (mean 22.9 years, SD = 3.5) were slightly, but not significantly, younger than males. None of the patients were under legal mandate to remain in treatment.

In the 6 months prior to intake, 32.4 % of the 108 patients had used a single drug, 28.7 % had used two drugs and 39.9 % had used three or more drugs. Cannabis was the most commonly used primary drug (38.9 %), followed by alcohol (18.5 %), amphetamine + cocaine (15.8 %), heroin (15.7 %) and other drugs (11.1 %). The average age of first use of the primary drug was 17 years, (results not shown) with 52.8 % of all patients being 15 years or younger when they first used their primary drug (Table 1).

At referral, all patients had a primary diagnosis of mental and behavioral disorders due to psychoactive substance use (ICD 10). Fifty-eight (53.7 %) of the patients were reported to have no psychiatric comorbid condition, 34 (31.5 %) had one, and 16 (14.8 %) had two or more. The most common of the comorbid conditions (results not shown) were behavioral disorders (36.2 %), followed by neurotic/stress (including post-traumatic stress disorder) disorders (34.8 %), mood disorders (20.3 %) and other disorders (8.7 %). Approximately 1 week after entry, 89 (82.4 %) patients' first Hopkins Symptom Check List 25 (HSCL-25) scores were equal to or above the psychosocial risk cutoff. Sixteen patients (14.8 %) were prescribed substitution medicine (15 buprenorphine, 1 methadone) during all or part of their treatment (Table 1).

HAT participation

Forty-three patients (39.8 %) received treatment as usual (non-HAT group) and 65 (60.2 %) had treatment as usual plus HAT (HAT intervention group). The intervention was well tolerated with no reported adverse treatment effect or injury arising from HAT. None of the patients were withdrawn from HAT for clinical reasons.

Although this was a naturalistic study, there were no major differences in baseline characteristics between the HAT group and the non-HAT group. However, significantly more HAT participants were aged 27 years or more (24.6 vs 9.3 %, p = 0.03) and their average age was slightly older than non-HAT participants (mean 23.7 years, SD = 3.4 vs mean 22.1 years, SD = 3.2, p < 0.02) (results not shown). They were also more likely than non-HAT

participants to have one or more temporary exits from treatment (49.2 vs 25.6 %, p = 0.05) (Table 1).

Thirty-seven (56.9 %) of HAT participants completed their treatment compared with only six (14.0 %) of non-HAT participants, p < 0.001 (Table 1).

Time in treatment

Days in treatment ranged from 1 to 555, (mean 113, SD = 92.7). Twenty-six (24.0 %) of the 108 patients remained in treatment for less than 30 days, 49 (21.3 %) for 30–89 days and 59 (54.6 %) for 90 days or more (results not shown). Forty-eight (44.4 %) remained in treatment for the mean 113 days or more, and 33 (76.7 %) of those completed treatment (Table 2).

HAT participants remained in treatment for a significantly longer period (p < 0.001) than those who did not participate in HAT (mean 141 days, SD = 93.6, vs mean 70 days, SD = 73.8). They were almost four times more likely to remain in treatment for 90 days or more (OR 3.9 CI 1.7–8.8, p = 0.001) (results not shown).

Treatment discharge status

At discharge, 43 (39.8 %) of the 108 patients in the study had completed treatment and 65 (60.3 %) had dropped out. Treatment completion was significantly associated with only HAT participation [χ^2 (1,108) = 19.9, p < 0.001] and length of time in treatment {for both mean days in treatment [χ^2 (1,108) = 30.2, p < 0.001] and the critical 90 days period [χ^2 (1,108) = 32.8, p < 0.001] (Table 2)}.

Prediction of treatment completion

Apart from the length of time in treatment, HAT participation was the only significant univariate predictor of treatment completion (OR 8.2, CI 3.0–22.0, p < 0.001) (results not shown). Excluding time in treatment, and after controlling for the potentially confounding influence of age, sex, education, number and severity of substances used, psychological distress and temporary exits, the adjusted odds ratio for HAT participants completing treatment was 8.4 (95 % CI 2.7–26.4, p < 0.001), (Table 3).

Discussion

This study found a statistically significant association between HAT participation and longer time in treatment, and between HAT participation and completion of treatment. Although not direct measures of substance use, both duration and completion of treatment are reported in previous studies to be predictors of positive treatment outcome for substance use disorders [3, 4, 8, 9].

Length of time in treatment was the strongest predictor of treatment completion. This is consistent with

Table 1 Comparison of patient characteristics: treatment as usual (not-horse assisted therapy) with intervention group (treatment as usual plus horse assisted therapy)

Variable	Item	Not-HAT[a] N = 43	HAT[a] N = 65	Total N = 108	% 100	Chi square
Discharge status	Dropped out	37 (86.0)	28 (43.1)	65	60.2	19.94, p < 0.001
	Completed	6 (14.0)	37 (56.9)	43	39.8	
Days in treatment						
Mean	<113 days	32 (74.4)	28 (43.1)	57	55.6	10.30, p = 0.001
	113+ days	11 (25.6)	37 (56.9)	51	44.4	
Critical period	<90 days	28 (65.1)	21 (32.3)	49	45.4	11.24, p = 0.001
	90+ days	15 (34.9)	44 (67.7)	59	54.6	
Gender	Female	8 (18.6)	22 (33.8)	30	27.8	2.10, p = 0.083
	Male	35 (81.4)	43 (66.2)	78	72.2	
Age	<20 years	9 (20.9)	5 (7.7)	14	13	6.80, p = 0.034
	20–26 years	30 (69.8)	44 (67.7)	74	68.5	
	27+ years	4 (9.3)	16 (24.6)	20	18.5	
Years of schooling	<10 years	7 (16.3)	11 (16.9)	18	16.7	2.42, p = 0.298
	10–12 years	31 (72.1)	39 (60.0)	70	64.8	
	13+ years	5 (11.6)	15 (23.1)	20	18.5	
Primary substance	Cannabis	20 (46.5)	22 (33.8)	42	38.9	6.31, p = 0.389
	Alchol	6 (14.0)	14 (21.5)	20	18.5	
	Heroin	6 (14.0)	11 (16.9)	17	15.7	
	Amphetamine	4 (9.3)	11 (16.9)	15	13.9	
	Benzodiazepine	3 (7.0)	5 (7.7)	8	7.4	
	GHB[b]	2 (4.7)	2 (3.1)	4	3.7	
	Cocaine	2 (4.7)	0 (0.0)	2	1.9	
No. of substances	1 substances	12 (27.9)	23 (35.4)	35	32.4	0.82, p = 0.662
	2 substances	14 (32.6)	17 (26.2)	31	28.7	
	3 substances	17 (39.5)	25 (38.5)	42	38.9	
Age of first use	<16 years	25 (58.1)	32 (49.2)	57	52.8	0.82, p = 0.364
	16+ years	18 (41.9)	33 (50.8)	51	47.2	
HSCL-25[c]	<1.75	9 (20.9)	10 (15.4)	19	17.6	0.55, p = 0.459
	1.75+	34 (79.1)	55 (84.6)	89	82.4	
Subsitution medicine[d]	No	38 (88.4)	54 (83.1)	92	85.2	0.58, p = 0.450
	Yes	5 (11.6)	11 (16.9)	16	14.8	
Psych. co-morbidity (at entry)	None diagnosed	21 (48.8)	37 (56.9)	58	53.7	1.10, p = 0.580
	1 diagnosed	16 (37.2)	18 (27.7)	34	31.5	
	2+ diagnosed	6 (14.0)	10 (15.4)	16	14.8	
Temporary exit	No exit	32 (74.4)	33 (50.8)	65	60.2	6.10, p = 0.05
	1 re-entry	6 (14.0)	18 (27.7)	24	22.3	
	2+ re-entries	5 (11.6)	14 (21.5)	19	17.6	

[a] Not horse assisted therapy/horse assisted therapy

[b] Gamma hydroxybutyrate ($C_4H_8O_3$)

[c] Hopkins Symptom Checklist-25

[d] Opioid pharmacotherapy

previously reported studies [1, 3, 13], but it may hide the influence of other patient or treatment variables [4, 10], such as HAT in our study. The optimal duration of treatment is debatable and may depend upon the individual needs of the patient and the type of treatment method [10]. However, 90 days is often identified as the minimum period for effective treatment [2, 3, 11–13].

HAT participants were significantly more likely than non-HAT participants to remain in treatment for 90 days or more and to complete their treatment.

Table 2 Comparison of discharge status: dropout or completed by patient characteristics

Variable	Item	Dropout N = 65	Completed N = 43	Total N = 108	% 100	Chi square
Participation in HAT	No	37 (56.9)	6 (14.0)	43	39.8	19.94, p < 0.001
	Yes	28 (43.1)	37 (86.0)	65	60.2	
Days in treatment						
Mean	<113 days	50 (76.9)	10 (23.3)	60	55.6	30.18, p < 0.001
	113+ days	15 (23.1)	33 (76.7)	48	44.4	
Critical period	<90 days	44 (67.7)	5 (11.6)	49	45.4	32.82, p < 0.001
	90+ days	21 (32.3)	38 (88.4)	59	54.6	
Gender	Female	16 (24.6)	14 (32.6)	30	27.8	0.81, p = 0.367
	Male	49 (75.4)	29 (67.4)	78	72.2	
Age	<20 years	12 (18.5)	2 (4.7)	14	13	4.81, p = 0.090
	20–26 years	43 (66.2)	31 (72.3)	74	68.5	
	27+ years	10 (15.4)	10 (23.3)	20	18.5	
Years of schooling	<10 years	13 (20.0)	5 (11.6)	18	16.7	1.96, p = 0.376
	10–12 years	42 (64.6)	28 (65.1)	70	64.8	
	13+ years	10 (15.4)	10 (23.3)	20	18.5	
Primary substance	Cannabis	23 (35.4)	19 (44.2)	42	38.9	4.75, p = 0.577
	Alchol	14 (21.5)	6 (14.0)	20	18.5	
	Heroin	12 (18.5)	5 (11.6)	17	15.7	
	Amphetamine	7 (10.8)	8 (18.6)	15	13.9	
	Benzodiazepine	5 (7.7)	3 (7.0)	8	7.4	
	GHB[a]	2 (3.1)	2 (4.7)	4	3.7	
	Cocaine	2 (3.1)	0 (0.0)	2	1.9	
No. of substances	1 substances	20 (30.8)	15 (34.9)	35	32.4	0.15, p = 0.292
	2 substances	16 (24.6)	15 (34.9)	31	28.7	
	3 substances	29 (44.6)	13 (30.2)	42	38.9	
Age of first use	<16 years	35 (53.8)	22 (51.2)	57	52.8	0.08, p = 0.785
	16+ years	30 (46.2)	21 (48.8)	51	47.2	
Substitution medicine[b]	No	55 (84.6)	37 (86.0)	92	85.2	0.42, p = 0.840
	Yes	10 (15.4)	6 (14.0)	16	14.8	
HSCL-25[c]	<1.75	12 (18.5)	7 (16.3)	19	17.6	0.09, p = 0.771
	1.75+	53 (81.5)	36 (83.7)	89	82.4	
Psych co-morbidity (at entry)	None diagnosed	32 (49.2)	26 (60.5)	58	53.7	2.25, p = 0.325
	1 diagnosed	24 (36.9)	10 (23.3)	34	31.5	
	2+ diagnosed	9 (13.8)	7 (16.3)	16	14.8	
Temporary exit	No exit	42 (64.6)	23 (53.5)	65	60.2	1.87, p = 0.393
	1 re-entry	14 (21.5)	10 (23.3)	24	22.3	
	2+ re-entries	9 (13.8)	10 (23.3)	19	17.6	

[a] Gamma hydroxybutyrate ($C_4H_8O_3$)

[b] Opioid pharmacotherapy

[c] Hopkins Symptom Checklist-25

However, they were also more likely to have had a temporary exit. This may seem anomalous with some regarding any unscheduled exit as negative. However, return to complete treatment is encouraged and it is possible that attachment to the horses may have made the decision to return a little easier for some. Further controlled studies are needed to clarify the causal relationship between HAT and temporary exit, duration and completion of treatment.

A major challenge in addiction treatment is to identify what treatment modality or other factors motivate patients to stay in treatment [6, 10, 43, 44]. Treatment factors (method, setting, duration, staff/patient ratio) and treatment process factors (motivation, alliance,

Table 3 Logistic regression predicting likelihood of completing treatment: a multivatiate model of all variables listed

Variable	Item	Total	%	p value	Odds ratio	Confid. lower	Interval upper
Participation in HAT	No (0)	43	39.8				
	Yes (1)	65	60.2	<0.01	8.42	2.7	26.4
Gender	Female (0)	30	27.8				
	Male (1)	78	72.2	0.84	0.90	0.3	2.6
Age	<20 years (0)	14	13	0.25			
	20–26 years (1)	74	68.5	0.11	4.37	0.7	26.0
	27+ years (2)	20	18.5	0.13	4.78	0.6	36.2
Years of schooling	<10 years (0)	18	16.7	0.41			
	10–12 years (1)	70	64.8	0.20	2.58	0.6	10.1
	13+ years (2)	20	18.5	0.30	2.40	0.5	11.3
No. of substances	3 substances (0)	42	38.9	0.25			
	2 substances (1)	31	28.7	0.09	2.66	0.9	8.4
	1 substances (2)	35	32.4	0.43	1.60	0.5	5.1
Substance severity[a]	Less severe (0)	62	57.4				
	More severe (1)	46	42.6	0.47	1.42	0.6	3.7
HSCL-25[b]	<1.75 (0)	19	17.6				
	1.75+ (1)	89	82.4	0.90	1.11	0.3	3.9
Temporary exit	2+ re-entries (0)	19	17.6	0.67			
	1 re-entry (1)	24	22.3	0.37	0.53	0.1	2.1
	No exit (2)	65	60.2	0.58	0.70	0.2	2.5

[a] Less severe (cannabis and alchol) more severe (heroin, amphetamine, benzodiazepine, Gamma hydroxybutyrate, cocaine)

[b] Hopkins Symptom Checklist

satisfaction, and interaction) are amongst the best predictors of treatment outcome [6, 44]. Furthermore, Simpson and colleagues suggest that use of therapeutic process and environmental influences as treatment enhancement may improve substance use outcomes [45]. HAT, in this study, is an innovative adjunct-treatment factor.

From the substance use and the HAT literature, we identified a number of possible explanations for why HAT participants may remain in and complete treatment. These include therapeutic alliance, the environment, physical activity, staff influence, individual attention and comorbidity.

Relational factors and therapeutic alliance can predict retention in treatment [1] and treatment outcome [44]. Premature termination of treatment and poor therapeutic alliance have been consistently reported in the scientific literature as predictors of negative treatment outcome [2–4, 6, 46]. Many HAT studies refer to the human–horse relationship as a positive motivating factor in therapy [16, 18, 20, 31, 47]. Burgon argues that building rapport with the horse increases comfort in the therapeutic relationship and leads to positive change and learning [25]. This may well be true, but we were unable to find substantiating quantitative studies of HAT and therapeutic alliance. It warrants further study.

As other experienced therapists report, many young patients respond better to the therapist in an active, less verbal environment than they do sitting in the more formal environment of a therapist's office [20, 43, 46, 47, 53]. Inclusion of an adjunct activity, such as gardening, music or art therapy, is also reported to be associated with successful treatment completion, as Decker et al. found in their pilot study of novel treatments [43].

A pleasant environment, physical activity and hobbies can have a beneficial impact in addiction and related psychological treatment [48–52]. HAT is a body-oriented psychotherapy with a range of physical activities, most of which occur outdoors in a pleasant, natural and quiet environment where therapeutic activities can be adapted to the seasons. Staff can also influence retention [2, 4, 5]. The HAT team works in a relaxed, non-judgmental atmosphere with patients, to explore and work on their issues.

Patients "are likely to continue in treatment longer … with individual attention and when seen in smaller groups in friendly comfortable environments" (Stark, 1992, p. 93) [3]. HAT sessions are conducted in small groups of not more than four patients with four staff, or in individual patient–therapist sessions. Patients can choose to work with their preferred horse, and most have a favorite. Other substance use studies have found focused personal attention, to be a key element in participants' retention in treatment [13, 43]. It is possible that the focused horse and human attention during HAT is a contributing factor to patients' retention in treatment.

Depression, anxiety, aggression, poor motivation and low self-esteem are among the most commonly cited psychological conditions associated with and responding to therapy with horses [16, 18, 21]. These conditions are also common elements of addiction comorbidity [54, 55]. The literature shows that distress scores on the HSCL-25 are very high at entry, because of the unstable condition at entry both emotionally (starting treatment) and because of the former drug use lifestyle. This may be one reason why we found no association between HSCL-25 and completion of treatment. Distress scores should be re-examined in a broader study of HAT and comorbidity.

Given the naturalistic study design, we cannot infer causality. Nor should the results be interpreted as an assessment of HAT as a therapeutic process (for substance use or for other psychological disorders). The purpose of the study was simply to examine whether, as some patients claimed, participation in the HAT program was associated with longer duration and completion of treatment. Further work is required to understand better HAT's therapeutic processes, and the underlying causes of, and impact on comorbidity and longer-term treatment effect.

Strengths and limitations
The size and relative homogeneity of the population studied is a strength when compared with other studies of therapy involving horses. However, there are limitations to both internal and external validity. Nonrandom assignment, including possible self-selection bias, is the most obvious limitation. The possible novelty effect of HAT is another. These shortcomings need to be addressed in large controlled studies that seek to clarify HAT's role, including causal inference, in substance use disorder therapy, in treatment outcomes and treatment effect.

HAT participation was voluntary. Because there were no data on why patients joined or did not join the HAT program, it was not possible to form an opinion on whether the HAT participants stayed in treatment longer because they participated in the HAT program or because of some other positive factor, which also led them to participate in HAT. Data on patients' motivation and program satisfaction (such as those used by Decker et al. [43]) might have been useful but were not available.

Dropout, the most frequently used measure of addiction treatment outcome, is fraught with definitional and other problems [3, 4, 6, 10]. There is no consistent definition of the term. Many studies fail to define how they have used it and/or omit discussion of the impact of temporary exits. We did not find any studies that included dropout as a measure of treatment outcome for HAT, and therefore comparisons were not possible.

Our findings are consistent with claims that HAT has a positive effect on psychosocial illness. However, we acknowledge this could be due, in whole or in part, to a variety of possible confounding factors that were not examined (such as, for example the "honeymoon" effect of a new program, the outdoor environment or the ambience around the stables). These factors lend themselves initially to qualitative investigation.

It is possible that a similar effect might be obtained more economically with another animal, such as a dog. Inclusion of dogs in substance misuse therapy has been found to improve therapeutic relationships [56]. However, we have found no studies which compare the use of horses with other animals as an adjunct therapy for substance misuse but note that Nurenberg [32] and colleagues in their comparison did find a significantly positive effect of therapy involving horses, but not dogs, when incorporated into psychotherapy for aggressive behavior.

Relevance
Ongoing care was not addressed in the study. However, HAT may have considerable potential as a community-based activity for outpatient treatment. If available from accredited public and private providers in community settings, it may enable engagement in healthy, pleasurable outdoor activities with a nonsubstance use peer group.

There is a continuous struggle to find what motivates substance use disorder patients to remain healthy. Rigorous evidence of safety and efficacy is required before HAT can become a conventionally accepted treatment with the associated provision of health insurance cover [57–59]. The positive findings from this treatment facility-based study, and HAT's broader community potential, prompt further investigation of both the underlying therapeutic processes and the longer-term impact of HAT on substance use disorder treatment.

Conclusion
This naturalistic study used intention-to-treat analysis to examine HAT in a substance use disorder treatment program for young adults. The objective was to assess whether HAT patients remained in treatment longer and were more likely to complete their agreed program of treatment than were non-HAT patients. It found statistically significant associations between HAT participation and duration and completion of treatment. These findings are consistent with the claims of patients and the growing body of equine therapy literature. However, the

study does not indicate whether either HAT or the horses per se might have accounted for the results. Investment is needed in larger controlled studies, in qualitative investigation of the patients' and clinicians' perspectives, and in the ethological study of the horses' actual contribution in the therapeutic process.

Authors' contributions

AKG did the literature review, conceived the study and designed it under supervision from ER and EA. AKG was responsible for HAT data extraction and interpretation, and performed the statistical analysis under supervision from ER and EA. AKG drafted the manuscript under supervision by ER. EW had access to all data and was responsible for the YATEP data collection, extraction and interpretation. EA and EW critically reviewed the manuscript. All authors read and approved the final manuscript.

Author details

[1] Department of Addiction Treatment, Oslo University Hospital, Sognsvannsveien 21, Building 22, 0424 Oslo, Norway. [2] Department of Psychology, University of Oslo, Oslo, Norway. [3] Norwegian Centre for Addiction Research (SERAF), University of Oslo, Oslo, Norway.

Acknowledgements

We thank the Oslo University Hospital stable therapists and support staff for their cooperation and Marie Isachsen, Ullevål Medical Library, Oslo University Hospital, for assistance with the literature review.

Competing interests

AKG is funded by the Norwegian Research Council and the Swedish-Norwegian Foundation for Equine Research. The funders had no role in the study design, data collection, analysis, data interpretation, or writing of the report. All other authors declare they have no conflict of interests.

Ethics committee approval

All necessary patient consent and data inspection authority approvals were obtained as part of the Youth Addiction Treatment Evaluation Project (YATEP). The study was reviewed and approved by the Norwegian Regional Committee for Medical Research Ethics and performed in accordance with their guidelines and the Helsinki Declaration.

References

1. Simpson DD, Joe GW, Rowan-Szal GA, Greener JM. Drug abuse treatment process components that improve retention. J Subst Abuse Treat. 1997;14(6):565–72.
2. McLellan AT. What we need is a system: creating a responsive and effective substance abuse treatment system. In: Miller WR, Carroll KM, editors. Rethinking substance abuse: What the science shows, and what we should do about it. New York: The Guilford Press; 2006.
3. Stark MJ. Dropping out of substance abuse treatment: a clinically oriented review. Clin Psychol Rev. 1992;12(1):93–116.
4. Baekeland F, Lundwall L. Dropping out of treatment: a critical review. Psychol Bull. 1975;82(5):738–83.
5. Craig RJ. Reducing the treatment drop out rate in drug abuse programs. J Subst Abuse Treat. 1985;2(4):209–19.
6. Brorson HH, Ajo Arnevik E, Rand-Hendriksen K, Duckert F. Drop-out from addiction treatment: a systematic review of risk factors. Clin Psychol Rev. 2013;33(8):1010–24.
7. Miller WR, Carroll KM, editors. Rethinking substance abuse: what the science shows, and what we should do about it. New York: The Guilford Press; 2006.
8. Ravndal E, Vaglum P, Lauritzen G. Completion of long-term inpatient treatment of drug abusers: a prospective study from 13 different units. Eur Addict Res. 2005;11(4):180–5.
9. Miller W, Carroll K. Drawing the science together: ten principles, ten recommendations. In: Miller WR, Carroll KM, editors. Rethinking substance abuse: what the science shows, and what we should do about it. New York: The Guilford Press; 2006.
10. Dalsbø1 TK, Hammerstrøm KT, Vist GE, Gjermo H, Smedslund G, Steiro A, Høie B. Psychosocial interventions for retention in drug abuse treatment. Cochrane Database Syst Rev. 2010. doi:10.1002/14651858.CD00822010.
11. Simpson DD. The relation of time spent in drug abuse treatment to post treatment outcome. Am J Psychiatry. 1979;136(11):1449–53.
12. Simpson DD. Treatment for drug abuse. Follow-up outcomes and length of time spent. Arch Gen Psychiatry. 1981;38(8):875–80.
13. Hser YI, Evans E, Huang D, Anglin DM. Relationship between drug treatment services, retention, and outcomes. Psychiatr Serv. 2004;55(7):767–74.
14. Ernst E. The role of complementary and alternative medicine. BMJ. 2000;321(7269):1133–5.
15. Anestis MD, Anestis JC, Zawilinski LL, Hopkins TA, Lilienfeld SO. Equine-related treatments for mental disorders lack empirical support: a systematic review of empirical investigations. J Clin Psychol. 2014;70(12):1115–32.
16. Hallberg L. Walking the way of the horse. Exploring the power of the horse-human relationship. Bloomington: iUniverse; 2008.
17. Selby A. A historical perspective on psychotherapy involving equines. Sci Educ J Ther Rid. 2011;17:5–19.
18. Fry NE. Equine-assisted therapy: an overview. In: Grassberger MSR, Gileva OS, Kim CMH, Mumcuoglu KY, editors. Biotherapy-history, principles and practice: a practical guide to the diagnosis and treatment of disease using living organismsedn. Dordrecht: Springer; 2013. p. 255–84.
19. Lavender DUMP. Equine-facilitated psychotherapy: dance with those that run with laughter. USA: Mrunalini Press; 2006.
20. Shambo L, Young D, Madera C. The listening heart. The limbic path beyond office therapy. USA: Human-Equine Alliance for Learning (HEAL); 2013.
21. Hamilton A. Zen mind Zen horse: the science and spirituality of working with horses. MA: Storey Publishing; 2011.
22. Lysell J. Bruk av hest i terapi (use of horses in therapy). In: Moe T, editor. Psykisk helsearbeid - mer enn medisiner og samtaleterapi (mental health work-more than medication and talk therapy). Bergen: Fagbokforlaget; 2011.
23. Mandrell PJ. Introduction to equine-assisted therapy. US: Xulon Press; 2006.
24. Hauge H, Braastad B, Berget B, Kvalem I, Engers-Slegers M. The effect of the horse on adolescents' self-efficacy, self-esteem and social skills. In: Berget BLL, Pálsdóttir AM, Sioni K, Thodberg K, editors. Green Care in the Nordic countries—a research field in progress. Report from the Nordic research workshop on Green Care. Trondheim: Norwegian University of Life Sciences; 2012. p. 28.
25. Burgon H. Equine-assisted therapy and learning with at-risk young people. London: Palgrave Macmillan; 2014.
26. Carlsson C, Nilsson-Ranta D, Træen B. Equine assisted social work as a mean for authentic relations between clients and their staff. Human Anim Interact Bull. 2014;2(1):19–38.
27. Dell CA, Chalmers D, Bresette N, Swain S, Rankin D, Hopkins C. A healing space: the experiences of first nations and inuit youth with equine-assisted learning (EAL). Child Youth Care For. 2011;40(4):319–36.
28. Burgon HL. 'Queen of the world': experiences of 'at-risk' young people participating in equine-assisted learning/therapy. J Soc Work Pract. 2011;25(02):165–83.
29. Trotter KS, Chandler CK, Goodwin-Bond D, Casey J. A comparative study of the efficacy of group equine assisted counseling with at-risk children and adolescents. J Creat Ment Health. 2008;3(3):254–84.
30. Vidrine M, Owen-Smith P, Faulkner P. Equine-facilitated group psychotherapy: applications for therapeutic vaulting. Issues Ment Health Nurs. 2002;23(6):587–603.
31. Selby A, Smith-Osborne A. A systematic review of effectiveness of complementary and adjunct therapies and interventions involving equines. Health Psychol. 2013;32(4):418–32.
32. Nurenberg JR, Schleifer SJ, Shaffer TM, Yellin M, Desai PJ, Amin R, Bouchard A, Montalvo C. Animal-assisted therapy with chronic psychiatric inpatients: equine-assisted psychotherapy and aggressive behavior. Psychiatr Serv. 2014;66(1):80–6.

33. Annual Report Equine assisted growth and learning association (EAGALA). 2015. http://www.eagala.org/EAGALA_Annual_Report. Accessed 29 April 2015.

34. Derogatis LR, Lipman RS, Rickels K, Uhlenhuth EH, Covi L. The Hopkins symptom checklist (HSCL): a self-report symptom inventory. Behav Sci. 1974;19(1):1–15.

35. Sandanger IMT, Ingebrigtsen G, Dalgard OS, Sorensen T, Bruusgaard D. Concordance between symptom screening and diagnostic procedure: the Hopkins symptom checklist-25 and the Composite International Diagnostic Interview. Soc Psychiatry Psychiatr Epidemiol. 1998;33(7):345–54.

36. Skårderud F, Sommerfeldt B. Miljøterapiboken. Mentalisering som holding og handling (Minding the milieu. Mentalization based practice). Oslo: Gyldendal akademisk; 2013.

37. Kern-Godal A. Riding Out of Addiction. In: HETI Newsletter May 2013. Federation of Horses in Education and Therapy International. http://www.frdi.net/pdfs/Newsletters/May2013_revised.pdf. Accessed 9 Oct 2015.

38. EAGALA. Fundamentals of EAGALA model practice. 5th ed. Santaquin: Equine Assisted Growth and Learning Association; 2006.

39. Forsling S. The girl and the horse. Images from a reform school. BookArt Productions ISBN. 2003. p. 91–631.

40. Kohanov L. Riding between the worlds: expanding our potential through the way of the horse. Novato: New World Library; 2007.

41. Kohanov L. The Tao of Equus: a woman's journey of healing and transformation through the way of the horse. Novato: New World Library; 2007.

42. Resnick C. Naked liberty. Amigo Publications, Incorporated; 2005.

43. Decker KP, Peglow SL, Samples CR. Participation in a novel treatment component during residential substance use treatment is associated with improved outcome: a pilot study. Addict Sci Clin Pract. 2014;9:7.

44. Miller WR, Moyers TB. The forest and the trees: relational and specific factors in addiction treatment. Addiction. 2014;110:401–13.

45. Simpson DD, Joe GW, Rowan-Szal GA. Drug abuse treatment retention and process effects on follow-up outcomes. Drug Alcohol Depend. 1997;47(3):227–35.

46. Palmer RS, Murphy MK, Piselli A, Ball SA. Substance user treatment dropout from client and clinician perspectives: a pilot study. Subst Use Misuse. 2009;44(7):1021–38.

47. Karol J. Applying a traditional individual psychotherapy model to equine-facilitated psychotherapy (EFP): theory and method. Clin Child Psychol Psychiatry. 2007;12(1):77–90.

48. Brosse AL, Sheets ES, Lett HS, Blumenthal JA. Exercise and the treatment of clinical depression in adults: recent findings and future directions. Sports Med. 2002;32(12):741–60.

49. Capaldi CA, Dopko RL, Zelenski JM. The relationship between nature connectedness and happiness: a meta-analysis. Front Psychol. 2014;5:976.

50. Belcastro AN, Morrison KS, Hicks E, Matta H. Cardiorespiratory and metabolic responses associated with children's physical activity during self-paced games. Can J Physiol Pharmacol. 2012;90(9):1269–76.

51. Davis DL, Maurstad A, Cowles S. 'Riding with Walls', up forrested mountain sides and in wide open spaces: developing an ecology of horse-human relationships. University of Waterloo-Wilfrid Laurier University. 2012.

52. Hickman C. Cheerfulness and tranquility: gardens in the Victorian asylum. Lancet Psychiatry. 2014;1(7):506–7.

53. Bizub AL, Joy A, Davidson L. "It's like being in another world": demonstrating the benefits of therapeutic horseback riding for individuals with psychiatric disability. Psychiatr Rehabil J. 2003;26(4):377–84.

54. Mueser KT, Drake RE, Turner W, McGovern M. Comorbid substance use disorders and psychiatric disorders. In: Miller WR, Carroll KM, editors. Rethinking substance abuse: what the science shows, and what we should do about it. New York: The Guilford Press; 2006.

55. Ekinci S, Kandemir H. Childhood trauma in the lives of substance-dependent patients: the relationship between depression, anxiety and self-esteem. J Psychiatry. 2015;18(2):1–5.

56. Wesley MC, Minatrea NB, Watson JC. Animal-assisted therapy in the treatment of substance dependence. Anthrozoös. 2009;22(2):137–48.

57. Angell M, Kassirer JP. Alternative medicine—the risks of untested and unregulated remedies. N Engl J Med. 1998;339(12):839–41.

58. Offit PA. Do you believe in magic? the sense and nonsense of alternative medicine. New York: HarperCollins; 2013.

59. Margolin A, Avants SK, Kleber HD. Investigating alternative medicine therapies in randomized controlled trials. JAMA. 1998;280(18):1626–8.

2

Contribution of *BDNF* and *DRD2* genetic polymorphisms to continued opioid use in patients receiving methadone treatment for opioid use disorder: an observational study

Monica Bawor[1,2,3], Brittany B. Dennis[2,3,4], Charlie Tan[5], Guillaume Pare[2,4,6], Michael Varenbut[7], Jeff Daiter[7], Carolyn Plater[7], Andrew Worster[4,7,8], David C. Marsh[7,9], Meir Steiner[10,11,12], Rebecca Anglin[8,10], Dipika Desai[2], Lehana Thabane[4,13,14] and Zainab Samaan[1,2,3,4,10,15]*

Abstract

Background: The heritability of opioid use disorder has been widely investigated; however, the influence of specific genes on methadone treatment outcomes is not well understood. The association between response to methadone treatment and genes that are involved in substance use behaviors and reward mechanisms is poorly understood, despite evidence suggesting their contribution to opioid use disorder. The aim of this study was to investigate the effect of brain-derived neurotrophic factor (*BDNF*) and dopamine receptor D2 (*DRD2*) polymorphisms on continued opioid use among patients on methadone treatment for opioid use disorder.

Methods: *BDNF* 196G>A (*rs6265*) and *DRD2*-241A>G (*rs1799978*) genetic variants were examined in patients with opioid use disorder who were recruited from methadone treatment clinics across Southern Ontario, Canada. We collected demographic information, substance use history, blood for genetic analysis, and urine to measure opioid use. We used regression analysis to examine the association between continued opioid use and genetic variants, adjusting for age, sex, ethnicity, methadone dose, duration in treatment, and number of urine screens.

Results: Among 240 patients treated with methadone for opioid use disorder, 36.3 percent (n = 87) and 11.3 percent (n = 27) had at least one risk allele for *rs6265* and *rs1799978*, respectively. These genetic variants were not significantly associated with continued opioid use while on methadone maintenance treatment [*rs6265*: odds ratio (OR) = 1.37, 95 % confidence interval (CI) = 0.792, 2.371, $p = 0.264$; *rs1799978*: OR 1.27, 95 % CI 0.511, 3.182, $p = 0.603$].

Conclusions: Despite an association of *BDNF* rs6265 and *DRD2* rs1799978 with addictive behaviors, these variants were not associated with continued illicit opioid use in patients treated with methadone. Problematic use of opioids throughout treatment with methadone may be attributed to nongenetic factors or a polygenic effect requiring further exploration. Additional research should focus on investigating these findings in larger samples and different populations.

Keywords: Opioid use disorder, Methadone maintenance treatment, Treatment response, BDNF, Val66Met, DRD2

*Correspondence: samaanz@mcmaster.ca
[15] Mood Disorders Program, St. Joseph's Healthcare Hamilton, 100 West 5th St., Hamilton, ON L8N 3K7, Canada
Full list of author information is available at the end of the article

Background

Rates of illicit opioid use are continuing to rise on a global scale, with North America being among the regions with most problematic levels of opioid use [1, 2]. Now identified as a growing public health problem, the use of illicit opioids is putting individuals at risk for opioid-related problems, including psychological and physical dependence. The development of opioid use disorder is influenced by a combination of environmental, behavioral, and biological factors, which contribute to the chronic and relapsing nature of the illness. Treatment for opioid use disorder with methadone, a synthetic opioid agonist, has been shown to be effective in reducing rates of relapse [3, 4]; however, there are a number of patients who continue to abuse opioids while in treatment, with little to no progress in their recovery.

The success of opioid agonist treatments is likely to be influenced by individual differences in gene profiles [5]. Evidence for the heritability of opioid use disorders has long been established [6–14], from which an interest in the specific genetic variability of opioid use disorder and methadone maintenance treatment (MMT) has evolved [5, 15]. Existing genetic studies have explored the therapeutic response to MMT, with a focus on opioid use relapse and methadone dosing. Opioid receptor genes, specifically OPRM1, and methadone metabolism genes, including ABCB1 and CYP450, are among the most commonly studied genes to date [16–22]. However, the association between methadone treatment response and other genes such as those involved in substance use behaviors and reward mechanisms remains unknown, despite evidence suggesting their contribution to opioid use disorder [23, 24].

The brain-derived neurotrophic factor (BDNF) gene encodes the neurotrophic protein, BDNF, which modulates neuron survival and neurotransmission [25]. Located on chromosome 11p13-15, BDNF has been identified as a strong candidate gene in multiple psychiatric and substance use disorders [26–29], including opioid use disorder [30–32], as well as for certain addictive behaviors such as drug seeking, impulsivity, polysubstance use, and cigarette smoking [33–35]. The BDNF 196G>A single nucleotide polymorphism (SNP) rs6265, also known as Val66Met, is found in the pro-BDNF region of the gene and inhibits secretion of the BDNF protein. Val66Met has been linked with deficits in neurotrophin and neurotransmitter release in specific areas that are responsible for behavior, learning, and memory [36, 37]. In the context of methadone treatment, BDNF has been explored in relation to BDNF plasma levels [30] and methadone dose [38], with only one study examining methadone treatment response to date [39]. In their study of 91 patients enrolled in an MMT program, de

Cid and colleagues found that a haplotype block in the BDNF genomic region (GenBank accession number NC_000011; including 21 polymorphisms in a 63.8 kb region of coding sequence, and 3′ and 5′ untranslated regions) containing this specific SNP was more frequent in nonresponders compared to responders. However, the generalizability of these findings is limited by small sample size, large confidence intervals (CIs), and short period of urinalysis testing (previous four urine screens) [39].

Similarly, the dopamine receptor D2 (DRD2) gene plays a major role in opioid use disorders because of its involvement in the reward–dependence pathway [40]. The DRD2 gene is localized to chromosome 11q23 and is responsible for the synthesis of dopamine D2 receptors, which are involved in many signaling and neurotransmission processes underlying addiction, including motivation, pleasure, and reward. A reduction in dopamine receptor signaling has been linked to reward deficiency syndrome, whereby continuous use of opioids acts to compensate for this inhibited dopamine release or "low reward" state [41]. The dopaminergic system mediates withdrawal and drug-related learning [42] and is therefore an important candidate gene for studying opioid use and methadone treatment response. To date, most of the addiction literature involving DRD2 has focused on the Taq1A (rs1800497) polymorphism [43–46]. There is also widespread evidence for an effect of Taq1A on methadone dose, metabolism, and response, which is most often associated with poor outcomes [24, 40, 43, 47, 48]. However, as the DRD2 gene is heavily involved in the activation of dopamine reward circuitry, it is likely that other SNPs that have not been investigated as extensively as Taq1A are associated with methadone treatment outcomes. A promising target polymorphism, DRD2-241A>G (rs1799978), is of particular interest, as it has shown preliminary evidence for an association with opioid use disorder and methadone dose in a sample of 85 German drug users admitted to an outpatient methadone treatment center [43].

Despite evidence for a strong association with addictive and reward behaviors, few studies of BDNF rs6265 and DRD2 rs1799978 in the context of opioid dependence and response to methadone treatment are available, and those are often limited by small samples or variation in the definitions of methadone treatment response. Based on existing literature, there is high potential for these SNPs to demonstrate an effect on methadone treatment response, which may have important implications for treatment prognosis. The current study aims to examine the genetic contribution to methadone treatment response (continued opioid use) in individuals with opioid use disorder, with a specific focus on addiction-related genes, BDNF and DRD2. We hypothesize that carriers of the minor alleles of both *rs6265* and *rs1799978* will be more likely to engage in continued illicit opioid use during methadone treatment, indicating poor treatment response.

Methods

We have reported detailed methods of this study sample previously [49]. Data used in this study were collected as part of the GENetics of Opioid Addiction (GENOA) research program, in collaboration with Canadian Addiction Treatment Centres (CATC; formerly known as Ontario Addiction Treatment Centres, or OATC) and the Population Genomics Program at McMaster University. This study is a cross-sectional analysis of men and women with a DSM-IV opioid dependence disorder, recruited consecutively from four outpatient methadone clinics across Southern Ontario between June and December of 2011. This study was approved by the Hamilton Integrated Research Ethics Board (HIREB), and written informed consent was obtained from each participant.

Participants were included in the study if they were ≥18 years of age, enrolled in a methadone treatment program at the CATC clinics, on a stabilized dose for the past 3 months, and able to provide consent and blood samples. We utilized the genetic information from 240 participant blood samples from the GENOA study in this investigation, in addition to substance use and medical history obtained through structured clinical interviews.

Illicit opioid use (referring to the use of illegal opioids, such as heroin, or using prescription painkillers that were not prescribed for the given individual/condition) was detected by regular urine screens (weekly/biweekly) and measured as the percentage of positive urine screens per total number of urine screens available. Participants with <80 % negative opioid urine screens were classified as using illicit opioids during treatment, or as treatment nonresponders. We also collected information on demographics, methadone treatment duration, methadone dose, age of initial opioid use, and psychiatric history.

SNP selection and genotyping

We selected the *BDNF* and *DRD2* genes on the basis of evidence supporting their involvement in opioid dependence and addictive behavior. The *rs6265* and *rs1799978* SNPs were the preferred choices for the purpose of this investigation because of their association with substance use and psychiatric disorders among various clinical populations [33–35, 50–52]. We isolated DNA from whole blood and performed genotyping using the Applied Biosystems® ViiA™ 7 Real-Time PCR System (Life Technologies Corp., Carlsbad, CA, USA) with Applied Biosystems TaqMan Genotyping Master Mix (Life Technologies

Corp.), as described previously [49]. The genotype call rates were 97.7 and 99.2 % for *BDNF rs6265* and *DRD2 rs1799978*, respectively.

Urine toxicology

All participants underwent qualitative and semi-quantitative urine analysis weekly/biweekly using the iMDx™ Analyzer and Prep Assay (NOVX Systems Inc., Richmond Hill, ON, Canada). The urine toxicology assays were implemented as part of the treatment model to monitor methadone adherence and to identify use of opioids. The iMDx™ test can differentiate between natural and synthetic opioids, allowing for easier identification of specific opioid use. Urine samples were collected and assayed at the respective methadone clinic sites.

Statistical analysis

Sample demographics were summarized using descriptive summary measures expressed as mean (standard deviation, SD) for continuous variables and number (percent) for categorical variables. Genotype and allele frequencies were computed and tested for Hardy–Weinberg equilibrium.

We performed univariate analysis on sample characteristics to evaluate differences between responders and nonresponders. Student's t test was used for mean differences, and Chi square was used for categorical variables. We chose to use the results from these comparisons and include significant variables as covariates in our logistic regression model. We performed multivariable logistic regression analysis, with opioid use as the binary dependent variable and the two genetic variants, *BDNF rs6265* (A/A vs. A/G vs. G/G) and *DRD2 rs1799978* (G/A vs. A/A), as independent categorical variables adjusting for age, sex, ethnicity, methadone dose (mg), and duration of treatment (months). We also adjusted for the total number of urine screens to eliminate any effect of more frequent urine sampling, suggesting problematic behavior throughout treatment (change in outcome per opioid screen). We classified continued opioid use as having <80 % negative opioid urine screens (treatment nonresponders). This classification was based on data from our current sample and from previous literature demonstrating that 30–80 % of opioid urine screens generally test negative throughout the course of methadone treatment [53–55]. Given the maximum value of this range, individuals with greater than 80 % negative screens (or alternatively, less than 20 % positive screens) are considered to be in good standing and, therefore, responding well to treatment. Given that 85 % of the participants were of self-reported European origin, we did not perform subgroup analyses based on ethnicity due to the small sample size of other ethnic groups in our study; this ethnic distribution is in keeping with our region population mix. In our regression, participants of European origin were compared to non-European origin, and men were compared to women.

Regression results, including model coefficients (odds ratio, OR), corresponding CIs, and associated p values are reported. The criterion for statistical significance was set at alpha $= 0.05$. There were no missing data in our analyses. We performed all statistics using STATA Version 12 (Stata-Corp LP, College Station, USA). The study is reported in adherence with the Strengthening the Reporting of Observational Studies in Epidemiology statement [56].

We confirmed the statistical power of this investigation post hoc using Quanto Version 1.2.4 (Morrison & Gauderman 2009, California, USA), with treatment response (continued opioid use) as the outcome variable. Using an additive, gene-only, unmatched case–control (1:2) model, including 240 methadone patients and a two-sided test with a $p = 0.05$ level of significance, we had 85 % power to evaluate the effect of *BDNF rs6265* (minor allele frequency, MAF: 0.20) on methadone treatment response, with an OR of 1.5; and 70 % power to examine the effect of *DRD2 rs1799978* (MAF: 0.05) on methadone treatment response, with an OR of 1.8.

Results

Sample demographics

Of the initial 260 participants recruited from methadone clinics, 20 participants were excluded from the study (duplicate entries $= 5$, buprenorphine treatment $= 3$, missing blood sample or urine data $= 8$, being prescribed opioids for chronic pain condition $= 4$). Therefore, 240 participants in total were included in the analysis (Fig. 1). The sample consisted of 144 (60.0 %) men and 96 (40.0 %) women, with a total mean age of 37.1 (SD $= 10.4$). Participants of European ethnicity made up 85 % of the sample. A majority of participants (81.3 %; n $= 195$) reported having a family history of mental illness or addiction. Responders and nonresponders were comparable across the majority of factors. Additional details of sample characteristics are shown in Table 1.

Genotypic profile

Genotype frequencies for *rs6265* and *rs1799978* are presented in Table 1. They did not deviate significantly from Hardy–Weinberg equilibrium ($p = 0.21$ for *rs6265*; $p = 0.36$ for *rs1799978*), and MAFs were consistent with previous literature (0.20 for *rs6265* and 0.05 for *rs1799978*). Among our sample of 240 methadone patients, 36.3 % (n $= 87$) had at least one *rs6265* risk allele, and 11.3 % (n $= 27$) had at least one *rs1799978* risk allele.

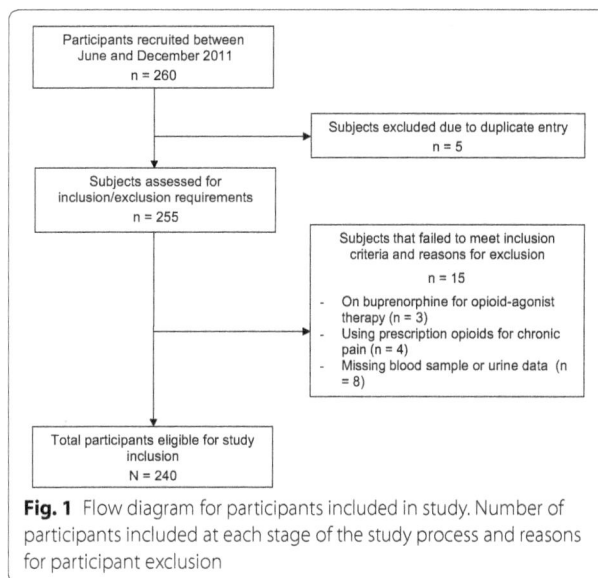

Fig. 1 Flow diagram for participants included in study. Number of participants included at each stage of the study process and reasons for participant exclusion

Genetic effect on opioid use during treatment

The continued use of opioids during methadone treatment was an indication of treatment nonresponse and can be measured objectively across samples. This allowed us to examine whether there was a genetic component to outcomes of methadone treatment. On average, 18.9 % (SD 24.1) of total urine screens throughout the duration of methadone treatment were positive for opioids in the total sample. Similar patterns were observed among genotype frequencies of responders and nonresponders (Table 1). Our logistic regression analysis showed that the minor alleles of *BDNF rs6265* and *DRD2 rs1799978* were not associated with continued opioid use during methadone treatment, while adjusting for age, sex, ethnicity, age of initial opioid use, methadone dose, duration of treatment, and total number of opioid urine screens (*rs6265*: OR 1.37, 95 % CI 0.792, 2.371, $p = 0.260$; *rs1799978*: OR 1.28, 95 % CI 0.511, 3.182, $p = 0.603$) (Table 2).

Discussion

Genetic association studies in addiction research aim to characterize genetic differences and variation in the processes that underly addiction and response to treatment. Patients with opioid use disorder have significant interindividual variability in their clinical response to treatment, which may be attributed in part to genetic factors. Variation in addiction-related genes (such as *BDNF* and *DRD2)* due to polymorphisms in the genetic sequence may confer susceptibility to continued opioid use while on methadone treatment for opioid use disorder.

Table 1 Characteristics of patients on methadone treatment for opioid use disorder

Characteristic	Total (N = 240)	Responders (n = 167)	Nonresponders (n = 73)	p value
Age in years; mean (SD)	37.1 (10.4)	37.1 (10.7)	36.9 (9.6)	0.868
Male; n (%)	144 (60.0)	105 (62.9)	39 (53.4)	0.169
Married/common law; n (%)	93 (38.8)	66 (39.5)	27 (37.0)	0.711
Employed; n (%)	72 (30.0)	53 (31.7)	19 (26.0)	0.375
Completed post-secondary education; n (%)	81 (33.8)	52 (31.1)	29 (39.7)	0.196
Ethnicity				
European; n (%)	203 (84.6)	139 (83.2)	64 (87.7)	0.381
Native North/South American; n (%)	19 (7.9)	14 (8.4)	5 (6.8)	0.686
Asian; n (%)	2 (0.8)	2 (1.2)	0 (0)	0.348
Persian; n (%)	1 (0.4)	1 (0.6)	0 (0)	0.508
Age of initial opioid use in years; mean (SD)	23.1 (9.2)	22.3 (8.8)	25.0 (9.8)	0.037
Current cigarette smokers; n (%)	214 (89.2)	145 (86.8)	69 (94.5)	0.210
Number of cigarettes smoked/day; mean (SD)	18.0 (10.1)	18.6 (10.5)	16.6 (9.2)	0.158
Psychiatric comorbidity, self-reported; n (%)	116 (48.3)	81 (48.5)	35 (47.9)	0.937
Family psychiatric history; n (%)	195 (81.3)	133 (79.6)	62 (84.9)	0.334
Alcohol use disorder; n (%)	42 (17.5)	29 (17.4)	13 (17.8)	0.934
Methadone dose (mg); mean (SD)	89.5 (60.8)	97.5 (67.5)	71.2 (35.9)	0.002
Duration of MMT (months); mean (SD)	40.5 (42.6)	44.2 (44.1)	31.8 (37.8)	0.042
Total number of opioid urine screens; mean (SD)	65.7 (23.7)	64.9 (20.7)	67.5 (29.6)	0.278
Opioid use (% positive urine screens); mean (SD)	18.9 (24.1)	5.4 (5.6)	49.8 (21.4)	<0.001
BDNF rs6265 genotype frequencies; n (%)				
G/G	153 (63.8)	110 (65.9)	43 (58.9)	0.302
A/G	81 (33.8)	52 (31.1)	29 (39.7)	0.196
A/A	6 (2.5)	5 (3.0)	1 (1.4)	0.458
DRD2 rs1799978 genotype frequencies; n (%)				
A/A	213 (88.8)	150 (89.8)	63 (86.3)	0.427
A/G	27 (11.3)	17 (10.2)	10 (13.7)	0.427

Frequency for DRD2 rs1799978 G/G genotype is 0 % in this sample; therefore, descriptive statistics are not available

BDNF brain-derived neurotrophic factor, DRD2 dopamine receptor D2, SD standard deviation, MMT methadone maintenance treatment

Table 2 Summary of multivariable regression results

Continued opioid use	OR	95 % CI	p value
Age: year	1.00	0.966, 1.038	0.928
Sex: male	0.64	0.349, 1.178	0.152
Ethnicity: European	1.83	0.715, 4.697	0.207
Age of initial opioid use: year	1.02	0.986, 1.060	0.235
Methadone dose: milligram	0.99	0.983, 0.998	0.016
Duration on treatment: month	1.00	0.987, 1.005	0.364
Total number of opioid screens	1.01	0.997, 1.024	0.148
BDNF rs6265: allele (A)	1.37	0.792, 2.371	0.260
DRD2 rs1799978: allele (G)	1.28	0.511, 3.182	0.603

LR χ^2 (7) = 20.23, Prob > χ^2 = 0.0165, Psuedo R^2 = 0.0728, Log likelihood = −128.822

BDNF brain-derived neurotrophic factor, DRD2 dopamine receptor D2, OR odds ratio, CI confidence interval

Summary of findings

In this study, we explored the effect of *BDNF rs6265* and *DRD2 rs1799978* polymorphisms on an important methadone treatment outcome, continued opioid use, which represents an objective measurement of response to treatment. In our sample of 240 methadone patients of primarily European origin, we were unable to confirm a role for these specific SNPs in continued opioid use during treatment.

Our findings are in line with a study by de Cid and colleagues, the only other study to examine the influence of *BDNF rs6265* in methadone treatment response [39]. They performed a haplotype analysis of 30 SNPs in the *BDNF* coding region, including *rs6265*, in a sample of 91 Caucasian individuals receiving methadone treatment for opioid use disorder. Grouping their sample into responders and nonresponders, they were unable to establish an effect of *rs6265* on response to methadone treatment [39], but found that a haplotype block containing this specific SNP appeared more frequently in nonresponders compared with responders. However, the generalizability of these findings is limited by small sample size, large CIs, and short period of urinalysis testing (previous four urine screens, or approximately 1 month) [39]. With respect to other methadone outcomes, another study demonstrated no effect of *rs6265* on methadone dose in a sample of 227 former heroin-dependent individuals in methadone treatment [38].

The *rs1799978* SNP of *DRD2* has only been examined in association with opioid dependence or methadone dose in two single-SNP and haplotype analyses. In both studies (by Hung et al. [40]; Doehring et al. [43]), the minor allele of *rs1799978* was more common in opioid users. However, Hung et al. [40] demonstrated that carriers of the minor llele also required higher methadone doses in their sample of 321 methadone patients, which was not a consistent finding in the study by Doehring and colleagues for a sample of 85 German drug users [43], thus suggesting a potential ancestral influence of *rs1799978* on methadone dose.

Although methadone dose was a significant predictor of continued opioid use in our regression analysis, this was an expected finding given the available evidence on methadone dosing in treatment [16, 57]. We included this variable to ensure that any effect found between the SNPs and continued opioid use was not explained by the relationship between methadone dose and continued opioid use.

Implications

Contrary to what the current literature suggests, although there may be a potential role for both *BDNF rs6265* and *DRD2 rs1799978* in susceptibility to opioid use disorder, the present study shows that these variants do not appear to exert large effects on continued illicit opioid use during treatment with methadone. Treatment response may, however, be influenced by the collective genetic risk conferred through multiple SNPs across several different genes (a polygenic effect). It is also possible that the continued illicit use of opioids during methadone treatment may be a result of other clinically relevant factors (i.e., medical or psychiatric comorbidity, social circumstances, life stressors, etc.).

Future directions

Given that there is little conclusive evidence to support a genetic impact on methadone treatment, there is a need for well-designed, powerful, genome-wide association studies to identify specific SNPs that are relevant

to methadone treatment response. Perhaps with this information, we will be able to simultaneously examine multiple candidate genes to understand the genetic composition of polygenic psychiatric disorders. Implementing the use of a gene score to assess an individual's genetic load may prove to be a promising approach to predicting and identifying those patients who require closer monitoring or alternate treatment strategies to overcome their continued opioid use.

Future research should focus on investigating these questions in larger samples and in various populations to ensure validity. Furthermore, a thorough examination of other nongenetic determinants of continued opioid use may prove useful for identifying problematic areas that require modifications in treatment delivery. Additionally, the genetic effects of withdrawal symptoms and adverse methadone events may be a promising area of study.

Strengths and limitations

To our knowledge, this is one of few studies to investigate the potential for an allelic effect of *BDNF rs6265* and *DRD2 rs1799978* on continued illicit opioid use among a large sample of methadone patients. These factors have not been thoroughly investigated in the context of methadone treatment response (as measured objectively through urine toxicology screens), which highlights a novel direction of research in the treatment of opioid use disorder with opioid-agonist treatments. Through this analysis, we aim to stimulate further research into potential polygenic influences on methadone treatment outcomes, as well as to confirm our findings in a larger sample of methadone patients. The uniformity of our cohort, attributed to consistency in delivery of treatment and standard of care across CATC clinics, ensures representativeness of the entire methadone patient population across Ontario, and likely throughout all of Canada. Our objective selection and definition of outcome measurements—specifically, continued opioid use—is also a noteable strength of this study.

Despite our negative findings, this study should be replicated in a larger sample using multiple genes in order to confirm a lack of association between *BDNF rs6265* or *DRD2 rs1799978* and methadone treatment response. Because the frequencies of the minor alleles were relatively low in our sample, a larger sample size may be required to estimate with confidence the effect of these variants on continued illicit opioid use.

In summary, the present study has demonstrated a lack of association between the two genetic variants (*BDNF rs6265* and *DRD2 rs1799978)* and MMT response, contrary to what previously had been believed about the role of these variants in psychiatric disorders and addictive behavior. Further research with larger samples is needed to re-evaluate this question, as well as to investigate multiple genes simultaneously to assess polygenic effects on susceptibility to poor treatment response. Nevertheless, this study elucidates the potential for other nongenetic determinants that may contribute to continued opioid use during methadone treatment; it also brings attention to further questions regarding the role of genetics in addiction research.

Abbreviations

MMT: methadone maintenance treatment; BDNF: brain-derived neurotrophic factor; SNP: single nucleotide polymorphism; DRD2: dopamine receptor D2; GENOA: GENetics of Opioid Addiction; CATC: Canadian Addiction Treatment Centres; OATC: Ontario Addiction Treatment Centres; HIREB: Hamilton Integrated Research Ethics Board; SD: standard deviation; OR: odds ratio; CI: confidence interval; MAF: minor allele frequency.

Authors' contributions

MB and ZS were responsible for the development of the research question, interpretation of data, manuscript writing, and critical revision of the manuscript. BD also contributed to manuscript writing and critical revision. CP, AW, MV, JD, DM, DD, and GP were jointly responsible for the process of data collection and communication with OATC clinics, as well as the clinical interpretation of results and critical revision of the manuscript. RA and MS were involved in the interpretation of data and critical revision of the manuscript. CT and GP performed genetic testing and assisted with interpretation of data and critical revision of the manuscript. LT assisted with statistical analysis, interpretation of data, and revision of the manuscript. All authors read and approved the final manuscript.

Author details

[1] MiNDS Neuroscience Program, McMaster University, Hamilton, ON, Canada. [2] Population Genomics Program, Chanchlani Research Centre, McMaster University, Hamilton, ON, Canada. [3] Peter Boris Centre for Addictions Research, St. Joseph's Healthcare Hamilton, Hamilton, ON, Canada. [4] Department of Clinical Epidemiology and Biostatistics, McMaster University, Hamilton, ON, Canada. [5] Michael G. DeGroote School of Medicine, McMaster University, Hamilton, ON, Canada. [6] Department of Pathology and Molecular Medicine, McMaster University, Hamilton, ON, Canada. [7] Canadian Addiction Treatment Centres (CATC), Richmond Hill, ON, Canada. [8] Department of Medicine, McMaster University, Hamilton, ON, Canada. [9] Northern Ontario School of Medicine, Laurentian Campus, Sudbury, ON, Canada. [10] Department of Psychiatry and Behavioural Neurosciences, McMaster University, Hamilton, ON, Canada. [11] Women's Health Concerns Clinic, St. Joseph's Healthcare Hamilton, Hamilton, ON, Canada. [12] Department of Obstetrics and Gynecology, McMaster University, Hamilton, ON, Canada. [13] Biostatistics Unit, Centre for Evaluation of Medicine, Hamilton, ON, Canada. [14] System Linked Research Unit, Hamilton, ON, Canada. [15] Mood Disorders Program, St. Joseph's Healthcare Hamilton, 100 West 5th St., Hamilton, ON L8N 3K7, Canada.

Acknowledgements

We would like to thank the CATC clinical staff for their efforts in recruitment and data collection and the patients who participated and generously donated their time, information, and samples; without them, this study would not have been possible. A special thank you also goes to the undergraduate students at McMaster University who volunteered a great deal of time to helping with data entry and genetic analysis. This study was supported by: a Canadian Institutes of Health Research (CIHR) Drug Safety and Effectiveness Network grant (Grant number: 126639) from Ottawa, Canada (ZS); an Innovation Award from the Department of Psychiatry and Behavioral Neurosciences at McMaster University (Grant number: 2-15311) in Hamilton, Canada (ZS); the Peter Boris Centre for Addictions Research at St. Joseph's Healthcare Hamilton; and the Chanchlani Research Centre at McMaster University, Hamilton, Canada. We also were supported by the CIHR Intersections of Mental Health

Perspectives and Addictions Research Training (IMPART) Fellowship (MB, BD). The funding sources had no role in the study design, collection, analysis, and interpretation of data, or the reporting of results.

Compliance with ethical guidelines

Competing interests

The authors declare that they have no competing interests.

References

1. Gomes T, Mamdani MM, Dhalla IA, Cornish S, Paterson JM, Juurlink DN. The burden of premature opioid-related mortality. Addiction. 2014;109(9):1482–8.
2. United Nations Office on Drugs and Crime: World Drug Report 2014. http://www.unodc.org/documents/wdr2014/World_Drug_Report_2014_web.pdf.
3. Oviedo-Joekes E, Brissette S, Marsh DC, Lauzon P, Guh D, Anis A, Schechter MT. Diacetylmorphine versus methadone for the treatment of opioid addiction. N Engl J Med. 2009;361(8):777–86.
4. Mattick RP, Breen C, Kimber J, Davoli M. Methadone maintenance therapy versus no opioid replacement therapy for opioid dependence. Cochrane Database Syst Rev. 2009; (3):CD002209.
5. Li Y, Kantelip JP, Gerritsen-van Schieveen P, Davani S. Interindividual variability of methadone response: impact of genetic polymorphism. Mol Diagn Ther. 2008;12(2):109–24.
6. Rounsaville BJ, Kosten TR, Weissman MM, Prusoff B, Pauls D, Anton SF, Merikangas K. Psychiatric disorders in relatives of probands with opiate addiction. Arch Gen Psychiatry. 1991;48(1):33–42.
7. Luthar SS, Anton SF, Merikangas KR, Rounsaville BJ. Vulnerability to substance abuse and psychopathology among siblings of opioid abusers. J Nerv Ment Dis. 1992;180(3):153–61.
8. Merikangas KR, Stolar M, Stevens DE, Goulet J, Preisig MA, Fenton B, Zhang H, O'Malley SS, Rounsaville BJ. Familial transmission of substance use disorders. Arch Gen Psychiatry. 1998;55(11):973–9.
9. Grove WM, Eckert ED, Heston L, Bouchard TJ Jr, Segal N, Lykken DT. Heritability of substance abuse and antisocial behavior: a study of monozygotic twins reared apart. Biol Psychiatry. 1990;27(12):1293–304.
10. Pickens RW, Svikis DS, McGue M, Lykken DT, Heston LL, Clayton PJ. Heterogeneity in the inheritance of alcoholism. A study of male and female twins. Arch Gen Psychiatry. 1991;48(1):19–28.
11. Kendler KS, Prescott CA. Cannabis use, abuse, and dependence in a population-based sample of female twins. Am J Psychiatry. 1998;155(8):1016–22.
12. Kendler KS, Prescott CA. Cocaine use, abuse and dependence in a population-based sample of female twins. Br J Psychiatry. 1998;173:345–50.
13. Cadoret RJ, Troughton E, O'Gorman TW, Heywood E. An adoption study of genetic and environmental factors in drug abuse. Arch Gen Psychiatry. 1986;43(12):1131–6.
14. Cadoret RJ, Yates WR, Troughton E, Woodworth G, Stewart MA. Adoption study demonstrating two genetic pathways to drug abuse. Arch Gen Psychiatry. 1995;52(1):42–52.
15. Haile CN, Kosten TA, Kosten TR. Pharmacogenetic treatments for drug addiction: alcohol and opiates. Am J Drug Alcohol Abuse. 2008;34:355–81.
16. Fonseca F, de la Torre R, Diaz L, Pastor A, Cuyas E, Pizarro N, Khymenets O, Farre M, Torrens M. Contribution of cytochrome P450 and ABCB1 genetic variability on methadone pharmacokinetics, dose requirements, and response. PLoS One. 2011;6(5):e19527.
17. Crettol S, Deglon JJ, Besson J, Croquette-Krokkar M, Gothuey I, Hammig R, Monnat M, Huttemann H, Baumann P, Eap CB. Methadone enantiomer plasma levels, CYP2B6, CYP2C19, and CYP2C9 genotypes, and response to treatment. Clin Pharmacol Ther. 2005;78(6):593–604.
18. Eap CB, Broly F, Mino A, Hammig R, Deglon JJ, Uehlinger C, Meili D, Chevalley AF, Bertschy G, Zullino D, Kosel M, Preisig M, Baumann P. Cytochrome P450 2D6 genotype and methadone steady-state concentrations. J Clin Psychopharmacol. 2001;21(2):229–34.
19. Dennis BB, Bawor M, Thabane L, Sohani Z, Samaan Z. Impact of ABCB1 and CYP2B6 genetic polymorphisms on methadone metabolism, dose and treatment response in patients with opioid addiction: a systematic review and meta-analysis. PLoS One. 2014;9:e86114.

20. Bunten H, Liang WJ, Pounder DJ, Seneviratne C, Osselton D. OPRM1 and CYP2B6 gene variants as risk factors in methadone-related deaths. Clin Pharmacol Ther. 2010;88(3):383–9.

21. Bunten H, Liang WJ, Pounder D, Seneviratne C, Osselton MD. CYP2B6 and OPRM1 gene variations predict methadone-related deaths. Addict Biol. 2011;16(1):142–4.

22. Bauer IE, Soares JC, Nielsen DA. The role of opioidergic genes in the treatment outcome of drug addiction pharmacotherapy: a systematic review. Am J Addict. 2015;24(1):15–23.

23. Dalley JW, Fryer TD, Brichard L, Robinson ES, Theobald DE, Laane K, Pena Y, Murphy ER, Shah Y, Probst K, Abakumova I, Aigbirhio FI, Richards HK, Hong Y, Baron JC, Everitt BJ, Robbins TW. Nucleus accumbens D2/3 receptors predict trait impulsivity and cocaine reinforcement. Science. 2007;315(5816):1267–70.

24. Lawford BR, Young RM, Noble EP, Sargent J, Rowell J, Shadforth S, Zhang X, Ritchie T. The D(2) dopamine receptor A(1) allele and opioid dependence: association with heroin use and response to methadone treatment. Am J Med Genet. 2000;96(5):592–8.

25. Russo SJ, Mazei-Robison MS, Ables JL, Nestler EJ. Neurotrophic factors and structural plasticity in addiction. Neuropharmacology. 2009;56(Suppl 1):73–82.

26. Beuten J, Ma JZ, Payne TJ, Dupont RT, Quezada P, Huang W, Crews KM, Li MD. Significant association of BDNF haplotypes in European-American male smokers but not in European-American female or African-American smokers. Am J Med Genet B Neuropsychiatr Genet. 2005;139B(1):73–80.

27. Itoh K, Hashimoto K, Shimizu E, Sekine Y, Ozaki N, Inada T, Harano M, Iwata N, Komiyama T, Yamada M, Sora I, Nakata K, Ujike H, Iyo M. Association study between brain-derived neurotrophic factor gene polymorphisms and methamphetamine abusers in Japan. Am J Med Genet B Neuropsychiatr Genet. 2005;132B(1):70–3.

28. Jockers-Scherubl MC, Danker-Hopfe H, Mahlberg R, Selig F, Rentzsch J, Schurer F, Lang UE, Hellweg R. Brain-derived neurotrophic factor serum concentrations are increased in drug-naive schizophrenic patients with chronic cannabis abuse and multiple substance abuse. Neurosci Lett. 2004;371(1):79–83.

29. Gratacòs M, González JR, Mercader JM, de Cid R, Urretavizcaya M, Estivill X. Brain-derived neurotrophic factor Val66Met and psychiatric disorders: meta-analysis of case-control studies confirm association to substance-related disorders, eating disorders, and schizophrenia. Biol Psychiatry. 2007;61(7):911–22.

30. Chen SL, Lee SY, Chang YH, Wang TY, Chen SH, Chu CH, Chen PS, Yang YK, Hong JS, Lu RB. The BDNF Val66Met polymorphism and plasma brain-derived neurotrophic factor levels in Han Chinese heroin-dependent patients. Sci Rep. 2015;5:8148.

31. Jia W, Shi JG, Wu B, Ao L, Zhang R, Zhu YS. Polymorphisms of brain-derived neurotrophic factor associated with heroin dependence. Neurosci Lett. 2011;495(3):221–4.

32. Cheng CY, Hong CJ, Yu YW, Chen TJ, Wu HC, Tsai SJ. Brain-derived neurotrophic factor (Val66Met) genetic polymorphism is associated with substance abuse in males. Brain Res Mol Brain Res. 2005;140(1–2):86–90.

33. Greenwald MK, Steinmiller CL, Sliwerska E, Lundahl L, Burmeister M. BDNF Val(66)Met genotype is associated with drug-seeking phenotypes in heroin-dependent individuals: a pilot study. Addict Biol. 2013;18(5):836–45.

34. Uhl GR, Liu QR, Walther D, Hess J, Naiman D. Polysubstance abuse-vulnerability genes: genome scans for association, using 1,004 subjects and 1,494 single-nucleotide polymorphisms. Am J Hum Genet. 2001;69(6):1290–300.

35. Lang UE, Sander T, Lohoff FW, Hellweg R, Bajbouj M, Winterer G, Gallinat J. Association of the met66 allele of brain-derived neurotrophic factor (BDNF) with smoking. Psychopharmacology. 2007;190(4):433–9.

36. Egan MF, Kojima M, Callicott JH, Goldberg TE, Kolachana BS, Bertolino A, Zaitsev E, Gold B, Goldman D, Dean M, Lu B, Weinberger DR. The BDNF val66met polymorphism affects activity-dependent secretion of BDNF and human memory and hippocampal function. Cell. 2003;112(2):257–69.

37. Angelucci F, Ricci V, Pomponi M, Conte G, Mathe AA. Attilio Tonali P, Bria P: Chronic heroin and cocaine abuse is associated with decreased serum concentrations of the nerve growth factor and brain-derived neurotrophic factor. J Psychopharmacol. 2007;21:820–5.

38. Levran O, Peles E, Randesi M, Shu X, Ott J, Shen PH, Adelson M, Kreek MJ. Association of genetic variation in pharmacodynamic factors with methadone dose required for effective treatment of opioid addiction. Pharmacogenomics. 2013;14(7):755–68.

39. de Cid R, Fonseca F, Gratacos M, Gutierrez F, Martin-Santos R, Estivill X, Torrens M. BDNF variability in opioid addicts and response to methadone treatment: preliminary findings. Genes Brain Behav. 2008;7(5):515–22.

40. Hung CC, Chiou MH, Huang BH, Hsieh YW, Hsieh TJ, Huang CL, Lane HY. Impact of genetic polymorphisms in ABCB1, CYP2B6, OPRM1, ANKK1 and DRD2 genes on methadone therapy in Han Chinese patients. Pharmacogenomics. 2011;12(11):1525–33.

41. Blum K, Braverman ER, Holder JM, Lubar JF, Monastra VJ, Miller D, Lubar JO, Chen TJ, Comings DE. Reward deficiency syndrome: a biogenetic model for the diagnosis and treatment of impulsive, addictive, and compulsive behaviors. J Psychoactive Drugs. 2000;32(Suppl i–iv):1–112.

42. Di Chiara G, Bassareo V, Fenu S, De Luca MA, Spina L, Cadoni C, Acquas E, Carboni E, Valentini V, Lecca D. Dopamine and drug addiction: the nucleus accumbens shell connection. Neuropharmacology. 2004;47(Suppl 1):227–41.

43. Doehring A, Hentig N, Graff J, Salamat S, Schmidt M, Geisslinger G, Harder S, Lotsch J. Genetic variants altering dopamine D2 receptor expression or function modulate the risk of opiate addiction and the dosage requirements of methadone substitution. Pharmacogenet Genomics. 2009;19(6):407–14.

44. Munafo M, Clark T, Johnstone E, Murphy M, Walton R. The genetic basis for smoking behavior: a systematic review and meta-analysis. Nicotine Tob Res. 2004;6:583–97.

45. Munafo MR, Matheson IJ, Flint J. Association of the DRD2 gene Taq1A polymorphism and alcoholism: a meta-analysis of case-control studies and evidence of publication bias. Mol Psychiatry. 2007;12(5):454–61.

46. Nacak M, Isir AB, Balci SO, Pehlivan S, Benlier N, Aynacioglu S. Analysis of dopamine D2 receptor (DRD2) gene polymorphisms in cannabinoid addicts. J Forensic Sci. 2012;57(6):1621–4.

47. Crettol S, Besson J, Croquette-Krokar M, Hammig R, Gothuey I, Monnat M, Deglon JJ, Preisig M, Eap CB. Association of dopamine and opioid receptor genetic polymorphisms with response to methadone maintenance treatment. Prog Neuropsychopharmacol Biol Psychiatry. 2008;32(7):1722–7.

48. Barratt DT, Coller JK, Somogyi AA. Association between the DRD2 A1 allele and response to methadone and buprenorphine maintenance treatments. Am J Med Genet B Neuropsychiatr Genet. 2006;141B(4):323–31.

49. Samaan Z, Bawor M, Dennis BB, Plater C, Varenbut M, Daiter J, Worster A, Marsh DC, Tan C, Desai D, Thabane L, Pare G. Genetic influence on methadone treatment outcomes in patients undergoing methadone maintenance treatment for opioid addiction: a pilot study. Neuropsychiatr Dis Treat. 2014;10:1503–8.

50. Hamidovic A, Dlugos A, Skol A, Palmer AA, de Wit H. Evaluation of genetic variability in the dopamine receptor D2 in relation to behavioral inhibition and impulsivity/sensation seeking: an exploratory study with d-amphetamine in healthy participants. Exp Clin Psychopharmacol. 2009;17:374–83.

51. Laucht M, Becker K, Frank J, Schmidt MH, Esser G, Treutlein J, Skowronek MH, Schumann G. Genetic variation in dopamine pathways differentially associated with smoking progression in adolescence. J Am Acad Child Adolesc Psychiatry. 2008;47:673–81.

52. Morton LM, Wang SS, Bergen AW, Chatterjee N, Kvale P, Welch R, Yeager M, Hayes RB, Chanock SJ, Caporaso NE. DRD2 genetic variation in relation to smoking and obesity in the prostate, lung, colorectal, and ovarian cancer screening trial. Pharmacogenet Genomics. 2006;16:901–10.

53. Schottenfeld RS, Pakes JR, Kosten TR. Prognostic factors in buprenorphine-versus methadone-maintained patients. J Nerv Ment Dis. 1998;186(1):35–43.

54. Mulvaney FD, Brown LS Jr, Alterman AI, Sage RE, Cnaan A, Cacciola J, Rutherford M. Methadone-maintenance outcomes for Hispanic and African-American men and women. Drug Alcohol Depend. 1999;54(1):11–8.

55. Jones HE, Fitzgerald H, Johnson RE. Males and females differ in response to opioid agonist medications. Am J Addict. 2005;14(3):223–33.

56. von Elm E, Altman DG, Egger M, Pocock SJ, Gotzsche PC, Vandenbroucke JP. The strengthening the reporting of observational studies in epidemiology (STROBE) statement: guidelines for reporting observational studies. Lancet. 2007;370(9596):1453–7.

57. Bao YP, Liu ZM, Epstein DH, Du C, Shi J, Lu L. A meta-analysis of retention in methadone maintenance by dose and dosing strategy. Am J Drug Alcohol Abuse. 2009;35:28–33.

3

Drinking to toxicity: college students referred for emergency medical evaluation

Sigmund J. Kharasch[1*], David R. McBride[2], Richard Saitz[3] and Ward P. Myers[4]

Abstract

Background: In 2009, a university adopted a policy of emergency department transport of students appearing intoxicated on campus. The objective was to describe the change in ED referrals after policy initiation and describe a group of students at risk for acute alcohol-related morbidity.

Methods: A retrospective cohort of university students during academic years 2007–2011 (September–June) transported to local ED's was evaluated. Data were compared 2 years prior to initiation of the policy and 3 years after and included total number of ED transports and blood or breath alcohol level.

Results: 971 Students were transported to local ED's. The mean number of yearly transports 2 years prior to policy initiation was 131 and 3 years after was 236 (56 % increase, p < 0.01). 92 % had a blood or breath alcohol level obtained. The mean alcohol level was 193 mg/dL. Twenty percent of students had alcohol levels greater than 250 mg/dL.

Conclusions: Adoption of a university alcohol policy was followed by a significant increase in ED transports of intoxicated students. College students identified as intoxicated frequently drank to toxicity.

Background

For more than five decades, surveys have documented the excessive and pervasive use of alcohol on U.S. college campuses [1–3]. The Office of the Surgeon General has characterized high-risk drinking among college students as a major public health problem [4] and nearly one-third meet the diagnostic criteria for alcohol use disorder [5]. It is estimated that 1700 college students die each year from alcohol related injuries [6].

Studies of alcohol use among college students have relied predominantly on self-report data, and objective measures of alcohol consumption among this group have infrequently been verified. The Harvard School of Public Health College Alcohol Surveys (CAS) conducted four times between 1993 and 2001 reported the sustained prevalence (40–45 %) of heavy episodic ("binge") drinking among college students nationwide and described the increased prevalence of impaired cognition, diminished

academic performance, alcohol-related injuries, engagement in vandalism, risky sexual activity, and drinking while driving among students who engaged in binge drinking [7]. Other national surveys have confirmed a similar prevalence of binge drinking among college students [8, 9].

In 2004, the National Institute of Alcohol Abuse and Alcoholism (NIAAA) defined a binge "as a pattern of drinking alcohol that brings blood alcohol concentration to 0.08 g percent or above and corresponds to the 4+/5+ level of consumption for females and males within about a 2 h period" [10]. However, studies have found that drinking at these levels in a college population frequently results in blood alcohol concentrations much lower than the 0.08 threshold [11]. Additionally, students often, poorly estimate the actual volume of a drink [12], adding further confusion as to the true nature of college drinking patterns and behaviors.

Blood alcohol concentration (BAC) or breath alcohol concentration (BrAC) to assess intoxication levels in a collegiate environment is an important adjunct to self-report surveys or interviews. Previous studies comparing BAC to BrAC have demonstrated near equivalency [13, 14]. Emergency departments (EDs) are uniquely situated

*Correspondence: skharasch@partners.org
[1] Division of Pediatric Emergency Medicine, Massachusetts General Hospital, Harvard Medical School, Zero Emerson Place, Suite 3B, Boston, MA 02114, USA
Full list of author information is available at the end of the article

to collect such objective data in order to elucidate the level of college drinking behavior. In previous ED studies of college students with alcohol intoxication at Vanderbilt University and the University of Virginia, the epidemiology of alcohol–related problems and intoxication among college students were described. At Vanderbilt University, 101 (16.4 %) of 616 undergraduate ED encounters over one academic year were alcohol related and 28 % presented with clinical or laboratory findings of severe alcohol intoxication. Four percent of students were hospitalized for medical complications and one student died of head trauma. Overall, it was estimated that 1 of every 15 undergraduates seen in the campus ED had alcohol-related problems. At the University of Virginia, 193 (13 %) of 1529 ED encounters over two academic years were alcohol related. Thirty-four percent presented with clinical or laboratory findings of severe alcohol intoxication and 53 % had associated trauma related to alcohol. Five percent of students were hospitalized for trauma or ventilator support for alcohol poisoning. However, alcohol levels were measured in only 21 and 16 % of students respectively, thereby limiting the scope of objective data collected [15, 16].

Several prevention practices and policies exist on college campuses to address alcohol-related problems. Binge drinking prevention initiatives at U.S. colleges and universities range from alcohol education, prohibitions on alcohol access, alcohol-free campus housing and activities, and restrictions on alcohol advertising [17–19]. However, few individual policies have been evaluated for their effectiveness [20] and implementation of specific policies varies by size and location of schools as well as by college administrators' perception of the importance of alcohol use as a problem on campuses [21]. Recently, two universities have implemented "arrest-first" policies for violations of alcohol laws [22]. Strict enforcement of existing policies may be associated with reductions of alcohol use among college students [23].

Additional research has focused on the student's role in assisting other students with alcohol intoxication or poisoning to try to avoid students not seeking help when needed, potentially avoiding preventable deaths. In a study of students at a Midwest university, 58 % of students indicated they had helped another student with symptoms of alcohol poisoning but did not seek outside help under such circumstances. Students more reluctant to seek help did not do so primarily due to their inability to distinguish symptoms of alcohol poisoning and their perception that help was not needed [24]. Increasingly, universities have adopted Good Samaritan or medical amnesty policies (MAP) to eliminate or reduce campus judicial consequences and encourage college students to seek help in cases of alcohol poisoning. At Cornell

University, calls to emergency medical services (EMS) for assistance with intoxicated students increased after initiation of MAP [25]. Combining alcohol-poisoning education with MAP has been found to have the greatest impact on help-seeking behavior of students [26].

Responding in part to highly publicized alcohol related tragedies in Massachusetts as well as ongoing feedback from our ED to University Student Health Services regarding alcohol levels, intoxication and poisoning among its student population, a large, local university in Boston instituted a policy of university police notification in 2009 with subsequent ED transport by EMS of college students on campus identified with presumed alcohol intoxication. For several years prior to implementation of this policy, it had been the practice of the University to intermittently transport intoxicated students to ED's. The purpose of the policy was to ensure the safety and well being of students and all members of the university community by requiring EMS transports to local ED's for medical evaluation of intoxicated students who might otherwise suffer serious health consequences or harm others. The purpose of this study was to evaluate the change in ED referral patterns from before to after adoption of a university-wide policy and to describe a large group of university students at risk for acute alcohol-related morbidity. It was hypothesized that adoption of such a policy would be followed by an increase in ED transports and that many of these identified students consume alcohol at potentially dangerous alcohol levels, as measured in blood or breath.

Methods

A retrospective cohort of university students transported to local ED's from academic years 2007–2011 was evaluated. Undergraduate students during the specified academic years were included in the study. The university health center and police maintain a list of all students brought to ED's with intoxication (EMS transports and ED contact person) for clinical follow-up purposes. Prior to the policy initiation in academic year 2009, the university notified (through group departmental meetings and emails) campus housing personnel, security, and resident advisors of the new protocol. Students exhibiting signs or symptoms of acute alcohol intoxication or poisoning on campus including ataxia, slurred speech, vomiting, disorientation, or alterations in consciousness by university personnel or calls for help by other students, had the university police called and subsequent EMS transport to local emergency rooms. Demographic data (name, date of birth, date of visit) were sent from the university health center to the Boston Medical Center (BMC) data warehouse, and de-identified clinical data were provided to the study investigators. Data were compared 2 years prior to initiation of the policy and 3 years after. Total number of ED transports and blood or breath alcohol levels were compared for the two time periods using a Welch t test, assuming unequal variance. Breath alcohol levels were obtained on patients presenting with clinical intoxication. For patients unable to provide a breath alcohol level (e.g., vomiting, diminished level of consciousness) a blood alcohol level was obtained. The distribution of alcohol levels was tested and confirmed to be normal using the Shapiro–Wilks test. Gender, age, length of stay, disposition and associated diagnosis were tabulated for the BMC group. Proportion of visits for males and females were compared using the exact binomial test. Alcohol levels for males and females were compared using a Welch t-test, assuming unequal variance. The Boston University Institutional Review Board approved the study protocol. Statistical analyses were performed in R [27].

Results

Between academic years 2007 and 2011, 971 students were transported to ED's for presumed alcohol intoxication. The mean number of yearly transports 2 years prior to policy initiation was 131 and 3 years after was 236 (Fig. 1, 56 % increase, $p < 0.01$). Despite a nearly two-fold increased in the number of students transported after policy initiation, the mean alcohol level did not significantly change (Fig. 1). During the five academic years, 679 students (70 %) were brought to the BMC ED. Of the BMC group, 55 % were female. The mean age was 19 years with 84 % being below the legal drinking age. The mean alcohol level was 193 and mean length of stay was 252.5 min. Males had a significantly higher mean alcohol level (199 vs. 188 mg/dL, $p < 0.05$), although this difference may not be clinically significant. Nine (1.3 %) students were hospitalized for trauma or medical conditions (including five closed head injuries, one diabetic

ketoacidosis, one vomiting/hypoglycemia, one incidental brain mass and one psychosis) and were eventually discharged. The mean alcohol level of admitted patients (236 mg/dL) was significantly greater than was the mean level for those not admitted (193 mg/dL) ($p < 0.01$). Nine percent had at least two repeat visits for alcohol intoxication within the study period.

Six hundred and twenty-six (92 %) of students had a BAC or BrAC level performed. Ninety-five percent had an alcohol level greater than 80 mg/dL. Seventy-three percent had a level between 100 and 250 mg/dL and 20 % had a level between 250 and 400 mg/dL (Fig. 2). Students with alcohol levels >250 mg/dL were significantly more likely to be male (57 vs. 41 %, $p < 0.01$), older (19.2 vs. 18.9 years, $p < 0.05$), have a longer length of stay (358 vs. 232 min, $p < 0.01$), more likely to be restrained (9 vs. 1 %, $p < 0.001$), and more likely to have an imaging study (10 vs. 3 %, $p < 0.01$).

Comment

Studies of alcohol use among college students have relied predominantly on self-report survey data and utilizing objective measures of alcohol consumption has been identified as an important research priority [28].

To our knowledge, the current study is the first comprehensive use of blood or breath alcohol screening among college students and provides an important window into alcohol consumption behaviors. Almost all university students transported to the emergency room in our data had a blood or breath alcohol level measured. The mean alcohol level was high and almost all (95 %) had alcohol levels greater than the NIAAA definition (80 mg/dL) for binge drinking and 70 % had alcohol concentrations two times (160 mg/dL) this level. In a previous study focusing on extreme drinking practices in college freshman,

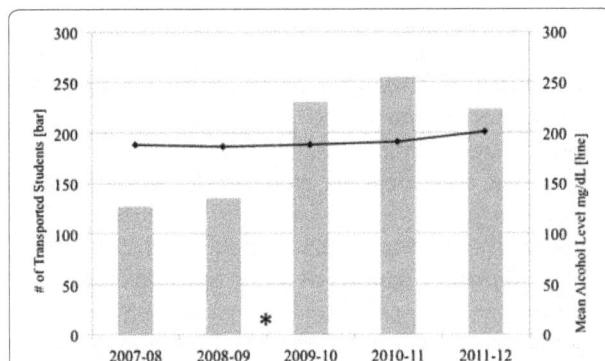

Fig. 1 Yearly number of transported students and mean alcohol levels. Policy initiation noted by *asterisk*. Change in transported students pre/post policy is significant at p < 0.01 level

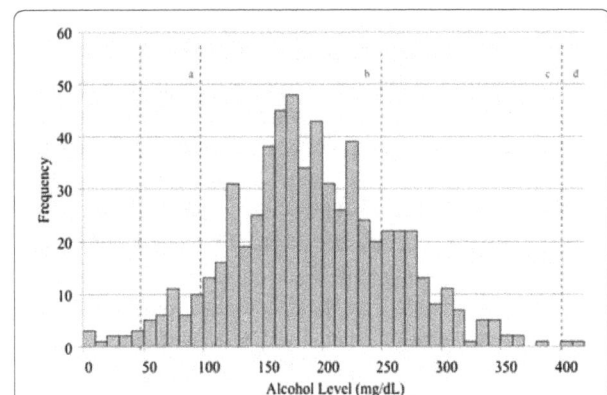

Fig. 2 Histogram of alcohol levels. *Notes*: levels typically associated with following symptoms. *a*—decreased judgment and coordination. *b*—ataxia slurred speech, vomiting. *c*—stupor or coma, incontinence. *d*—loss of protective airway reflexes, hypothermia, death

50 % of males and 24 % of females categorized as binge drinkers drank at levels at least twice the binge threshold (10 + males, 8 + females) [29]. Students that engage in extreme drinking practices have a significantly increased risk of alcohol related injuries compared to those that drink at the 4+/5+ threshold [30].

Most students in our study had between 100 and 250 mg/dL, levels where clinical effects of cerebellar and vestibular dysfunction (ataxia, slurred speech, diplopia, nystagmus), confusion, nausea and vomiting and stupor may occur; a substantial minority had alcohol levels between 250 and 400 mg/dL, levels that have been associated with respiratory depression, stupor, coma, and death [31].

Binge drinking among 18–22 year olds not enrolled in college decreased significantly though by a small absolute amount from 2002 (39 %) to 2010 (36 %). However, among college students 18–22 years of age, binge drinking has remained relatively stable from 2002 (44 %) to 2010 (42.2 %) [32]. While adoption of the policy in the current study was followed by a 56 % increase in ED transports, we cannot infer a cause-effect relationship due to the lack of a comparison group. For example, at the university evaluated in this study, alcohol education and assessment programs for students (BASICS, e-CHUG) and other efforts informing students of the dangers of heavy alcohol consumption occurred simultaneously and following policy adoption. While it was beyond the scope of the current study to assess the impact of such programs on alcohol transports, increased student awareness as to the dangers of alcohol intoxication or poisoning could have influenced calls for assistance for such students and hence EMS transports.

Nevertheless, the finding that blood or breath alcohol concentrations were not significantly different before or after policy initiation highlights the potentially effective practice of behavioral identification of intoxicated students by university personnel; presumably many of such students in prior years would not have presented for care and could have suffered consequences. While adoption of such a policy is not an alcohol prevention practice per se, it is perhaps better viewed as an alcohol safety policy. The fact that 20 % of students had alcohol levels greater than 250 mg/dL, underscores the toxic level of drinking behaviors among college students and subsequent potential for disastrous health consequences. While most students were eventually discharged, they can be safely monitored and treated in an ED environment for potential airway complications (respiratory depression, aspiration), trauma, on-going fluid losses and other complications of acute alcohol intoxication.

Our study had important strengths, primarily in the use of objective measures to verify the levels of drinking behavior in a college population that has not been previously described. Ninety-two percent of students in the current study had blood or breath alcohol level obtained which provides additional new and important information in our understanding of alcohol use among college students. The toxic level of drinking described in our study highlights the importance of studies of campus policies that focus on early identification and medical evaluation of students that engage in high-risk drinking in order to avoid dire health consequences.

Limitations

Our study had several important limitations. First, although most were, not all students were brought to the BMC ED. However, we have no reason to believe that students brought to other EDs in Boston were clinically different than the BMC group. Second, the experience described here is limited to only one university and may not be generalizable to others. Additionally, other efforts at the university as discussed above may have influenced the increase in EMS transports of intoxicated students. Lastly, the students transported to EDs in Boston may represent only the minority of students that were identified as engaging in extreme drinking practices on a college campus and certainly raises concerns regarding selection bias. Nevertheless, we believe that the current study provides objective criteria to better understand the potentially dangerous aspect of college students drinking practices.

Conclusions

Our study findings demonstrate that college students identified as intoxicated and brought to an emergency department frequently drink to toxicity as measured by blood or breath alcohol levels. Medical amnesty policies, arrest first policies and alcohol poisoning education are potential areas of study and policy development that may impact the safety and well being of college students. Such studies should go beyond single universities, involve quasi-experimental designs, and consider other policies and practices implemented.

Despite the limitations in the current study, we do believe that these data are sufficient for universities to consider such approaches as part of comprehensive alcohol strategies, perhaps evaluating such policies as they are put in place. Adoption of a university alcohol policy that identifies intoxicated students with subsequent EMS transport to an ED, may provide an important safety measure to reduce alcohol morbidity and mortality among college students.

Authors' contributions
SK, DM, RS and WM participated in designing the study, collecting data, interpreting results and drafting the manuscript. WM was responsible for the statistical analysis. All authors read and approved the final manuscript.

Author details
[1] Division of Pediatric Emergency Medicine, Massachusetts General Hospital, Harvard Medical School, Zero Emerson Place, Suite 3B, Boston, MA 02114, USA. [2] Division of Student Affairs, University of Maryland, College Park, Campus Drive, Building 140, College Park, MD 20742, USA. [3] Department of Community Health Sciences, Boston University School of Public Health, 801 Massachusetts Ave, 4th Floor, Boston, MA 02118, USA. [4] Department of Emergency Medicine, Boston Medical Center, Boston University School of Medicine, One Boston Medical Center Place, Boston, MA 02118, USA.

Acknowledgements
The study was not funded.

Competing interests
The authors declare that they have no competing interests.

References
1. Straus R, Bacon SD. Drinking in college. New Haven: Yale University Press; 1953.
2. Wechsler H, Isaac N. "Binge" drinkers at Massachusetts's colleges. Prevalence, drinking style, time trends and associated problems. JAMA. 1992;267:2929–31.
3. Wechsler H, Davenport A, Dowdall G, Moeykens B, Castillo S. Health and behavioral consequences of binge drinking in college. A national survey of students at 140 campuses. JAMA. 1994;272:1672–7.
4. Office of the Surgeon General. The surgeon general's call to action to prevent and reduce underage drinking. Rockville: Office of the Surgeon General, Department of Health and Human Services; 2007.
5. Knight JK, Wechsler H, Kuo M, Seibring M, Weitzman ER, Schockit MA. Alcohol abuse and dependence among U.S. college students. J Stud Alcohol. 2002;63:263–70.
6. Hingson R, Heeren T, Winter M, Wechsler H. Magnitude of alcohol-related mortality and morbidity among U.S. college students ages 18–24: changes from 1998–2001. Ann Rev Publ Health. 2005;26:259–79.
7. Wechsler H, Lee JE, Kuo M, Seibring M, Nelson TF, Lee H. Trends in college binge drinking during a period of increased prevention efforts: findings from 4 Harvard School of Public Health College Alcohol Study surveys: 1993–2001. J Am Coll Health. 2002;50:203–17.
8. Hingson RW, Wenxing Z, Weitzman ER. Magnitude of and trends in alcohol-related mortality and morbidity among U. S. college students ages 18–24, 1998–2005. J Stud Alcohol Drugs. 2009;16:12–20.
9. Johnston LD, O'Malley PM, Bachman JG, Schulenberg JE. Monitoring the future national survey results on drug use, 1975–2011, vol. II: College Students and Adults Ages 19–50. Ann Arbor: Institute for Social Research, the University of Michigan; 2012.
10. National Institute on Alcohol, Abuse and Alcoholism. NIAAA council approves definition of binge drinking. (p. 3). NIAAA Newsletter. NIH Publication No. 04-5346, Bethesda MD; 2004.
11. Thombs DL, Scott Olds R, Snyder BM. Field assessment of BAC data to study late-night college drinking. J Stud Alcohol. 2003;64:322–30.
12. Kerr WC, Stockwell T. Understanding standard drinks and drinking guidelines. Drug Alcohol Rev. 2012;31:200–5.
13. Grubb D, Rasmussen B, Linet K, Olsson SG, Lindberg L. Breath alcohol analysis incorporating standardization to water vapor is as precise as blood alcohol analysis. Forensic Sci Int. 2012;216:88–91.
14. Lindberg L, Braur S, Wollmer P, Goldberg L, Jones AW, Olsson SG. Breath alcohol concentration determined with a new analyzer using free exhalation predicts almost precisely the arterial blood alcohol concentration. Forensic Sci Int. 2007;168:200–7.
15. Turner JC, Shu J. Serious health consequences associated with alcohol use among college students: demographic and clinical characteristics of patients seen in an emergency department. J Stud Alcohol. 2004;65:179–83.
16. Wright SW, Slovis CM. Drinking on campus. Undergraduate intoxication requiring emergency care. Arch Pediatr Adolesc Med. 1996;150:699–702.
17. Lenk KM, Erickson DJ, Nelson TF, Winters KC, Toomey TL. Alcohol policies and practices among four-year colleges in the United States: prevalence and patterns. J Stud. Alcohol Drugs. 2012;73:361–7.
18. Nelson TF, Toomey TL, Lenk KM, Erickson DJ, Winters KC. Implementation of NIAAA college drinking task force recommendations: How are colleges doing 6 years later? Alcohol Clin Exp Res. 2010;24:1687–93.
19. Wechsler H, Kelley K, Weitzman ER, Giovanni JPS, Seibring M. What colleges are doing about student binge drinking. A survey of college administrators. J Am Coll Health. 2000;48:219–26.
20. Toomey TL, Lenk KM, Wagenaar A. Environmental policies to reduce college drinking: an update of research findings. J Stud Alcohol Drugs. 2007;68:208–19.
21. Wechsler H, Seibring M, Liu IC, Ahl M. Colleges respond to student binge drinking: reducing student demand or limiting access. J Am Coll Health. 2004;52:159–68.
22. Barlow R. Boston police move to arrest –first policy for alcohol laws. Retrieved from BU Today. 2013. http://www.bu.edu/today/2013/boston-police-move-to-arrest-first-policy-for-alcohol-laws.
23. Harris SK, Sherritt L, Hook SV, Wechsler H, Knight JR. Alcohol policy enforcement and changes in student drinking rates in a statewide public college system: a follow-up study. Sub Abuse Treat Prev Pol. 2010;5:1–11.
24. Oster-Aaland L, Lewis MA, Neighbors C, Vangsness J, Larimer E. Alcohol poisoning among college students turning 21: Do they recognize the symptoms and how do they help? J Stud Alcohol Drugs. 2009;16:122–30.
25. Lewis DK, Marchell TC. Safety first: a medical amnesty approach to alcohol poisoning at a U.S. university. Int J Drug Policy. 2006;17:329–38.
26. Oster-Aaland L, Thompson K, Eighmy M. The impact of an online educational video and a medical amnesty policy on college student's intentions to seek help in the presence of alcohol poisoning symptoms. JSARP. 2011;48:147–64.
27. R Core Team. R: A language and environment for statistical computing. R Foundation for Statistical Computing. Vienna, Austria; 2013. http://www.R-project.org.
28. Dowdall GW, Wechsler H. Studying college alcohol use: widening the lens, sharpening the focus. J Stud Alcohol Suppl. 2002;14:14–22.
29. White AM, Kraus CL, Swartzwelder HS. Many college freshmen drink at levels far beyond the binge threshold. Alcohol Clin Exp Res. 2006;30:1006–10.
30. Mundt MP, Zakleskaia LI, Fleming MF. Extreme college drinking and alcohol-related injury risk. Alcohol Clin Exp Res. 2009;33:1532–8.
31. White A, Hingson R. The burden of alcohol use: excessive alcohol consumption and related consequences among college students. Alcohol Res. 2014;35:201–18.
32. Substance Abuse and Mental Health Services Administration. Results from the 2011 National Survey on Drug Use and Health: Summary of National Findings. NSDUH Series H-44, HHS Publication No. (SMA) 12-4713. Rockville MD; 2012.

4

Validation of the AUDIT-C in adults seeking help with their drinking online

Zarnie Khadjesari[1,2]●, Ian R. White[3], Jim McCambridge[4], Louise Marston[1*], Paul Wallace[1], Christine Godfrey[4] and Elizabeth Murray[1]

Abstract

Background: The abbreviated Alcohol Use Disorder Identification Test for Consumption (AUDIT-C) is rapidly becoming the alcohol screening tool of choice for busy practitioners in clinical settings and by researchers keen to limit assessment burden and reactivity. Cut-off scores for detecting drinking above recommended limits vary by population, setting, country and potentially format. This validation study aimed to determine AUDIT-C thresholds that indicated risky drinking among a population of people seeking help over the Internet.

Method: The data in this study were collected in the pilot phase of the Down Your Drink trial, which recruited people seeking help over the Internet and randomised them to a web-based intervention or an information-only website. Sensitivity, specificity, and positive and negative likelihood ratios were calculated for AUDIT-C scores, relative to weekly consumption that indicated drinking above limits and higher risk drinking. Receiver-operating characteristic (ROC) curves were created to assess the performance of different cut-off scores on the AUDIT-C for men and women. Past week alcohol consumption was used as the reference-standard and was collected via the TOT-AL, a validated online measure of past week drinking.

Results: AUDIT-C scores were obtained from 3720 adults (2053 female and 1667 male) searching the internet for help with drinking, mostly from the UK. The area under the ROC curve for risky drinking was 0.84 (95% CI 0.80, 0.87) (female) and 0.80 (95% CI 0.76, 0.84) (male). AUDIT-C cut-off scores for detecting risky drinking that maximise the sum of sensitivity and specificity were ≥ 8 for women and ≥ 8 for men; whereas those identifying the highest proportion of correctly classified individuals were ≥ 4 for women and ≥ 5 for men. AUDIT-C cut-off scores for detecting higher risk drinking were also calculated.

Conclusions: AUDIT-C cut-off scores for identifying alcohol consumption above weekly limits in this largely UK based study population were substantially higher than those reported in other validation studies. Researchers and practitioners should select AUDIT-C cut-off scores according to the purpose of identifying risky drinkers and hence the relative importance of sensitivity and/or specificity.

Keywords: Alcohol, AUDIT-C, Validation, Past week drinking, Online

Background

Early identification of people drinking at risky levels followed by brief intervention is the key individual-level intervention approach for reducing alcohol intake to safer levels [1, 2], with efficacy demonstrated in a range of settings including primary care, emergency departments, higher education and the workplace [3–8]. From the 1980s onwards the World Health Organisation (WHO) developed the Alcohol Use Disorders Identification Test (AUDIT), a 10-item screening questionnaire for detecting hazardous, harmful and dependent drinking in primary care [9]. There is now a substantial literature demonstrating the validity of the AUDIT in settings beyond primary care, such as inpatient hospital wards, emergency departments, universities, workplaces, outpatient settings and psychiatric services [10]. Above the basic threshold score

*Correspondence: l.marston@ucl.ac.uk
[1] Department of Primary Care and Population Health, UCL Royal Free Campus, Upper Third Floor, Rowland Hill Street, London NW3 2PF, UK
Full list of author information is available at the end of the article

of 8, the AUDIT guidance offers cut-off scores that indicate the severity of a person's drinking, which in turn can be matched to the help they require, i.e. simple advice (score 8–15), simple advice plus brief counselling and continued monitoring (score 16–19), or referral to a specialist for assessment and treatment (score 20–40) [9]. These higher cut-offs are based on expert opinion rather than validation data.

Since the development of the AUDIT there have been a number of abbreviated versions that allow screening to take place in busy environments where time is limited [11]. The AUDIT-C is an abbreviated version of the AUDIT that has been advocated for use in both research and practice settings where there is insufficient time to administer the full AUDIT [11]. It consists of the first three questions of the AUDIT that relate to alcohol intake, where 'C' indicates 'Consumption' [12]. The AUDIT-C demonstrates similar accuracy to the full AUDIT [13, 14], however, the cut-off scores used to identify risky drinking, i.e. consumption above recommended limits, have varied in previous studies.

In 2007, a review of abbreviated versions of the AUDIT recommended an AUDIT-C cut-off score of ≥3 (women) and ≥4 (men) for detecting hazardous or harmful drinking [13]. This recommendation was based on a narrative review of 10 studies, of which four were in primary care patients, two in veteran populations, two in the general population [15, 16], one in hospitalised patients and one in psychiatric patients. Two studies included in this review found 'optimal' AUDIT-C scores (defined as those that maximise the sum of sensitivity and specificity) for detecting drinking above recommended limits in the general population of ≥5 in Germany [15] and ≥5 (men) and ≥3 (women) in the US [16]. Another review published the following year, identified four studies that tested the accuracy (i.e. the highest overall proportion of true positives and false negatives) of the AUDIT-C in detecting risky drinking in European general population samples, with cut-off scores of ≥5 and ≥6 [15, 17–19], where prevalence ranged from 5 to 37% [14]. Surprisingly few studies published since these reviews have validated the AUDIT-C in general population samples. One recently published study based in the adult general population in Sweden found the 'optimal' AUDIT-C cut-off score for detecting drinking above recommended limits (termed "risk drinking") was ≥6 (men) and ≥4 (women) [20]. The AUDIT-C has not been validated for identifying risky drinking in adults from the United Kingdom.

There may be many reasons for the heterogeneity in findings in previous studies including differences in populations, settings and cultures, where both prevalence and recommended drinking limits vary. Validation studies use different reference standards and forms

of measurement for determining hazardous or harmful drinking, e.g. time-line follow-back, 10-item AUDIT, International Classification of Diseases (ICD-10 criteria) and the Diagnostic and Statistical Manual of Mental Disorders (DSM-III-R, DSM-IV) [13, 14]. There are also differences in the type of cut-off scores selected, depending on the use to which the test is put.

Screening and brief intervention delivered over the Internet has grown in popularity over the past decade and is now a substantial field of research [21]. Electronic screening enables instantaneous data collection and eliminates the need for manual data entry, thereby reducing errors that this process may introduce. Alcohol screening tests, which are conventionally delivered in-person or in paper-based format, appear to retain their psychometric properties when delivered online [22–26]. There is also some evidence that being self-administered, online screening is likely to generate more honest reporting of risky alcohol use, in comparison with a face-to-face interview [27, 28]. The AUDIT-C has been used to screen for eligibility in two trials of web-based alcohol screening and brief intervention delivered to students in New Zealand (≥4 for men and women) [29, 30] and two trials of facilitated access to an online intervention delivered in primary care in Italy and Spain (≥5 for men and ≥4 women) [31, 32]. These trials did not validate the AUDIT-C for use online, and were not conducted in general population samples.

The purpose of this study was to determine a suitable cut-off score for the AUDIT-C for identifying risky drinkers in a general population sample of people seeking online help with their drinking. Objectives were to determine the sensitivity, specificity, likelihood ratios and area under the Receiver-operating characteristic (ROC) curves of different cut-off scores for the AUDIT-C, with a goal of identifying people drinking above the recommended UK weekly consumption limits. To the best of our knowledge, this is the first study that seeks to validate the AUDIT-C in a population of people seeking help with their drinking over the Internet.

Methods
The data for this study were collected during the eight month pilot phase (February to October 2007) of an online randomised controlled trial investigating the effectiveness of an internet-based intervention (called Down Your Drink—DYD [33] for people looking for help or information on their drinking [34, 35]. One of the objectives of this pilot trial was to determine a suitable AUDIT-C cut-off score for identifying people drinking above UK weekly limits advocated by the Royal Colleges of General Practitioners and Psychiatrists and Department of Health [36, 37] for use in recruiting to the main

trial phase of Down Your Drink [34]. Ethical approval for the DYD pilot trial was obtained from UCL Research Ethics Committee. The Down Your Drink website was identified via Internet searches for help or information on drinking, or from the home page of Alcohol Concern, the UK's largest alcohol charity; no further advertising was needed to meet the sample size for the pilot trial. The DYD homepage asked visitors to "find out if you are drinking too much" by directing them to the AUDIT-C questionnaire. In order to gain access to the Down Your Drink website, people were required to enter an online trial and provide informed consent, if aged 18 years or above. Visitors subsequently registered with the website and completed baseline data before being randomised. The first baseline questionnaire, following the initial screen with the AUDIT-C, was an online measure of past week drinking (the TOT-AL, detailed below), which was followed by other validated measures of alcohol problems and dependence [34].

AUDIT-C

The AUDIT-C constitutes the following three questions:

1. How often do you have a drink containing alcohol? Answer: Never (score 0), Monthly or less (score 1), 2–4 times per month (score 2), 2–3 times per week (score 3), 4+ times per week (score 4);
2. How many units of alcohol do you drink on a typical day when you are drinking? Answer: 1–2 (score 0), 3–4 (score 1), 5–6 (score 2), 7–9 (score 3), 10+ (score 4);
3. How often have you had 6 or more units if female, or 8 or more if male, on a single occasion in the last year? Answer: Never (score 0), Less than monthly (score 1), Monthly (score 2), Weekly (score 3), Daily or almost daily (score 4).

Reference standard

Our reference standard is the TOT-AL measure of past week drinking, which is used here to identify two conditions: (1) risky drinking, and (2) higher risk drinking.

1. Weekly drinking limits recommended by the Royal Colleges of General Practitioners and Psychiatrists [36] and previously by the Department of Health [37] were used as the reference standards to evaluate the performance of the AUDIT-C:

- 14 units of alcohol per week for women;
- 21 units of alcohol per week for men, where (1 UK unit is 8 grams of ethanol). At the time of writing there was a consultation on reducing this to 14 units [38].

2. We were also interested in evaluating performance against the accepted UK threshold for a level of heavy drinking at which problems are likely to be occurring. These "higher risk" thresholds were:

- 35 units of alcohol per week for women;
- 50 units of alcohol per week for men.

The TOT-AL is a reliable and valid online measure that presents drop-down menus on the type, brand, size and quantity of alcohol consumed on each of the past seven days and calculates total units of alcohol consumed (measured in UK units) [39]. There is a strong correlation between repeated measurements of the TOT-AL ($r = 0.99$; 95% CI 0.98, 0.99) and between the units calculated by the TOT-AL and a face-to face interview ($r = 0.97$; 95% CI 0.95, 0.99). A high level of agreement between measurements was also observed in a Bland–Altman analysis [39]. The TOT-AL was completed by all participants. Data were entered anonymously by participants from a computer with Internet access from any location.

Analyses

The sensitivity and specificity of cut-off scores between two and ten on the AUDIT-C were examined separately for males and females using the recommended weekly drinking limits (measured by the TOT-AL) as the reference-standard. Positive and negative likelihood ratios were calculated to estimate how different cut-off scores change the odds of being a risky drinker and a higher risk drinker, where positive likelihood ratios = sensitivity/(1 − specificity), and negative likelihood ratios = (1 − sensitivity)/specificity. Receiver-operating characteristic (ROC) curves were created to assess the performance of different cut-off scores on the AUDIT-C for men and women. ROC curves plot the sensitivities of different cut-off scores against 1-specificities (known as the false positive rate). The area under the ROC curve quantifies the ability of the AUDIT-C to discriminate between those people drinking above and within weekly drinking limits. A perfect test is indicated by an area under the ROC curve of 1.0, whereas a worthless test is indicated by 0.5. Analyses were conducted in Stata V13 [40].

Validation studies of the AUDIT-C in general population settings tend to report a cut-off score that maximises the sum of sensitivity and specificity. We refer to this as an 'optimal' cut-off score [41]. This cut-off score is used when the sensitivity and specificity of a test are of equal importance. In addition to these 'optimal' cut-off scores, our study also presents 'accuracy' cut-off scores which identify the highest overall proportion of correctly classified risky and lower-risk drinkers.

When the same data are used both to select a cut-off score and to evaluate performance (sensitivity, specificity, likelihood ratios or accuracy) at the cut-off, performance tends to be over-estimated—a phenomenon known as "optimism" or "overfitting" [42]. To avoid this, the data were randomly split into two subsets. The cut-offs were re-estimated in one subset and their performance was evaluated in the other subset, and vice versa, and the estimated performances were averaged to give an "optimism-adjusted" performance. This procedure was not needed in evaluating performance at fixed cut-offs.

Results
Baseline characteristics
A total of 3720 participants completed baseline measures in the pilot trial. All participants included in this study had data for both TOT-AL and AUDIT-C measures, there was no drop out or withdrawals. Participants were mostly female (55%), with an average age of 37 years (SD 11), mostly 'White British' (84%) and living in the UK (89%). Participants living outside the UK were most commonly from other Anglophone countries (highest U.S. n = 108, Canada n = 40) with small numbers from other countries (highest France n = 28). Half of all participants were educated to university degree level or above (51%). Average (geometric mean − given the skewed distribution of the data) alcohol intake at baseline was 38 UK units in the past week (SD 4) and the mean AUDIT-C score was 8 (SD 2), for distribution of AUDIT-C scores in men and women see Fig. 1. The mean number of drinking days in past week was 5 (SD 2) and mean number of days drinking >6 ♀/>8 ♂ units of alcohol in past week, was 3 (SD 2). Baseline characteristics are reported separately by gender in Table 1.

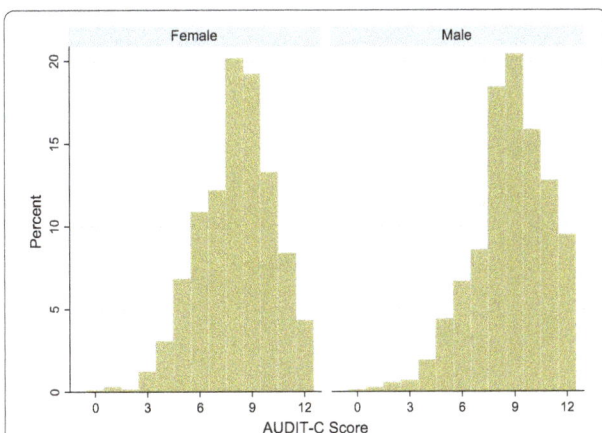

Fig. 1 Distribution of AUDIT-C scores in female and male participants

Drinking above recommended weekly limits
The area under the ROC curve was 0.84 (95% CI 0.80, 0.87) for females and 0.80 (95% CI 0.76, 0.84) for males (Fig. 2).

The 'optimal' AUDIT-C cut-off scores for identifying people drinking above weekly limits were found to be ≥8 (female) and ≥8 (male). Performance at optimal cut-offs are reported in Table 6 without and with adjustment for optimism, but the optimism-adjusted values are described here. Estimated sensitivity was 76% (95% CI 74, 78) and specificity 73% (95% CI 66, 79) for women, and sensitivity was 85% (95% CI 83, 87) and specificity of 58% (95% CI 50, 65) for men. The positive likelihood ratios corresponding to a cut-off score of ≥8 were 2.81 (95% CI 2.56, 3.08) for women and 2.02 (95% CI 1.78, 2.29) for men; the negative likelihood ratios were 0.32 (95% CI 0.25, 0.41) for women and 0.26 (95% CI 0.21, 0.32) for men (Tables 2, 3, 6).

The most accurate AUDIT-C cut-off scores for identifying people drinking above weekly limits were ≥4 (female) and ≥5 (male), with corresponding sensitivity of 99% (95% CI 98, 99) and specificity of 25% (95% CI 19, 33) for females, and sensitivity of 99% (95% CI 99, 100) and specificity of 25% (95% CI 19, 32) for males. These cut-off scores led to a high proportion of participants correctly identified as drinking above recommended limits for both females (92%) and males (91%). The positive likelihood ratios corresponding to a cut-off score of ≥4 was 1.32 (95% CI 1.03, 1.70) for women and ≥5 was 1.33 (95% CI 1.03, 1.71) for men; the negative likelihood ratios were 0.05 (95% CI 0.03, 0.07) for women and 0.03 (95% CI 0.02, 0.05) for men (Tables 2, 3, 6).

Higher risk drinking
The area under the ROC curve was 0.79 (95% CI 0.77, 0.81) for females and 0.78 (95% CI 0.76, 0.81) for males (Fig. 3).

The 'optimal' AUDIT-C cut-off scores for identifying higher risk drinkers, i.e. more than 35 units/week for women and more than 50 units/week for men) was found to be ≥8 for women and ≥9 for men, with corresponding sensitivity of 70% (95% CI 67, 73) and specificity of 71% (95% CI 67, 74) for women, and sensitivity of 77% (95% CI 74, 79) and specificity of 65% (95% CI 61, 69) for men. The positive likelihood ratios corresponding to a cut-off score of ≥8 was 2.39 (95% CI 2.26, 2.53) for women and ≥9 was 2.19 (95% CI 2.05, 2.34) for men; the negative likelihood ratios were 0.42 (95% CI 0.37, 0.48) for women and 0.36 (95% CI 0.31, 0.42) for men (Tables 4, 5, 6).

The most accurate AUDIT-C cut-off scores for identifying higher risk drinkers were also found to be ≥8 for women and ≥9 for men (Tables 4, 5, 6). These cut-off scores identified the highest proportion of participants

Table 1 Demographics

Demographic variables	Female N = 2053	Male N = 1667
Age (years): mean (SD)	37 (11)	38 (11)
Educated at least to degree level: n (%)	1039 (50)	853 (51)
White British: n (%)	1785 (86)	1363 (82)
Living in UK: n (%)	1883 (91)	1439 (86)
AUDIT-C: mean (SD)	8 (2)	9 (2)
Past week's alcohol consumption in units: arithmetic mean (SD)[a]	48 (30)	64 (42)
Past week's alcohol consumption in units: geometric mean (approx. SD[b])[a]	35 (4)	43 (5)
Number of drinking days in past week: mean (SD)[a]	5 (2)	5 (2)
Number of days drinking >6 ♀/>8 ♂ units of alcohol in past week: mean (SD)[a]	3 (2)	3 (2)
Drinking >14 ♀/>21 ♂ units of alcohol in past week: n (%)[a,c]	1901 (91)	1486 (89)
Drinking >35 ♀/>50 ♂ units of alcohol in past week: n (%)[a,d]	1298 (62)	937 (56)

[a] Drinking measures using data collected by the TOT-AL

[b] Approximate SD back-calculated from the log-scale

[c] Above weekly limits

[d] Higher risk drinking

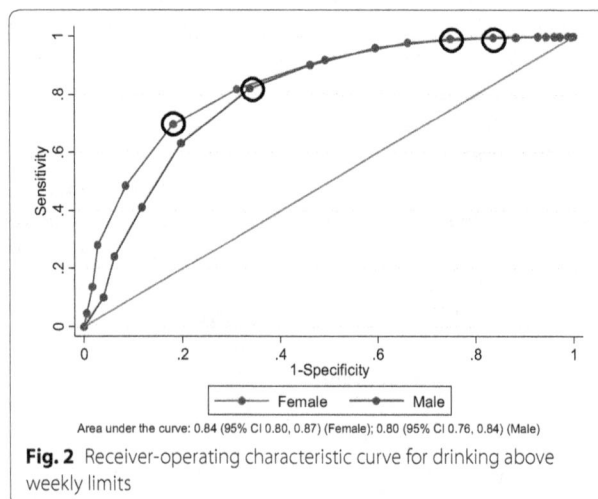

Area under the curve: 0.84 (95% CI 0.80, 0.87) (Female); 0.80 (95% CI 0.76, 0.84) (Male)

Fig. 2 Receiver-operating characteristic curve for drinking above weekly limits

correctly identified as drinking at higher risk levels for both women (70%) and men (72%).

Discussion

This study identified AUDIT-C thresholds that indicated risky and higher risk drinking among adults seeking online help with their drinking. This study found that 'optimal' AUDIT-C cut-off scores, defined as those that maximise the sum of sensitivity and specificity, for identifying drinking above recommended weekly limits were ≥8 for women and ≥8 for men; whereas the most accurate AUDIT-C cut-off scores, i.e. those with the highest proportion of individuals correctly classified as risky, were ≥4 for women and ≥5 for men. Optimal and accurate AUDIT-C cut-off scores for identifying higher risk drinkers were equal at ≥8 for women and ≥9 for men.

Table 2 AUDIT-C threshold for drinking above weekly limits (female)

AUDIT-C score	Sensitivity % (95% CI)	Specificity % (95% CI)	LR+[a] (95% CI)	LR−[b] (95% CI)	Sensitivity + specificity	% Correctly classified (95% CI)
≥2	99.95 (99.70, 100.0)	3.95 (1.60, 7.98)	1.04 (0.50, 2.15)	0.01 (0.00, 0.07)	103.90	91.67 (90.39, 92.83)
≥3	99.95 (99.70, 100.0)	5.65 (2.74, 10.14)	1.06 (0.58, 1.94)	0.01 (0.00, 0.07)	105.60	91.82 (90.55, 92.97)
≥4*	99.63 (99.23, 99.85)	16.38 (11.26, 22.68)	1.19 (0.85, 1.66)	0.02 (0.01, 0.04)	116.01	92.45 (91.22, 93.56)
≥5	97.92 (97.17, 98.52)	33.90 (26.97, 41.38)	1.48 (1.20, 1.82)	0.06 (0.04, 0.08)	131.82	92.40 (91.17, 93.51)
≥6	92.06 (90.74, 93.24)	50.85 (43.24, 58.43)	1.87 (1.62, 2.16)	0.16 (0.13, 0.20)	142.91	88.50 (87.05, 89.85)
≥7	81.88 (80.06, 83.60)	68.93 (61.55, 75.66)	2.63 (2.38, 2.91)	0.26 (0.20, 0.33)	150.81	80.76 (78.99, 82.44)
≥8**	69.78 (67.64, 71.85)	81.92 (75.45, 87.29)	3.86 (3.58, 4.16)	0.37 (0.27, 0.51)	151.70	70.82 (68.80, 72.78)
≥9	48.61 (46.33, 50.90)	91.53 (86.41, 95.18)	5.74 (5.38, 6.12)	0.56 (0.34, 0.91)	140.14	52.31 (50.13, 54.49)
≥10	28.14 (26.12, 30.24)	97.18 (93.53, 99.08)	9.96 (9.23, 10.75)	0.74 (0.31, 1.76)	125.32	34.10 (32.05, 36.19)

Drinking >14 units of alcohol in past week

*The most accurate AUDIT-C cut-off score for identifying risky drinkers

**The 'optimal' AUDIT-C cut-off score for identifying risky drinkers

[a] LR+ positive likelihood ratio

[b] LR− negative likelihood ratio

Table 3 AUDIT-C threshold for drinking above weekly limits (male)

AUDIT-C score	Sensitivity % (95% CI)	Specificity % (95% CI)	LR+[a] (95% CI)	LR−[b] (95% CI)	Sensitivity + specificity	% Correctly classified (95% CI)
≥2	99.93 (99.62, 100.0)	2.81 (0.92, 6.43)	1.03 (0.43, 2.44)	0.02 (0.00, 0.14)	102.74	89.35 (87.75, 90.81)
≥3	99.86 (99.50, 99.98)	7.30 (3.95, 12.17)	1.08 (0.64, 1.82)	0.02 (0.01, 0.08)	107.16	89.78 (88.21, 91.21)
≥4	99.66 (99.20, 99.89)	11.80 (7.45, 17.47)	1.13 (0.76, 1.69)	0.03 (0.01, 0.07)	111.46	90.09 (88.53, 91.49)
≥5*	99.18 (98.56, 99.57)	25.28 (19.08, 32.33)	1.33 (1.03, 1.71)	0.03 (0.02, 0.05)	124.46	91.13 (89.64, 92.46)
≥6	96.09 (94.96, 97.02)	40.45 (33.17, 48.05)	1.61 (1.35, 1.92)	0.10 (0.08, 0.13)	136.54	90.02 (88.47, 91.44)
≥7	90.25 (88.61, 91.72)	53.93 (46.32, 61.42)	1.96 (1.71, 2.25)	0.18 (0.14, 0.22)	144.18	86.29 (84.53, 87.92)
≥8**	82.14 (80.08, 84.08)	66.29 (58.84, 73.19)	2.44 (2.19, 2.72)	0.27 (0.21, 0.34)	148.43	80.42 (78.41, 82.31)
≥9	63.19 (60.65, 65.67)	80.34 (73.73, 85.91)	3.21 (2.96, 3.49)	0.46 (0.34, 0.62)	143.53	65.06 (62.69, 67.37)
≥10	41.21 (38.67, 43.79)	88.20 (82.53, 92.55)	3.49 (3.22, 3.79)	0.67 (0.45, 1.00)	129.41	46.33 (43.89, 48.78)

Drinking >21 units of alcohol in past week

*The most accurate AUDIT-C cut-off score for identifying risky drinkers

**The 'optimal' AUDIT-C cut-off score for identifying risky drinkers

[a] LR+ positive likelihood ratio

[b] LR− negative likelihood ratio

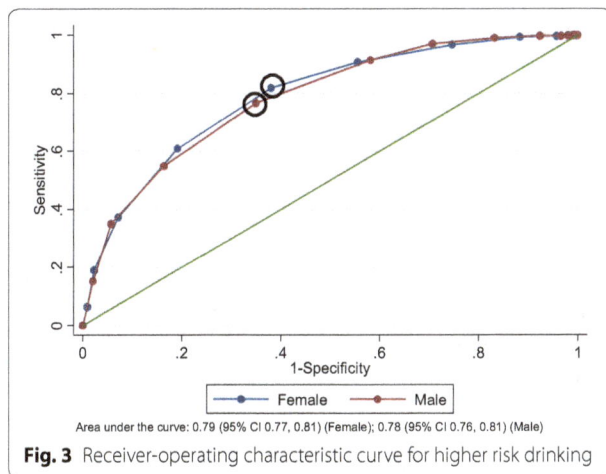

Area under the curve: 0.79 (95% CI 0.77, 0.81) (Female); 0.78 (95% CI 0.76, 0.81) (Male)

Fig. 3 Receiver-operating characteristic curve for higher risk drinking

These findings relate to a largely UK based population of adults seeking online help with their drinking.

The optimal cut-off scores for identifying people drinking above advocated weekly limits were substantially higher in this study of online help seekers predominantly from the UK than in other validation studies in general population samples. Online help seekers are a novel population in this field of study. Studies in the US, Germany and Scandinavia identified in the small number of reviews in this field [13, 14] have validated the AUDIT-C for detecting risky drinking in the general population, all of which administered measures in-person. The optimal AUDIT-C scores found in the present study are higher than those previously identified which is a potentially important finding, particularly for researchers evaluating

Table 4 AUDIT-C thresholds for higher risk drinking (female)

AUDIT-C score	Sensitivity % (95% CI)	Specificity % (95% CI)	LR+[a] (95% CI)	LR−[b] (95% CI)	Sensitivity + specificity	% Correctly classified (95% CI)
≥2	99.92 (99.56, 100.0)	0.90 (0.36, 1.85)	1.01 (0.48, 2.11)	0.09 (0.01, 0.64)	100.82	62.45 (60.31, 64.55)
≥3	99.92 (99.56, 100.0)	1.29 (0.62, 2.35)	1.01 (0.55, 1.87)	0.06 (0.02, 0.24)	101.21	62.59 (60.46, 64.69)
≥4	99.76 (99.31, 99.95)	4.25 (2.94, 5.91)	1.04 (0.74, 1.45)	0.06 (0.02, 0.19)	104.01	63.61 (61.49, 65.70)
≥5	99.37 (98.77, 99.73)	11.71 (9.54, 14.18)	1.13 (0.93, 1.37)	0.05 (0.03, 0.10)	111.08	66.20 (64.10, 68.24)
≥6	96.71 (95.58, 97.62)	25.35 (22.33, 28.57)	1.30 (1.15, 1.47)	0.13 (0.10, 0.18)	122.06	69.70 (67.66, 71.69)
≥7	90.83 (89.11, 92.36)	44.40 (40.87, 47.98)	1.63 (1.50, 1.77)	0.21 (0.17, 0.25)	135.23	73.26 (71.29, 75.16)
≥8*	81.90 (79.67, 83.97)	61.90 (58.39, 65.33)	2.15 (2.02, 2.28)	0.29 (0.25, 0.34)	143.80	74.33 (72.38, 76.21)
≥9	60.97 (58.23, 63.66)	80.82 (77.88, 83.53)	3.18 (3.01, 3.36)	0.48 (0.41, 0.56)	141.79	68.49 (66.43, 70.49)
≥10	37.38 (34.72, 40.10)	92.79 (90.74, 94.51)	5.19 (4.82, 5.59)	0.67 (0.52, 0.87)	130.17	58.35 (56.19, 60.50)

Drinking >35 units of alcohol in past week

*The 'optimal' and most accurate AUDIT-C cut-off score for identifying higher risk drinkers

[a] LR+ positive likelihood ratio

[b] LR− negative likelihood ratio

Table 5 AUDIT-C thresholds for higher risk drinking (male)

AUDIT-C score	Sensitivity % (95% CI)	Specificity % (95% CI)	LR+[a] (95% CI)	LR−[b] (95% CI)	Sensitivity + specificity	% Correctly classified (95% CI)
≥2	100.00 (99.60, 100.0)	0.84 (0.31, 1.82)	1.01 (0.46, 2.24)	0.00	100.84	56.61 (54.17, 59.03)
≥3	99.89 (99.40, 100.0)	1.96 (1.07, 3.26)	1.02 (0.61, 1.71)	0.06 (0.01, 0.43)	101.85	57.04 (54.60, 59.45)
≥4	99.78 (99.22, 99.97)	3.36 (2.16, 4.95)	1.03 (0.70, 1.53)	0.06 (0.02, 0.24)	103.14	57.59 (55.15, 60.00)
≥5	99.78 (99.22, 99.97)	7.69 (5.85, 9.90)	1.08 (0.84, 1.39)	0.03 (0.01, 0.12)	107.47	59.49 (57.06, 61.88)
≥6	99.02 (98.15, 99.55)	16.78 (14.12, 19.73)	1.19 (1.01, 1.40)	0.06 (0.03, 0.12)	115.8	63.04 (60.64, 65.38)
≥7	96.95 (95.63, 97.97)	29.37 (26.05, 32.86)	1.37 (1.22, 1.54)	0.10 (0.07, 0.14)	126.32	67.38 (65.05, 69.65)
≥8	91.40 (89.40, 93.14)	41.82 (38.17, 45.53)	1.57 (1.44, 1.72)	0.21 (0.17, 0.26)	133.22	69.71 (67.41, 71.93)
≥9*	76.71 (73.84, 79.41)	65.03 (61.41, 68.53)	2.19 (2.05, 2.34)	0.36 (0.31, 0.42)	141.74	71.60 (69.35, 73.78)
≥10	54.84 (51.56, 58.09)	83.64 (80.72, 86.27)	3.35 (3.13, 3.58)	0.54 (0.45, 0.65)	138.48	67.44 (65.11, 69.71)

Drinking >50 units of alcohol in past week

*The 'optimal' and most accurate AUDIT-C cut-off score for identifying higher risk drinkers

[a] LR+ positive likelihood ratio

[b] LR− negative likelihood ratio

the effectiveness of brief alcohol interventions accessible over the Internet, as thresholds that are set too low may underestimate intervention impact if they are not appropriately targeted.

This study included a sample of people who were web-browsing and visited the Down Your Drink site. Some, at least, will have been actively seeking help, and they may therefore display different characteristics to opportunistically-recruited non-help seeking populations in primary care and other settings in which brief intervention studies usually take place. Participants were concerned enough to think about or change their drinking. These 'e-help' seekers consumed higher levels of alcohol than the general (non-help seeking) population, with almost the entire sample drinking above recommended limits (91% female, 89% male). DYD participants also differ from the general population as a whole by reporting fewer problems with mobility, self-care, usual activities and pain because they were younger. However, they were more likely to report experiencing anxiety and/or depression (57% DYD vs. 21% general population) [43]. The nature of this study population thus warrants careful consideration in relation to study findings and the generalisability of these data.

When selecting a suitable threshold for the identification of risky drinkers there are various factors that need to be considered, such as prevalence, the regularity of screening, and any physical, psychological and economic costs related to the identification of false positives or false negatives [44]. For example, when screening for risky drinking in primary care settings, it has been suggested that sensitivity may be more important than specificity due to the relative ease and low cost of further assessment [12]. Contrary to this, the US Department of Veteran

Affairs medical centres use an AUDIT-C threshold of ≥5 for men and women as a means of minimising burden of false positives on primary care providers, where recommended thresholds in this setting are typically lower [45]. It is important to note that the present study was conducted with an online help-seeking population and should be used to inform screening of populations identified in a similar manner. In the DYD trial, we used the most accurate cut-off scores to screen adults for risky and higher risk drinking. In this context we wanted to maximise the number of correctly screened individuals, with no particular emphasis on sensitivity—no harm was associated with false positives, and no particular emphasis on specificity—the intervention was delivered online with no time or financial restraints on its delivery. Rather, it was important that the test was credible in detecting whether people were at risk from their drinking or not. It has been suggested that 'optimal' cut-off scores, which maximise sensitivity and specificity, are nonsensical as they often combine accuracy data from thresholds that are not clinically relevant [46]. We suggest that researchers, practitioners and policy makers think carefully about the context and implications of alcohol screening before selecting or advocating an AUDIT-C cut-off score.

Strengths and limitations

One of the key strengths of this study is the use of past week drinking data as the reference-standard with which the AUDIT-C scores were compared. In using a very detailed online measure of past week drinking (the TOTAL), we were able to determine the AUDIT-C cut-off score at which participants were drinking above the recommended UK weekly limits of 14 units per week for women, and 21 units per week for men. Many of the studies

Table 6 Optimal and most accurate AUDIT-C thresholds

Drinking category	Selected thresholds by sex, evaluations with and without optimism		Sensitivity (%) (95% CI)	Specificity (%) (95% CI)	LR+[c] (95% CI)	LR−[d] (95% CI)	Sensitivity + specificity	% Correctly classified (95% CI)
Above weekly limits[a]	Optimal	Female ≥8	With optimism	69.78 (67.64, 71.85)	81.92 (75.45, 87.29)	3.86 (3.58, 4.16)	0.37 (0.27, 0.51)	151.7	70.82 (68.80, 72.78)
			Optimism-adjusted	76.33 (74.34, 78.24)	72.88 (65.70, 79.28)	2.81 (2.56, 3.08)	0.32 (0.25, 0.41)	149.21	76.04 (74.13, 77.87)
		Male ≥8	With optimism	82.14 (80.08, 84.08)	66.29 (58.84, 73.19)	2.44 (2.19, 2.72)	0.27 (0.21, 0.34)	148.43	80.42 (78.41, 82.31)
			Optimism-adjusted	85.10 (83.16, 86.89)	57.87 (50.25, 65.21)	2.02 (1.78, 2.29)	0.26 (0.21, 0.32)	142.97	82.13 (80.18, 83.96)
	Most accurate	Female ≥4	With optimism	99.63 (99.23, 99.85)	16.38 (11.26, 22.68)	1.19 (0.85, 1.66)	0.02 (0.01, 0.04)	116.01	92.45 (91.22, 93.56)
			Optimism-adjusted	98.61 (97.98, 99.09)	25.42 (19.19, 32.50)	1.32 (1.03, 1.70)	0.05 (0.03, 0.07)	124.03	92.30 (91.07, 93.42)
		Male ≥5	With optimism	99.18 (98.56, 99.57)	25.28 (19.08, 32.33)	1.33 (1.03, 1.71)	0.03 (0.02, 0.05)	124.46	91.13 (89.64, 92.46)
			Optimism-adjusted	99.18 (98.56, 99.57)	25.28 (19.08, 32.33)	1.33 (1.03, 1.71)	0.03 (0.02, 0.05)	124.46	91.13 (89.64, 92.46)
Higher risk drinking[b]	Optimal	Female ≥8	With optimism	81.90 (79.67, 83.97)	61.90 (58.39, 65.33)	2.15 (2.02, 2.28)	0.29 (0.25, 0.34)	143.80	74.33 (72.38, 76.21)
			Optimism-adjusted	81.90 (79.67, 83.97)	61.90 (58.39, 65.33)	2.15 (2.02, 2.28)	0.29 (0.25, 0.34)	143.80	74.33 (72.38, 76.21)
		Male ≥9	With optimism	76.71 (73.84, 79.41)	65.03 (61.41, 68.53)	2.19 (2.05, 2.34)	0.36 (0.31, 0.42)	141.74	71.60 (69.35, 73.78)
			Optimism-adjusted	76.71 (73.84, 79.41)	65.03 (61.41, 68.53)	2.19 (2.05, 2.34)	0.36 (0.31, 0.42)	141.74	71.60 (69.35, 73.78)
	Most accurate	Female ≥8	With optimism	81.90 (79.67, 83.97)	61.90 (58.39, 65.33)	2.15 (2.02, 2.28)	0.29 (0.25, 0.34)	143.80	74.33 (72.38, 76.21)
			Optimism-adjusted	81.90 (79.67, 83.97)	61.90 (58.39, 65.33)	2.15 (2.02, 2.28)	0.29 (0.25, 0.34)	143.80	74.33 (72.38, 76.21)
		Male ≥9	With optimism	76.71 (73.84, 79.41)	65.03 (61.41, 68.53)	2.19 (2.05, 2.34)	0.36 (0.31, 0.42)	141.74	71.60 (69.35, 73.78)
			Optimism-adjusted	76.71 (73.84, 79.41)	65.03 (61.41, 68.53)	2.19 (2.05, 2.34)	0.36 (0.31, 0.42)	141.74	71.60 (69.35, 73.78)

[a] Above weekly limits >14 units of alcohol in past week (women); >21 units of alcohol in past week (men)

[b] Higher risk drinking >35 units of alcohol in past week (women); >50 units of alcohol in past week (men)

[c] LR+ positive likelihood ratio

[d] LR− negative likelihood ratio

investigating different cut-off scores for abbreviated versions of the AUDIT have used the full AUDIT as their reference-standard which "violates the independence of data assumption underlying the use of these statistical tests" p. 22 [26]. Furthermore, the AUDIT-C is a measure of alcohol consumption, not harm, therefore, we deemed a measure of consumption as a more suitable reference standard than a combined measure of consumption and harm.

The TOT-AL measures past week consumption, known as actual or exact recall, which leads to easier and more accurate recall due to the recency of consumption, and avoids difficulties in attempts to estimate average consumption [41, 47]. This helps minimise task-related errors, though the nature of the behaviour being reported upon is intrinsically difficult to measure retrospectively, as recall must contend with variations in drinking patterns over time [41, 47]. In addition, short-term measurement does not accurately reflect alcohol consumption among infrequent drinkers due to inadequate time sampling [41, 47].

The use of weekly limits as a reference-standard is also arguably a weakness. Despite the focus of the AUDIT-C on consumption, it was principally developed as a screening tool for problematic drinking [12]. As such, one limitation of this study, notwithstanding the strong population-level correlation between consumption and problems, is that we are unable to classify participants as problematic drinkers, in the absence of any individual-level information on alcohol-related harm or problems. This also limits the generalisability of this study, if one is interested in identifying people who are experiencing current problems and may be more receptive to interventions than those who are not [48]. Note also that levels of consumption or compliance with weekly drinking limits per se provide information on risk (i.e. possible future problems), whereas the AUDIT was originally designed as a clinical instrument concerned with need for brief intervention [9]. Further limitations include the small student sample in which the TOT-AL was validated, and that past-week consumption may not reflect average consumption, and therefore differs from the AUDIT-C in that respect.

This study did not investigate whether different AUDIT-C scores were necessary for identifying risky drinking in different age groups as participants were aged 18 years or above, and due to the online nature of the DYD trial, older people may have been under-represented. Previous research has found that lower cut-off scores may be necessary in younger age groups [49], and the Royal College of Psychiatrists have advocated that lower recommended limits are introduced for people over the age of 65 [50]. Previous research findings are mixed as to the need for different cut-off scores for different ethnicities [51, 52]. This study constituted a largely 'White British' population (84%), therefore exploration of suitability for different ethnic groups was not possible.

Conclusion

The 'optimal' AUDIT-C scores for identifying people drinking above recommended weekly drinking limits were substantially higher in this study than in any previous study undertaken in any form of general population sample. This is one of the few studies that has validated the AUDIT-C in an adult UK population, and the web browsing nature of this sample is emphasised in interpreting these data. Researchers should consider carefully the basis for selecting AUDIT-C cut-off scores according to the purposes of identifying risky drinkers, the relative importance of sensitivity and/or specificity, and the setting in which screening is undertaken.

Authors' contributions
EM, IRW, JM and ZK conceived the study. ZK prepared the protocol and all authors contributed to the study design. LM undertook the statistical analysis, supported by IRW. ZK wrote the first draft of the manuscript. All authors read and approved the final manuscript.

Author details
[1] Department of Primary Care and Population Health, UCL Royal Free Campus, Upper Third Floor, Rowland Hill Street, London NW3 2PF, UK. [2] Health Service and Population Research Department, Centre for Implementation Science, Institute of Psychiatry, Psychology and Neuroscience, King's College London, De Crespigny Park, London SE5 8AF, UK. [3] MRC Biostatistics Unit, Cambridge Institute of Public Health, Forvie Site, Robinson Way, Cambridge Biomedical Campus, Cambridge CB2 0SR, UK. [4] Department of Health Sciences, Seebohm Rowntree Building, University of York, Heslington, York YO10 5DD, UK.

Acknowledgements
Not applicable.

Competing interests
PW has intellectual property rights for www.downyourdrink.org.uk, is Chief Medical Advisor to the UK charity Drinkaware and has provided private consultancy on the topic of screening and brief interventions to several agencies. All other authors declare that they have no competing interests.

Funding
Zarnie Khadjesari was funded by an NIHR School for Primary Care Research fellowship (October 2011 to September 2014). Zarnie is currently a King's Improvement Science postdoctoral fellow at King's College London. King's Improvement Science is part of the Centre for Implementation Science at the National Institute for Health Research (NIHR) Collaboration for Leadership in Applied Health Research and Care South London.

References
1. World Health Organisation. Global strategy to reduce the harmful use of alcohol. Italy: World Health Organisation; 2010.

2. Miller WR, Wilbourne PL. Mesa Grande: a methodological analysis of clinical trials of treatments for alcohol use disorders. Addiction. 2002;97:265–77.

3. Kaner EFS, Dickinson HO, Beyer FR, Campbell F, Schlesinger C, Heather N, Saunders JB, Burnand B, Pienaar ED. Effectiveness of brief alcohol interventions in primary care populations. Cochrane Database Syst Rev 2007;(2), Art No. CD004148. doi:10.1002/14651858.CD004148.pub3.

4. O'Donnell A, Anderson P, Newbury-Birch D, Schulte B, Schmidt C, Reimer J, Kaner E. The impact of brief alcohol interventions in primary healthcare: a systematic review of reviews. Alcohol Alcohol. 2014;49:66–78.

5. Webb G, Shakeshaft A, Sanson-Fisher R, Havard A. A systematic review of work-place interventions for alcohol-related problems. Addiction. 2009;104:365–77.

6. Havard A, Shakeshaft A, Sanson-Fisher R. Systematic review and meta-analyses of strategies targeting alcohol problems in emergency departments: interventions reduce alcohol-related injuries. Addiction. 2008;103:368–76 **(discussion 377–368)**.

7. Schulte B, O'Donnell AJ, Kastner S, Schmidt CS, Schäfer I, Reimer J. Alcohol screening and brief intervention in workplace settings and social services: a comparison of literature. Front Psychiatry. 2014;5:131.

8. Carey KB, Scott-Sheldon LA, Carey MP, DeMartini KS. Individual-level interventions to reduce college student drinking: a meta-analytic review. Addict Behav. 2007;32:2469–94.

9. Babor TF, Higgins-Biddle JC, Saunders JB, Monteiro MG. AUDIT—the alcohol use disorders identification test: guidelines for use in primary care. Second edition edition. Geneva: World Health Organization; 2001.

10. Berner MM, Kriston L, Bentele M, Harter M. The alcohol use disorders identification test for detecting at-risk drinking: a systematic review and meta-analysis. J Stud Alcohol Drugs. 2007;68:461–73.

11. NICE Public Health Guidance 24. Alcohol-use disorders: preventing the development of hazardous and harmful drinking. London: National Institute for Health and Clinical Excellence; 2010.

12. Bush K, Kivlahan DR, McDonell MB, Fihn SD, Bradley KA. The AUDIT alcohol consumption questions (AUDIT-C): an effective brief screening test for problem drinking. Ambulatory Care Quality Improvement Project (ACQUIP). Alcohol Use Disorders Identification Test. Arch Intern Med. 1998;158:1789–95.

13. Reinert DF, Allen JP. The alcohol use disorders identification test: an update of research findings. Alcohol Clin Exp Res. 2007;31:185–99.

14. Kriston L, Holzel L, Weiser AK, Berner MM, Harter M. Meta-analysis: are 3 questions enough to detect unhealthy alcohol use? Ann Intern Med. 2008;149:879–88.

15. Rumpf HJ, Hapke U, Meyer C, John U. Screening for alcohol use disorders and at-risk drinking in the general population: psychometric performance of three questionnaires. Alcohol Alcohol. 2002;37:261–8.

16. Dawson DA, Grant BF, Stinson FS, Zhou Y. Effectiveness of the derived Alcohol Use Disorders Identification Test (AUDIT-C) in screening for alcohol use disorders and risk drinking in the US general population. Alcohol Clin Exp Res. 2005;29:844–54.

17. Selin KH. Alcohol Use Disorder Identification Test (AUDIT): what does it screen? Performance of the AUDIT against four different criteria in a Swedish population sample. Subst Use Misuse. 2003;41:1881–99.

18. Aalto M, Tuunanen M, Sillanaukee P, Seppa K. Effectiveness of structured questionnaires for screening heavy drinking in middle-aged women. Alcohol Clin Exp Res. 2006;30:1884–8.

19. Tuunanen M, Aalto M, Seppa K. Binge drinking and its detection among middle-aged men using AUDIT, AUDIT-C and AUDIT-3. Drug Alcohol Rev. 2007;26:295–9.

20. Lundin A, Hallgren M, Balliu N, Forsell Y. The use of alcohol use disorders identification test (AUDIT) in detecting alcohol use disorder and risk drinking in the general population: validation of AUDIT using schedules for clinical assessment in neuropsychiatry. Alcohol Clin Exp Res. 2015;39:158–65.

21. Dedert EA, McDuffie JR, Stein R, McNiel JM, Kosinski AS, Freiermuth CE, Hemminger A, Williams JW Jr. Electronic interventions for alcohol misuse and alcohol use disorders: a systematic review. Ann Intern Med. 2015;163:205–14.

22. Thomas BA, McCambridge J. Comparative psychometric study of a range of hazardous drinking measures administered online in a youth population. Drug Alcohol Depend. 2008;96:121–7.

23. Kypri K, Gallagher SJ, Cashell-Smith ML. An internet-based survey method for college student drinking research. Drug Alcohol Depend. 2004;76:45–53.

24. McCabe SE, Boyd CJ, Young A, Crawford S, Pope D. Mode effects for collecting alcohol and tobacco data among 3rd and 4th grade students: a randomized pilot study of Web-form versus paper-form surveys. Addict Behav. 2005;30:663–71.

25. Miller ET, Neal DJ, Roberts LJ, Baer JS, Cressler SO, Metrik J, Marlatt GA. Test-retest reliability of alcohol measures: is there a difference between internet-based assessment and traditional methods? Psychol Addict Behav. 2002;16:56–63.

26. McCambridge J, Thomas BA. Short forms of the AUDIT in a Web-based study of young drinkers. Drug Alcohol Rev. 2009;28:18–24.

27. Tourangeau R, Smith TW. Asking sensitive questions—the impact of data collection mode, question format, and question context. Public Opinion Quarterly. 1996;60:275–304.

28. Wight RG, Rotheram-Borus MJ, Klosinski L, Ramos B, Calabro M, Smith R. Screening for transmission behaviors among HIV-infected adults. AIDS Educ Prev. 2000;12:431–41.

29. Kypri K, McCambridge J, Vater T, Bowe SJ, Saunders JB, Cunningham JA, Horton NJ. Web-based alcohol intervention for Maori university students: double-blind, multi-site randomized controlled trial. Addiction. 2013;108:331–8.

30. Kypri K, Vater T, Bowe SJ, Saunders JB, Cunningham JA, Horton NJ, McCambridge J. Web-based alcohol screening and brief intervention for university students: a randomized trial. JAMA. 2014;311:1218–24.

31. Lopez-Pelayo H, Wallace P, Segura L, Miquel L, Diaz E, Teixido L, Baena B, Struzzo P, Palacio-Vieira J, Casajuana C, et al. A randomised controlled non-inferiority trial of primary care-based facilitated access to an alcohol reduction website (EFAR Spain): the study protocol. BMJ Open. 2014;4:e007130.

32. Struzzo P, Scafato E, McGregor R, Della Vedova R, Verbano L, Lygidakis C, Tersar C, Crapesi L, Tubaro G, Freemantle N, Wallace P. A randomised controlled non-inferiority trial of primary care-based facilitated access to an alcohol reduction website (EFAR-FVG): the study protocol. BMJ Open. 2013;3:e002304.

33. Linke S, McCambridge J, Khadjesari Z, Wallace P, Murray E. Development of a psychologically enhanced interactive online intervention for hazardous drinking. Alcohol Alcohol. 2008;43:669–74.

34. Murray E, McCambridge J, Khadjesari Z, White IR, Thompson SG, Godfrey C, Linke S, Wallace P. The DYD-RCT protocol: an on-line randomised controlled trial of an interactive computer-based intervention compared with a standard information website to reduce alcohol consumption among hazardous drinkers. BMC Public Health. 2007;7:306.

35. Wallace P, Murray E, McCambridge J, Khadjesari Z, White IR, Thompson SG, Kalaitzaki E, Godfrey C, Linke S. On-line randomized controlled trial of an internet based psychologically enhanced intervention for people with hazardous alcohol consumption. PLoS ONE. 2011;6:e14740.

36. Royal Colleges. Alcohol and the heart in perspective: sensible drinking reaffirmed. Report of a Joint Working Group of the Royal College of Physicians, the Royal College of Psychiatrists and the Royal College of General Practitioners. London: Royal College of Physicians; 1995.

37. Department of Health. The health of the nation: a strategy for health in England. London: HMSO; 1992.

38. Department of Health. UK Chief Medical Officers' alcohol guidelines review. Summary of the proposed new guidelines London: Department of Health; 2016.

39. Khadjesari Z, Murray E, Kalaitzaki E, White IR, McCambridge J, Godfrey C, Wallace P. Test-retest reliability of an online measure of past week alcohol consumption (the TOT-AL), and comparison with face-to-face interview. Addict Behav. 2009;34:337–42.

40. StataCorp. Stata Statistical Software: Release 13. College Station, TX: StataCorp LP; 2013.

41. Dawson DA. Methodological issues in measuring alcohol use. Alcohol Res Health. 2003;27:18–29.

42. Smith GC, Seaman SR, Wood AM, Royston P, White IR. Correcting for optimistic prediction in small data sets. Am J Epidemiol. 2014;180:318–24.

43. Essex HN, White IR, Khadjesari Z, Linke S, McCambridge J, Murray E, Parrott S, Godfrey C. Quality of life among hazardous and harmful drinkers: EQ-5D over a 1-year follow-up period. Qual Life Res. 2014;23:733–43.

44. Alberg AJ, Park JW, Hager BW, Brock MV, Diener-West M. The use of "overall accuracy" to evaluate the validity of screening or diagnostic tests. J Gen Intern Med. 2004;19:460–5.

45. Bradley K, Berger D. Screening for unhealthy alcohol use. In: Saitz R, editor. Addressing unhealthy alcohol use in primary care. New York: Springer; 2013. p. 7–28.

46. Mallett S, Halligan S, Thompson M, Collins GS, Altman DG. Interpreting diagnostic accuracy studies for patient care. BMJ. 2012;345:e3999.

47. Rehm J. Measuring quantity, frequency, and volume of drinking. Alcohol Clin Exp Res. 1998;22:4S–14S.

48. McCambridge J, Rollnick S. Should brief interventions in primary care address alcohol problems more strongly? Addiction. 2014;109:1054–8.

49. Knight JR, Sherritt L, Harris SK, Gates EC, Chang G. Validity of brief alcohol screening tests among adolescents: a comparison of the AUDIT, POSIT, CAGE, and CRAFFT. Alcohol Clin Exp Res. 2003;27:67–73.

50. Older Persons' Substance Misuse Working Group of the Royal College of Psychiatrists. Our invisible addicts: College Report CR165. London: Royal College of Psychiatrists; 2011.

51. Steinbauer JR, Cantor SB, Holzer CE 3rd, Volk RJ. Ethnic and sex bias in primary care screening tests for alcohol use disorders. Ann Intern Med. 1998;129:353–62.

52. Frank D, DeBenedetti AF, Volk RJ, Williams EC, Kivlahan DR, Bradley KA. Effectiveness of the AUDIT-C as a screening test for alcohol misuse in three race/ethnic groups. J Gen Intern Med. 2008;23:781–7.

53. Murray E, Khadjesari K, Wallace P. Pilot and main trial data from the Down Your Drink Trial [Dataset]. 2014. doi:10.14324/49.3.

5

A pilot study comparing in-person and web-based motivational interviewing among adults with a first-time DUI offense

Karen Chan Osilla[1*], Susan M. Paddock[1], Thomas J. Leininger[2], Elizabeth J. D'Amico[1], Brett A. Ewing[1] and Katherine E. Watkins[1]

Abstract

Background: Driving under the influence (DUI) is a significant problem, and there is a pressing need to develop interventions that reduce future risk.

Methods: We pilot-tested the acceptance and efficacy of web-motivational interviewing (MI) and in-person MI interventions among a diverse sample of individuals with a first-time DUI offense. Participants (N = 159) were 65 percent male, 40 percent Hispanic, and an average age of 30 (SD = 9.8). They were enrolled at one of three participating 3-month DUI programs in Los Angeles County and randomized to usual care (UC)-only (36-h program), in-person MI plus UC, or a web-based intervention using MI (web-MI) plus UC. Participants were assessed at intake and program completion. We examined intervention acceptance and preliminary efficacy of the interventions on alcohol consumption, DUI, and alcohol-related consequences.

Results: Web-MI and in-person MI participants rated the quality of and satisfaction with their sessions significantly higher than participants in the UC-only condition. However, there were no significant group differences between the MI conditions and the UC-only condition in alcohol consumption, DUI, and alcohol-related consequences. Further, 67 percent of our sample met criteria for alcohol dependence, and the majority of participants in all three study conditions continued to report alcohol-related consequences at follow-up.

Conclusions: Participants receiving MI plus UC and UC-only had similar improvements, and a large proportion had symptoms of alcohol dependence. Receiving a DUI and having to deal with the numerous consequences related to this type of event may be significant enough to reduce short-term behaviors, but future research should explore whether more intensive interventions are needed to sustain long-term changes.

Keywords: DUI, Motivational interviewing, Brief intervention, Computer and web intervention, Alcohol dependence

Background

Driving under the influence (DUI) is a significant problem. Injury from alcohol-related motor vehicle crashes is a leading cause of premature death and disability [1]. Even after individuals with a first offense attend required alcohol education programs, rates of recidivism are high [2, 3]. Despite a decline in recidivism between 1990 and 1996 in California, rates of DUI incidents in the state have remained stable since 2010.

In California, individuals with a first-time DUI conviction must complete a state-licensed DUI program in order to regain their driver's license [4]. Programs are didactic and lecture-based and provide strategies to reduce drinking and driving, education about alcohol, and presentations by panels of victims whose lives have been affected by a DUI incident [5]. Unfortunately, DUI programs have had only modest effects on recidivism [4]. In 2011, there was no significant difference in the rates of 1-year crash and DUI incidents in California between

*Correspondence: karenc@rand.org
[1] RAND Corporation, 1776 Main Street, Santa Monica, CA 90407-2138, USA
Full list of author information is available at the end of the article

individuals with a DUI conviction who were court-assigned to a DUI program and those who were not [6]. This finding is consistent with the general literature showing that educational-type lectures do not have any effect on behavior change among individuals with alcohol use disorders [7–9].

A more effective approach towards behavior change may be a counseling method that focuses on exploring an individual's reasons for change and helping them develop a change plan that is meaningful for them. Motivational interviewing (MI) is a collaborative counseling style that strives to strengthen a client's commitment to change [10]; it is grounded in theories of self-determination [11] and self-efficacy [12]. Treatment approaches grounded in these theories empower an individual's motivation to change, reaffirm their autonomy, and guide people toward change if they are ready. MI could be particularly acceptable among individuals with DUI convictions who may vary considerably in their motivation to change. For example, some individuals may be ambivalent about changing their drinking and driving behaviors, whereas others may be very motivated to change because of the adverse event or "teachable moment" they experienced [13, 14].

MI is flexible and tailors the intervention content based on the individual's readiness to change. Counselors use processes such as engaging (establishing a connection), focusing (establishing goals such as behavior change), evoking (eliciting the client's motivations to change), and planning (committing to change and developing a plan) to individualize sessions [10]. Within the context of a DUI program, individuals who are not ready to change may benefit most from counselors who spend time engaging the individual and establishing rapport; individuals in later stages or those who are already moving toward change may be better helped by planning when to use problem-solving strategies and in ways to increase their commitment to action [10, 15].

Although many studies have shown the effectiveness of MI in other settings (e.g., college, primary care, substance abuse treatment) compared to no treatment [16], in-person interventions are limited by the availability of trained counselors, training costs, and the challenge of implementing the approach uniformly [17]. For example, research shows that counselors attending MI workshops often lose MI proficiency over time unless they receive ongoing feedback and coaching post-training [18, 19]. Thus, it is important to think about ways to utilize MI that may be more cost-effective and consistent. Web-based interventions that utilize MI principles (web-MI) may be a promising approach.

Web-MI makes it possible to disseminate evidenced-based approaches with high fidelity because the content is programmed and automated. Web-MI has been shown to be effective in reducing at-risk drinking among college students [20, 21] and adults in the general population and military [22, 23]. Web-MI has also been effective in reducing smoking among English and Spanish speakers [24], as well as drug use among postpartum women [25]. While some web-MIs are being explored in criminal justice settings [26], web-MI has not been tested in DUI settings. Few studies have compared the effectiveness of web-MI to active comparison groups (i.e., other interventions that include alcohol content) [27]. Existing research studies have typically compared the effects of a stand-alone web-MI to an assessment-only group [28], and they generally show small effect sizes at short-term follow-up [29]. Although even small effects may be clinically meaningful, more research is needed to improve their comparative effectiveness and determine whether these interventions may serve as an adjunct to more intensive approaches.

The current study evaluated the acceptance and efficacy of web-MI and in-person MI interventions among a diverse sample of individuals with a first-time DUI offense. This Stage 1b trial focused on determining participant acceptance of the intervention and intervention feasibility, and predicting the likely size of intervention effects for future trials [30]. We randomly assigned individuals enrolled in a DUI program to usual-care (UC-only), in-person MI plus UC, or web-MI plus UC. Given the pilot nature of this work, our primary aims were to evaluate the acceptance and efficacy of these MI interventions on alcohol-related outcomes compared to UC-only. We hypothesized that participants in the in-person and web-MI interventions would have greater acceptance and reduced alcohol consumption and alcohol-related consequences compared to UC-only.

Methods/design
Setting and design
Project REACH (Rethinking Avenues for Change; in Spanish, *REtomondo Avenidas para el Cambio Hoy*) was conducted in collaboration with the Los Angeles County Alcohol and Drug Program Administration (ADPA) and three private DUI programs under ADPA's regulatory authority. All clients received UC. Consenting clients were randomized to one of three conditions: UC-only, UC plus in-person MI, or UC plus web-MI using randomized block sampling with equally-sized blocks of six.

All procedures were approved by the institution's IRB. Because of the sensitivity of collecting data while clients were enrolled in the DUI program, participants were told that our Certificate of Confidentiality protected their privacy from any civil, criminal, administrative, legislative, or other proceeding at the federal, state, or local level and that participation in the study would not affect the services to which they were entitled.

Study conditions
Usual care
UC consisted of nine 2-h group sessions, twelve 1-h educational classes, and six community-based 12-step meetings. The 2-h group sessions were unstructured support groups that encouraged participants to examine their own personal attitudes and behavior and receive support for their alcohol or drug problems [31]. In the beginning of the study, we conducted focus groups with UC clients who reported that sessions were focused mainly on the consequences of DUI and heavy drinking [32].

Intervention conditions
We conducted focus groups with DUI program staff and clients to develop the in-person MI intervention for this population. Next, we adapted the in-person intervention for the web, and then conducted individual usability testing interviews with web-MI clients who were already enrolled in the DUI program [32]. We used the usability feedback to iteratively revise the interventions. We developed the interventions simultaneously in English and Spanish in order to create interventions that were culturally equivalent. The current pilot study evaluates the final revised intervention created from these formative assessment procedures.

Both the in-person MI and web-MI interventions consisted of one 45-min individual session and two 10-min booster sessions that were delivered by the same facilitator. Each session was different. The goals of the MI interventions were to reduce drinking and alcohol-related problems. The content of both the in-person and the web-MI intervention was adapted from earlier MI work [33–35] and covered similar content, but the efficacy of the revised interventions had not been tested until the current pilot study. The first session included normative personalized feedback in the following areas: (1) how their drinking and estimates of others' drinking compared to other men/women their age [36]; (2) their positive beliefs about drinking and the balanced placebo design experiment, which describes how alcohol expectancies (i.e., actual vs. expected effects) can influence drinking [37]; (3) their negative consequences from drinking, including their estimated blood alcohol content values; and (4) strategies for avoiding consequences in the future. Participants who were ready to change their drinking were asked to discuss a drinking-related goal they wanted to work on before the next booster session. We then used rulers to assess their confidence and willingness to work on that related goal. If the participant

was not ready to change, the facilitator went straight to the rulers.

The in-person and web-MI booster sessions were formatted similarly and included a check-in about the participant's drinking and goals from the previous session (e.g., "Last session, you said that you would try to stop your drinking by not going to happy hour. How did that go for you?"). Booster sesssions provided an opportunity to talk about new strategies to stop drinking, if they were willing, and to discuss their confidence and willingness to change using rulers with a 1–10 scale (e.g., not confident to very confident).

The style of the MI interventions was as important as the content. Both web-MI and in-person MI interventions used core MI skills, such as open-ended questions, affirmations, reflective statements, and summaries to convey a nonjudgmental and non-confrontational style [10]. For example, the in-person MI manual had examples of open-ended questions and reflective statements that facilitators could use, and these same statements were used by the narrator in the web-MI intervention. Both interventions emphasized the underlying spirit of MI (e.g., collaboration, evocation, acceptance, compassion).

While the web-MI intervention incorporated the same sections of the in-person MI intervention, we used artificial intelligence (e.g., automatic responses tailored to the participant's responses) and personalized feedback to tailor the intervention to the participant so that each session was interactive. For example, we used audio recordings and videos to share personalized feedback from the participant's baseline survey (e.g., "We asked you what your drinking was like and you said you drank 4 days a week."); asked questions that participants could respond to and receive tailored audios/videos based on those responses [e.g., "What do you think of this information?" (participant clicks "I'm surprised"); "It is very common to be surprised by this information and wonder if the numbers are correct..."]; used interactive exercises ("Click a number that best describes your mood when you start to drink. What happens to your mood as you continue to drink?"); and elicited change talk (e.g., "For the confidence ruler, why a 4 and not a 0?"). The web-MI intervention was narrated by a female Latina, and text captions were also available at the bottom of the screen. It was programmed at a 5th-grade reading level.

Participants and recruitment
Participants were individuals 21 and older convicted of a first-time DUI offense and who had entered one of the three participating 3-month DUI programs. Upon enrolling in the program, program staff asked clients if they could be contacted about a research study.

Interested clients completed a consent-to-contact form. Consenting clients were contacted and screened for 5th-grade completion (because of the nature of our self-report instruments) and at-risk drinking, using a score of 3 or higher for women or 5 or higher for men on the Alcohol Use Disorders Identification Test consumption questions (AUDIT-C; [38]). These cut points perform well, with high sensitivity and specificity in screening for at-risk drinking in the general population (men: >90 %, women: 80 %; [39]). Approximately 52 percent were ineligible for the study based on low AUDIT-C score and education (see Fig. 1).

Participants (N = 159) were randomized to one of the three conditions. Participants assigned to either of the two MI interventions were asked to complete their first individual session by the third week of entering the DUI program, and their booster sessions by their ninth and eleventh week in the DUI program, respectively. The timing of these intervention sessions was meant to correspond with the beginning, middle, and end of a participant's 3-month DUI program. As noted earlier, participants in both MI interventions had the same number of sessions as participants in the UC-only condition because their MI sessions replaced two 12-step meetings. All MI intervention sessions were delivered in a private office at the DUI program where UC groups took place. A total of 138 participants were successfully assessed at follow-up (86.8 %).

Procedures

Client data collection

We used in-person interviews to assess DSM-IV criteria for past-year alcohol abuse and dependence. Participants also completed web-based surveys at baseline, after the first session, and 3 months after baseline or at program termination. Participants received a $25 gift card for the Alcohol Use Disorder and Associated Disabilities Interview schedule (AUDADIS; [40]), $25 for the baseline survey, $10 for a satisfaction survey immediately after their first session, and $50 for the 3-month follow-up. All clients were followed in our intent-to-treat analyses, regardless of whether they completed all intervention sessions.

Facilitator training and supervision

Three bilingual facilitators received 40 h of MI training that included a one-day MI workshop delivered by authors KCO and EJD, who are clinical psychologists affiliated with the Motivational Interviewing Network of Trainers. In addition, facilitators received additional coaching and feedback after each session from KCO, who listened to audio recordings of sessions.

Intervention fidelity data collection and coding

In-person MI sessions were audio recorded. Two independent coders received 40 h of coding training [41], which included a half-day training on the Motivational Interviewing Treatment Integrity (MITI) scale [42] and

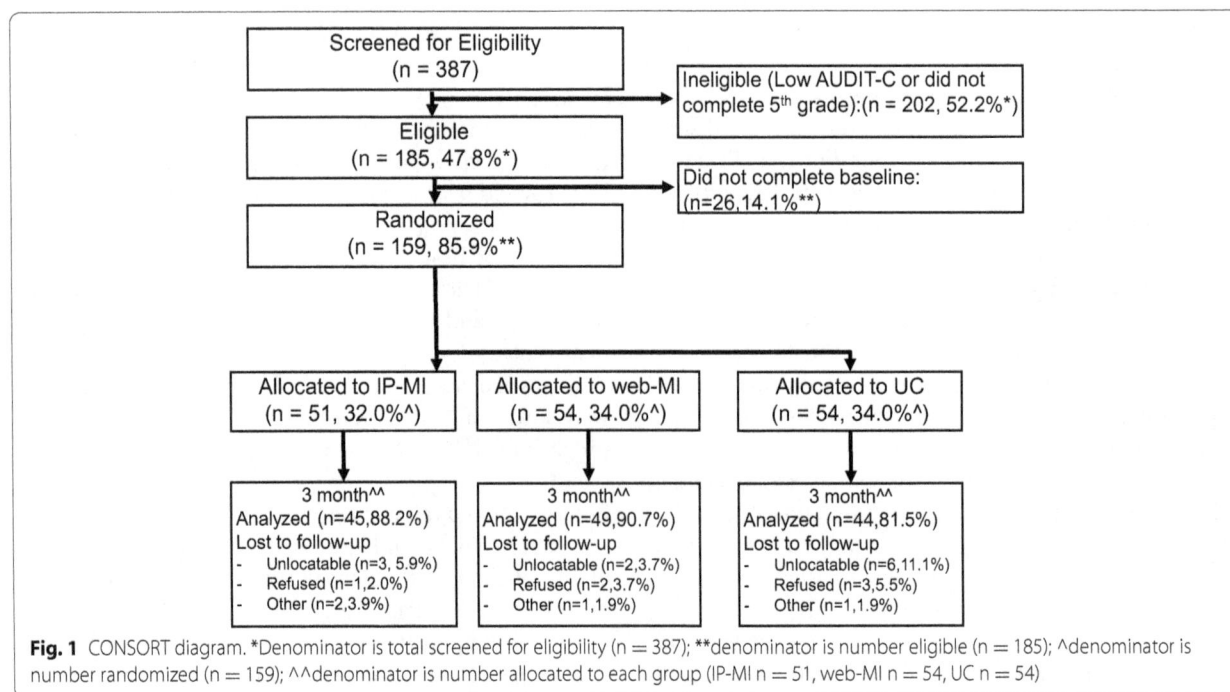

Fig. 1 CONSORT diagram. *Denominator is total screened for eligibility (n = 387); **denominator is number eligible (n = 185); ^denominator is number randomized (n = 159); ^^denominator is number allocated to each group (IP-MI n = 51, web-MI n = 54, UC n = 54)

several MITI practice assignments with pre-coded audio recordings [43]. Raters met weekly to discuss coding discrepancies and reconcile questions to maintain inter-rater agreement. UC sessions were not coded because not all individuals attending these groups were enrolled in the study, so it was not possible to record these sessions.

To monitor web-MI intervention fidelity, our web program measured the number of minutes each participant spent in each session. A facilitator was present in the room to address any problems that might have emerged, which may have also helped to ensure that the participant completed the session.

Measures

At baseline, we collected demographics and alcohol abuse and dependence information using AUDADIS and AUDIT-C [38, 40]. We collected client acceptance/satisfaction data immediately following the first session. At baseline and at 3-month follow-up, we collected data on alcohol use.

Client ratings of quality and satisfaction

Participants in all three conditions answered questions about the quality of and their satisfaction with the experience. Participants were asked, "How would you rate the quality of your session?" on a 4-point Likert scale, with a higher score representing higher quality. Satisfaction was measured using 22 items that were averaged (e.g., This program was respectful of my background; I felt the program respected where I was at with my alcohol and that any change was up to me; The program valued my opinion). Additional items included questions about the usefulness, quality, impact, and helpfulness of the session. They also were asked nine questions rating their session facilitator [44].

MI intervention fidelity

MITI 3.1 was used to code competency and adherence to in-person MI, and integrity was measured through global scores and behavioral counts [42]. The MITI 3.1 has five global scales (evocation, collaboration, autonomy/support, direction, and empathy) that are scored from 1 (low) to 5 (high), with a score of 3.5 indicating beginning proficiency and 4 indicating competency. The rater also counts the number of specific behaviors that occur during each coded segment, including the number of open questions and closed-ended questions, MI-adherent and nonadherent statements, and simple and complex reflections. Whereas global scores have a limited range (1–5), behavioral counts utilize a running tally with no upper end on the scale; thus, these scores can vary by session.

Twenty percent of the in-person MI sessions (n = 10) were randomly selected for double-coding. We calculated

prevalence-adjusted, bias-adjusted kappa (PABAK; [45] to assess inter-rater agreement for each global score by dichotomizing the 1–5 scale into 1–3 (MI beginning proficiency) and 4–5 (MI competent). The PABAK scores for the global scores of evocation, collaboration, autonomy/support, direction, and empathy were 0.6, 0.2, 0.6, 1.0, and 0, respectively, while the agreement averaged 72 percent across the global scores. We also calculated intraclass correlations (ICCs) between raters for each behavioral count. These ICCs ranged from 0.30 (MI-adherent) to 0.91 (closed questions), and averaged 0.69 across the behavioral counts. Since the distribution of MI-nonadherent behavioral counts was skewed toward 0 (with only one value among the coders that was neither 0 nor 1), a kappa statistic was computed instead to assess inter-rater agreement for reporting any versus no MI-nonadherent behaviors (PABAK = 0.2).

Client outcomes

Outcomes included changes in drinking behaviors and related consequences in the past 3 months. We examined the intensity and frequency of drinking in the past 3 months [46]. Drinking frequency was measured by asking how often participants drank alcohol in the past 3 months. Reponses ranged from 0 ('Never') to 10 ('Every day'). We converted these response categories to a pseudo-continuous variable to easily interpret the results as the number of days. Drinking frequency ranged from 0 to 90 days (e.g., 'Never' = 0 days, 'Less than Once a Month' = 2 days). Drinking quantity was measured by asking the respondent the typical number of drinks on a given occasion. Days of reported heavy drinking, defined as four or more drinks for women and five or more drinks for men, was also transformed from a categorical variable to a pseudo-continuous variable ranging from 0 to 90 days, as described above for drinking frequency. Drinking and driving in the past 3 months was reported on a categorical scale ranging from 0 ('Never') to 10 ('Every day'). Due to the skewed distribution of this variable, we created a dichotomous version to indicate any drinking while driving in the past 3 months. We assessed negative consequences from alcohol use using the Shortened Inventory of Problems Modified for Alcohol and Drug Use [47]. Finally, marijuana use frequency was assessed by asking participants how often they used marijuana in the past 3 months. Reponses were transformed to a continuous variable ranging from 0 to 90 days.

Analytic strategy
Client ratings of session quality and satisfaction

Client quality and satisfaction data were analyzed for differences across the three conditions using ANOVA and pair-wise t-tests.

Preliminary intervention efficacy

We first examined whether there was significant change over time in the outcomes within each study condition by conducting Wilcoxon signed-rank tests on the difference scores of continuous outcomes. We conducted a McNemar's test to assess a significant change in the rate of obtaining a DUI and experiencing negative consequences (none vs. any) in the past 3 months between baseline and follow-up, within study condition. Pseudo-continuous variables were treated as continuous, given the assumption that each variable reflected an underlying continuum [48, 49]. The treatment of these variables as continuous were expected to result in low bias when measuring more than seven categories and the measure had a bell-shape [50]. When the latter condition was not met, we ran sensitivity analyses with the ordinal outcome to confirm that conclusions did not differ under the two model specifications.

We next conducted analyses to test for a significant intervention effect. All outcomes were analyzed using an intent-to-treat approach. To compare the baseline characteristics of clients assigned to each condition, we used Chi squared tests for categorical variables and one-way ANOVAs for continuous variables. Longitudinally, each outcome was modeled with generalized, linear, mixed-effects regression modeling using the GLIMMIX procedure in SAS software (Version 9.2). Covariates included in the model were those characteristics identified as significant ($p < 0.1$) in bivariate analyses with the outcomes. These included days of marijuana use in the last 3 months and average number of drinks [46]. The baseline value of the outcome was included as a covariate in all models to control for any important differences among conditions and to improve the precision of the intervention-effect estimates [51]. Dummy variables for web-MI and in-person MI, with the comparison condition as the hold-out category, were included in all models. When the distribution of the pseudo-continuous measures was not bell-shaped, ordinal logistic regressions were conducted on the original ordinal measure as a sensitivity analysis to confirm that analytic conclusions did not differ under the two model specifications.

Results

Client acceptance

Approximately 57 percent attended all three in-person MI sessions, 14 percent attended two sessions, and 29 percent attended one session. Approximately 65 percent attended all three web-MI sessions, 17 percent attended two sessions, and 18 percent attended one session. We did not have data on the number of UC sessions attended. Participants' ratings of session quality varied significantly across conditions [$F(2135) = 6.93$,

$p = 0.0014$]. On average, in-person MI participants rated the quality of their session highest compared to web-MI and UC-only, and there were no differences in ratings by facilitator. Quality ratings were next highest for participants in the web-MI, and then the UC-only condition. Participants in the in-person MI intervention rated their satisfaction with the sessions significantly higher than participants from the other two conditions. There were no significant differences in satisfaction between web-MI and UC participants.

Intervention fidelity

Facilitators of the in-person MI scored a mean of 4.2 on the MITI global scores ($SD = 0.1$; range: 3.9–4.5), which indicates MI competency. Behavioral counts ranged between 5.5 (giving information), 9.5 (simple reflections), and 11.1 (MI-adherent statements, complex reflections), suggesting high frequency of MI-consistent behaviors.

Intervention efficacy
Sample characteristics

Sixty-five percent of the participants were male, 40 percent were Hispanic/Latino/a, 87 percent were born in the United States (excluding Puerto Rico), 91 percent had at least a high school education, and 64 percent were fully employed. Participants were 30.0 (SD = 9.8) years of age (Table 1).

Overall, 92 percent of the sample met diagnostic criteria for past-year alcohol abuse. Sixty-seven percent met diagnostic criteria for dependence. Diagnoses of alcohol abuse and dependence were not significantly different across the three conditions (for abuse, $X^2(2) = 1.52$, $p = 0.468$; for dependence, $X^2(2) = 2.00$, $p = 0.368$).

At baseline, web-MI clients reported more drinks on the occasion they drank the most compared to UC-only or in-person MI clients [see Table 1; $F(2156) = 3.39$, $p = 0.036$]. Clients receiving in-person MI also reported more days of marijuana use in the past 3 months compared to UC-only and web-MI clients [$F(2156) = 3.97$, $p = 0.021$]. Only one participant in our sample was monolingual Spanish-speaking, and was assigned to the web-MI intervention and included in analyses. There were no significant differences in outcomes by ethnicity.

Alcohol-related outcomes

Table 2 shows differences in within-group outcomes between baseline and follow-up. Overall, participants from all three conditions reported reduced drinking quantity, alcohol-related consequences, and drinking and driving between baseline and 3-month follow-up (p < 0.05). Regarding drinking outcomes, all participants drank about one drink less on a typical occasion compared to baseline amounts (p < 0.05) and reported fewer and less frequent consequences (3- to 4-point reduction

Table 1 Baseline characteristics of the study sample

	UC (N = 54)		In-person MI (N = 51)		Web-MI (N = 54)	
	Mean (%)	SD	Mean (%)	SD	Mean (%)	SD
Male	64.81		68.63		62.96	
Race						
Hispanic/Latino	38.89		41.18		40.74	
African American	9.26		9.80		11.11	
White	35.19		39.22		31.48	
Asian/PI	7.41		5.88		11.11	
Place of birth						
US, except Puerto Rico	85.19		92.16		85.19	
Other	14.81		7.84		14.81	
Education						
<HS/GED	3.70		5.88		3.70	
HS/GED	3.70		3.92		5.56	
>HS	92.59		90.20		90.74	
Employment						
Full/part time	66.67		64.71		59.26	
Unemployed	9.26		9.80		20.37	
Other work situation	24.07		25.49		20.37	
Age at time of DUI	29.56	8.96	29.75	10.18	30.56	10.40
Alcohol use measures						
Negative consequences (SIP)	8.70	8.26	10.06	11.08	10.76	10.14
Past 12 Months						
AUDADIS alcohol dependence^	64.15		64.71		74.07	
AUDADIS alcohol abuse^	88.68		96.08		90.74	
Past 3 months						
Alcohol use # of days	25.03	24.73	31.18	28.56	25.99	23.53
# Drinks on typical occasion	4.35	2.30	4.37	1.91	5.02	3.27
Heavy drinking # of days	10.19	12.87	13.93	18.39	10.55	13.09
Drink and drive past 3 months	51.85		49.02		48.15	
# Drinks on heaviest occasion*	7.98	4.03	8.98	3.99	10.56	24.07
Marijuana use	42.59		50.98		44.44	
Marijuana use in days*	16.11	31.22	27.74	28.77	10.56	24.07
Any other drug use	3.70		9.80		12.96	

* $p < 0.05$; ^ 1 UC participant did not complete the AUDADIS

roughly translates to experiencing several problems weekly to experiencing problems a few times in the past 3 months). Web-MI participants reported drinking 4.58 fewer days in the past 3 months at follow-up compared to baseline ($p = 0.036$). UC-only and in-person MI clients did not report a significant decrease in drinking days.

While there were within-group reductions in alcohol-related consequences, participants in all three groups continued to report alcohol-related consequences at follow-up. The proportions of participants who reported having at least one consequence at baseline and subsequently reported at least one consequence at follow-up were 61 percent of in-person MI, 78 percent of UC-only, and 81 percent of web-MI individuals.

Participants also reported within-group changes in their drinking and driving in the past 3 months ($p < 0.0001$). Across the three groups, 40–56 percent of participants reported not drinking and driving at follow-up. We were specifically interested in seeing the proportion of participants who reported drinking and driving behavior at baseline and whether they continued this behavior at follow-up. Across all conditions, about 50 percent of participants reported drinking and driving in the 3 months prior to baseline.[1] Of those participants, about 8 percent of them reported drinking and driving at

---

[1] In some cases, individuals might enter the DUI program more than 3 months after their DUI arrest.

Table 2 Differences in within-group outcomes between baseline and follow-up

Variable	UC				In-person MI				Web-MI			
	Difference (SD)	Test stat*	d^+	p	Difference (SD)	Test stat*	d^+	p	Difference (SD)	Test stat*	d^+	p
Negative conse-quences (SIP)	3.82 (8.81)	186.50	0.46	0.013	3.24 (6.10)	233.00	0.29	0.001	3.20 (5.86)	326.50	0.32	<0.0001
Alcohol use # of days	2.63 (19.12)	35.50	0.11	0.474	3.54 (17.49)	66.50	0.12	0.132	4.58 (14.30)	126.50	0.19	0.036
# Drinks on typi-cal occasion	0.61 (1.97)	111.50	0.27	0.049	0.82 (2.10)	115.50	0.43	0.014	1.08 (3.33)	143.00	0.33	0.011
Heavy drinking # of days	2.03 (15.46)	40.00	0.16	0.442	1.70 (10.90)	69.50	0.09	0.218	0.61 (13.21)	24.00	0.05	0.742

* Wilcoxon signed rank test for continuous variables

$^+$ Effect size is computed as Cohen's d: difference/within-group baseline standard deviation

follow-up. Also important to note, of participants who reported no drinking and driving within 3 months of baseline, 96 percent of them continued to report no drinking and driving at follow-up.

Table 3 shows the estimated intervention effect of each MI + UC condition compared to UC-only. After adjusting for baseline levels, there were no significant group differences between the MI conditions and the UC-only condition in alcohol consumption (number of typical and heavy drinking days, average number of drinks) and risk behaviors (alcohol-related negative consequences and drinking and driving). Further, estimates of the effect sizes were small (Cohen's $d = 0$–0.12) for typical and heavy drinking days, average number of drinks, and alcohol-related consequences. For drinking and driving in the past 3 months, the width of the confidence intervals indicates that substantial variability exists in our estimates.

Discussion

This pilot study takes an important first look at the acceptance and efficacy of new in-person MI and web-MI interventions added to DUI UC compared to UC-only for a diverse sample of individuals enrolled in a first-time DUI program. Participants in both the in-person and web-MI intervention conditions rated the quality of and satisfaction with their session higher than participants in the UC-only condition, suggesting that clients were more receptive to the MI interventions. Clients viewed the in-person MI more favorably than web-MI, which may be related to the stronger therapeutic alliance often found in

Table 3 Intervention effect estimates of outcomes compared to usual care at 3 months post-baseline

Outcome	Estimate	Confidence interval		t statistic (132 df)	p value	$d*$
Negative consequences (SIP)						
Web-MI	1.13	−1.42	3.69	0.88	0.382	0.12
In-person MI	1.13	−1.47	3.72	0.86	0.392	0.12
Alcohol use # of days						
Web-MI	0.03	−6.15	6.20	0.01	0.993	0.00
In-person MI	0.48	−5.79	6.75	0.15	0.880	0.04
# Drinks on typical occasion						
Web-MI	0.00	−0.81	0.81	0.00	0.998	0.00
In-person MI	−0.01	−0.82	0.81	−0.01	0.988	0.00
Heavy drinking # of days						
Web-MI	1.29	−3.31	5.90	0.56	0.580	0.08
In-person MI	1.20	−3.47	5.87	0.51	0.612	0.09
	Log-odds ratio	**Confidence interval**		**t statistic (132 df)**	**p value**	**Odds ratio**
Drink and drive past 3 months						
Web-MI	−1.39	−12.78	10.00	−0.24	0.810	0.25
In-person MI	−1.99	−13.43	9.46	−0.34	0.732	0.14

* Cohen's d = estimate/pooled standard deviation across the two comparison conditions

the in-person interactions compared to web-based inter-actions [52]. However, we did not find statistically signifi-cant differences in outcomes between the MI conditions and UC-only condition. In fact, regardless of study condi-tion, participants reported significant reductions in both alcohol consumption and risk behaviors. Thus, at pro-gram completion, participants from all three study con-ditions reported reduced alcohol consumption, DUI, and fewer alcohol-related consequences.

There were at least two unexpected results from our study. First, despite recruiting individuals with a first-time offense into the study, 67 percent of our sample met criteria for alcohol dependence, and the majority of par-ticipants in all three study conditions continued to report alcohol-related consequences at follow-up. From our previous discussions with DUI providers, we anticipated a larger percentage of at-risk versus dependent drinkers, and therefore designed the MI intervention for an at-risk population rather than a population with dependence. Our second unexpected result was that participants from each of the MI interventions did not report differences in their outcomes when compared to UC-only. We had hypothesized that because our MI interventions were focused on exploring behavioral change and developing a change plan, we would see significant improvements in individuals who received the MI interventions compared to individuals who only received UC.

There are several possible explanations for these find-ings. First, the extensiveness of UC services (i.e., 36 program hours) in these DUI programs may have been sufficient to improve outcomes in the short term, and an additional 3-session MI (i.e., about 65 min) may not have had an additive effect on outcomes. Second, our follow-up timeframe was short. We were only able to measure outcomes at the conclusion of clients' 3-month DUI program. Receiving a DUI and having to deal with the numerous financial, emotional, and social consequences (e.g., vehicle impoundment, jail time, probation, injury) related to this type of event may be significant enough to reduce a client's alcohol-related behaviors in the short term, but might not be enough to sustain long-term changes such as reductions in recidivism (D'Amico et al. [13]). This speaks to the challenge of conducting research in DUI programs that have strong behavioral expecta-tions and high sanctions for failing those expectations. Longer follow-up assessments (e.g., 6 months to one year after program completion) may be needed to better understand whether MI interventions and UC are differ-entially associated with sustained behavior change after a client completes a DUI program. Finally, MI interven-tions may not be the best fit for individuals with a first-time DUI offense, given the high levels of dependence that were reported in this study. Future studies should

evaluate whether alcohol dependence is as common in other first-time DUI offense programs. If dependence rates are similarly high in other programs, more intensive treatment approaches such as cognitive behavioral ther-apy or medication-assisted therapy may be more effective [53–58]. MI interventions may still be used to enhance engagement prior to these more intensive and long-term approaches [59] or they may be a better fit as a preventive intervention with individuals who are at risk for a future DUI but who have not yet been convicted. Determining which therapy or combination of therapies is associated with long-term changes should be the subject of future research.

In conducting community-based work, it is always important to examine lessons learned to help inform future research. Although MI is an evidence-based treat-ment that has been successful as a brief intervention in a variety of settings, it may be important to have more sessions for this more severe population. The population and providers were very receptive to MI [32], and it could perhaps be integrated into the lengthy UC treatment and provided in this group setting as with other man-dated populations [13]. Given that clients felt that the MI intervention was of higher quality and were more satis-fied with it than UC, integrating MI into UC could help standardize services provided to clients, help make the program more acceptable to them, and perhaps increase attendance, which could lead to better outcomes.

Our sample was recruited from DUI programs in California and may not be representative of clients in DUI programs nationally. Of note, about 52 percent of our sample was excluded mostly due to low AUDIT-C at program entry, which also affects generalizability. In addition, inter-rater agreement on the MITI was low for five measures, suggesting improvements in measure per-formance and/or the process for coding those items are needed for future studies. It is also important to note that under-reporting of DUI behaviors might be an issue, given the setting. The limitations of self-report data are well-known, although much research has shown that self-report is valid when procedures such as those used in the current study are implemented (e.g., establishing rapport and discussing confidentiality) [60].

This pilot study addresses an important policy ques-tion by examining whether individuals with a first-time DUI offense find MI interventions acceptable in a DUI setting and whether clients who receive an MI interven-tion have improved outcomes relative to UC. Findings suggest that participants from all three conditions expe-rienced improved outcomes, regardless of study condi-tion. Although it is possible that a longer follow-up may provide insights into whether within-group differences are sustained, we hypothesize based on our effect sizes and confidence intervals that between-group differences in a larger future trial with this population are not supported by the data. Instead, given that individuals with a first-time DUI offense are likely a unique population of individuals who may be experiencing consequences related to alcohol dependence, future research is needed to better understand the potential heterogeneity of this population and to determine the most appropriate level of care for these high-risk individuals to reduce long-term recidivism.

Authors' contributions
KCO, KEW, EJD, and SMP conceptualized the study and obtained funding. KCO, EJD, and KEW designed the interventions. KCO had overall responsibility for executing the MI interventions, data collection, analyses, and reporting. SMP, TJL, and BAE performed quantitative data analyses. All authors read and approved the final manuscript.

Author details
[1] RAND Corporation, 1776 Main Street, Santa Monica, CA 90407-2138, USA. [2] Department of Statistical Science, Duke University, Box 90251, Durham, NC 27708-0251, USA.

Acknowledgements
This research was supported by grants from NIAAA awarded to Katherine E. Watkins (RC1AA019034) and Susan M. Paddock (R01AA019663). The content is solely the responsibility of the authors and does not necessarily represent the official views of NIAAA or the National Institutes of Health. The authors would like to thank Jeannette and Jim Gilmore for their administrative support, along with DUI program staff Kramer Ruppe, Tarquino Ubidia, and Carlos Ubidia. We would also like to thank our intervention facilitators, Marylou Gilbert, Claudia Diaz Fuentes, Blanca Dominguez, Rob Reaugh, and our data collection staff, Kirsten Becker, Jen Parker, and Jeni Catch. Portions of this paper were presented as a poster at 2014's Research Society on Alcoholism conference in Bellevue, Washington.

Compliance with ethical guidelines

Competing interests
The authors declare that they have no competing interests.

References
1. World Health Organization: Alcohol fact sheet. http://www.who.int/mediacentre/factsheets/fs349/en/ (2011). Accessed April 1 2014.
2. Ahlin EM, Zador PL, Rauch WJ, Howard JM, Duncan GD. First-time DWI offenders are at risk of recidivating regardless of sanctions imposed. J Crim Justice. 2011;39:137–42.
3. National Highway Traffic Safety Administration, Traffic Tech: Technology Transfer Series: Repeat DWI Offenders Are an Elusive Target. Washington, DC: US Department of Transportation; 2000. http://www.nhtsa.gov/people/outreach/traftech/pub/tt217.html. Accessed April 1 2014.
4. Daoud SO, Tashima HN: Annual Report of the California DUI Management Information System. Sacramento: California Department of Motor Vehicles; 2007. http://ntis.library.gatech.edu/handle/123456789/9560.
5. Cavaiola A, Wuth C. Assessment and treatment of the DUI offender. New York: Haworth; 2002.
6. Daoud SO, Tashima HN. 2013 annual report of the California DUI management information system. Sacramento: California Department of Motor Vehicles; 2013.
7. Davis DA, Thomson MA, Oxman AD, Haynes RB. Changing physician performance. A systematic review of the effect of continuing medical education strategies. JAMA. 1995;274:700–5.
8. Kaminer Y, Burleson JA, Goldberger R. Cognitive-behavioral coping skills and psychoeducation therapies for adolescent substance abuse. J Nerv Ment Dis. 2002;190:737–45.
9. Miller WR, Wilbourne PL, Hettema JE. What works? A summary of alcohol treatment outcome research. In: Hester RK, Miller WR, editors. Handbook of alcoholism treatment approaches: effective alternatives. 3rd ed. Boston: Allyn and Bacon; 2003. p. 13–63.
10. Miller WR, Rollnick S. Motivational interviewing: helping people change. 3rd ed. New York: Guilford Press; 2012.
11. Markland D, Ryan RM, Tobin VJ, Rollnick S. Motivational interviewing and self–determination theory. J Social Clin Psychol. 2005;24:811–831. http://guilfordjournals.com/doi/abs/10.1521/jscp.2005.24.6.811.
12. Bandura A. Self-efficacy: the exercise of control. New York: W.H. Freeman; 1997.
13. D'Amico EJ, Hunter SB, Miles JN, Ewing BA, Osilla KC. A randomized controlled trial of a group motivational interviewing intervention for adolescents with a first time alcohol or drug offense. J Subst Abuse Treat. 2013;45:400–8.
14. Spirito A, Sindelar-Manning H, Colby SM, Barnett NP, Lewander W, Rohsenow DJ, Monti PM. Individual and family motivational interventions for alcohol-positive adolescents treated in an emergency department: results of a randomized clinical trial. Arch Pediatr Adolesc Med. 2011;165:269–74.
15. DiClemente CC, Velasquez MM. Motivational interviewing and the stages of change. In: Miller WR, Rollnick S, editors. Motivational interviewing: preparing people for change. 2nd ed. New York: Guilford Press; 2002. p. 201–16.
16. Smedslund G, Berg RC, Hammerstrom KT, Steiro A, Leiknes KA, Dahl HM, Karlsen K: Motivational interviewing for substance abuse. Cochrane Database Syst Rev. 2011;5: CD008063.
17. Carroll KM, Rounsaville BJ. A vision of the next generation of behavioral therapies research in the addictions. Addiction. 2007;102:850–62 **(discussion 863–869)**.
18. Miller WR, Yahne CE, Moyers TB, Martinez J, Pirritano M. A randomized trial of methods to help clinicians learn motivational interviewing. J Consul Clin Psychol. 2004;72:1050–62.
19. Moyers TB, Manuel JK, Wilson PG, Hendrickson SML, Talcott W, Durand P. A randomized trial investigating training in motivational interviewing for behavioral health providers. Behavioural and Cognitive Psychotherapy. 2008;36:149–62.
20. Collins SE, Kirouac M, Lewis MA, Witkiewitz K, Carey KB. Randomized controlled trial of web-based decisional balance feedback and personalized normative feedback for college drinkers. J Stud Alcohol Drugs. 2014;75:982–92.
21. Hester RK, Delaney HD, Campbell W. The college drinker's check-up: outcomes of two randomized clinical trials of a computer-delivered intervention. Psychol Addict Behav. 2012;26:1–12.
22. Hester RK, Squires DD, Delaney HD. The Drinker's Check-up: 12-month outcomes of a controlled clinical trial of a stand-alone software program for problem drinkers. J Subst Abuse Treat. 2005;28:159–69.
23. Pemberton MR, Williams J, Herman-Stahl M, Calvin SL, Bradshaw MR, Bray RM, Ridenhour JL, Cook R, Hersch RK, Hester RK, Mitchell GM. Evaluation of two web-based alcohol interventions in the U.S. military. J Stud Alcohol Drugs. 2011;72:480–9.
24. Muñoz RF, Barrera AZ, Delucchi K, Penilla C, Torres LD, Perez-Stable EJ. International Spanish/English internet smoking cessation trial yields 20% abstinence rates at 1 year. Nicotine Tob Res. 2009;11:1025–34.
25. Ondersma SJ, Svikis DS, Schuster CR. Computer-based brief intervention: a randomized trial with postpartum women. Am J Prev Med. 2007;32:231–8.
26. Walters ST, Ondersma SJ, Ingersoll KS, Rodriguez M, Lerch J, Rossheim ME, Taxman FS. MAPIT: development of a web-based intervention targeting substance abuse treatment in the criminal justice system. J Subst Abuse Treat. 2014;46:60–5.
27. Carey KB, Scott-Sheldon LA, Elliott JC, Bolles JR, Carey MP. Computer-delivered interventions to reduce college student drinking: a meta-analysis. Addiction. 2009;104:1807–19.
28. Khadjesari Z, Murray E, Hewitt C, Hartley S, Godfrey C. Can stand-alone computer-based interventions reduce alcohol consumption? A systematic review. Addiction. 2011;106:267–82.

29. Riper H, Blankers M, Hadiwijaya H, Cunningham J, Clarke S, Wiers R, Ebert D, Cuijpers P. Effectiveness of guided and unguided low-intensity internet interventions for adult alcohol misuse: a meta-analysis. PLoS One. 2014;9:e99912.

30. Rounsaville BJ, Carroll KM, Onken LS. A stage model of behavioral therapies research: getting started and moving on from stage I. Clin Psychol-Sci Pr. 2001;8:133–42.

31. California Department of Alcohol & Drug Programs. Title 9, California code of regulations, Division 4, Chapter 3. http://www.adp.ca.gov/Criminal_Justice/DUI/laws.shtml (2012). Accessed April 1, 2014.

32. Osilla KC, D'Amico EJ, Diaz-Fuentes CM, Lara M, Watkins KE. Multicultural web-based motivational interviewing for clients with a first-time DUI offense. Cultur Divers Ethnic Minor Psychol. 2012;18:192–202.

33. D'Amico EJ, Edelen MO. Pilot test of Project CHOICE: a voluntary afterschool intervention for middle school youth. Psychol Addict Behav. 2007;21:592–8.

34. D'Amico EJ, Miles JN, Stern SA, Meredith LS. Brief motivational interviewing for teens at risk of substance use consequences: a randomized pilot study in a primary care clinic. J Subst Abuse Treat. 2008;35:53–61.

35. Osilla KC, Zellmer SP, Larimer ME, Neighbors C, Marlatt GA. A brief intervention for at-risk drinking in an employee assistance program. J Stud Alcohol Drugs. 2008;69:14–20.

36. Chan KK, Neighbors C, Gilson M, Larimer ME, Marlatt G. Epidemiological trends in drinking by age and gender: providing normative feedback to adults. Addict Behav. 2007;32:967–76.

37. Marlatt GA, Rohsenow DJ. Cognitive processes in alcohol use: expectancy and the balanced placebo design. In: Mello NK, editor. Advances in Substance abuse: behavioral and biological research. Greenwich: JAI Press; 1980. p. 159–99.

38. Babor TF, Higgins-Biddle JC, Saunders J, Monteiro MG. AUDIT The alcohol use disorders identification test: guidelines for use in primary care. Geneva: World Health Organization; 2001.

39. Dawson DA, et al. Effectiveness of the derived alcohol use disorders identification test (AUDIT-C) in screening for alcohol use disorders and risk drinking in the US general population. Alcohol Clin Exp Res 2005;29(5):844–54.

40. Grant BF, Dawson DA, Stinson FS, Chou PS, Kay W, Pickering R. The Alcohol Use Disorder and Associated Disabilities Interview Schedule-IV (AUDADIS-IV): reliability of alcohol consumption, tobacco use, family history of depression and psychiatric diagnostic modules in a general population sample. Drug Alcohol Depend. 2003;71:7–16.

41. D'Amico EJ, Osilla KC, Miles JN, Ewing B, Sullivan K, Katz K, Hunter SB. Assessing motivational interviewing integrity for group interventions with adolescents. Psychol Addict Behav. 2012;26:994–1000.

42. Moyers TB, Martin T, Manuel JK, Miller WR, Ernst D: Revised Global Scales: Motivational Interviewing Treatment Integrity 3.1.1 (MITI 3.1.1). University of New Mexico: Center on Alcoholism, Substance Abuse, and Addictions; 2010.

43. University of Mexico, Center on Alcoholism, Substance Abuse, and Addictions. Coding Instruments. 2013. http://casaa.unm.edu/codinginst.html. Accessed February 18, 2014.

44. Hatcher RL, Gillaspy JA. Development and validation of a revised short version of the working alliance inventory. Psychother Res. 2006;16:12–25.

45. Byrt T, Bishop J, Carlin JB. Bias, prevalence and kappa. J Clin Epidemiol. 1993;46:423–9.

46. Unknown: PhenX Toolkit. RTI International; 2014. http://www.phenx-toolkit.org.

47. Tonigan JS, Miller WR. The inventory of drug use consequences (InDUC): test-retest stability and sensitivity to detect change. Psychol Addict Behav. 2002;16:165–8.

48. Hox JJ. Multilevel analysis: techniques and applications. 2nd edn. (Quantitative Methodology Series). New York: Routledge; 2010.

49. Miles J, Shevlin M. Applying regression and correlation: a guide for students and researchers. Sage; 2001.

50. Bauer DJ, Sterba SK. Fitting multilevel models with ordinal outcomes: performance of alternative specifications and methods of estimation. Psychol Methods. 2011;16:373–90. doi:10.1037/a0025813.

51. Tsiatis AA, Davidian M, Zhang M, Lu X. Covariate adjustment for two-sample treatment comparisons in randomized clinical trials: a principled yet flexible approach. Stat Med. 2008;27:4658–77.

52. Greene CJ, Morland LA, Macdonald A, Frueh BC, Grubbs KM, Rosen CS. How does tele-mental health affect group therapy process? Secondary analysis of a noninferiority trial. J Consult Clin Psychol. 2010;78:746–50.

53. Project MATCH Research Group. Matching patients with alcohol disorders to treatments: Clinical implications from project MATCH. J Mental Health. 1998;7:589–602.

54. Garbutt JC, West SL, Carey TS, Lohr KN, Crews FT. Pharmacological treatment of alcohol dependence: a review of the evidence. JAMA. 1999;281:1318–25.

55. Longabaugh R, Morgenstern J. Cognitive-behavioral coping-skills therapy for alcohol dependence. Current status and future directions. Alcohol Res Health. 1999;23:78–85.

56. Morgenstern J, Morgan TJ, McCrady BS, Keller DS, Carroll KM. Manual-guided cognitive-behavioral therapy training: a promising method for disseminating empirically supported substance abuse treatments to the practice community. Psychol Addict Behav. 2001;15:83–8.

57. Moore KA, Harrison M, Young MS, Ochshorn E. A cognitive therapy treatment program for repeat DUI offenders. J Criminal Just. 2008;36:539–45. doi:10.1016/j.jcrimjus.2008.09.004.

58. Donovan DM, Salzberg PM, Chaney EF, Queisser HR, Marlatt GA. Prevention skills for alcohol-involved drivers. Alcohol, Drugs & Driving. 1990;6:169–88.

59. Carroll KM, Ball SA, Nich C, Martino S, Frankforter TL, Farentinos C, Kunkel LE, Mikulich-Gilbertson SK, Morgenstern J, Obert JL, Polcin D, Snead N, Woody GE. Motivational interviewing to improve treatment engagement and outcome in individuals seeking treatment for substance abuse: a multisite effectiveness study. Drug Alcohol Depend. 2006;81:301–12.

60. Chan D. So why ask me? Are self-report data really that bad? In: Lance CE, Vandenberg RJ, editors. Statistical and methodological myths and urban legends: doctrine, verity and fable in the organizational and social sciences. New York: Taylor & Francis; 2009. p. 309–36.

6

A systematic review of health economic models of opioid agonist therapies in maintenance treatment of non-prescription opioid dependence

Mersha Chetty[1], James J. Kenworthy[2], Sue Langham[1], Andrew Walker[3] and William C. N. Dunlop[2*]

Abstract

Background: Opioid dependence is a chronic condition with substantial health, economic and social costs. The study objective was to conduct a systematic review of published health-economic models of opioid agonist therapy for non-prescription opioid dependence, to review the different modelling approaches identified, and to inform future modelling studies.

Methods: Literature searches were conducted in March 2015 in eight electronic databases, supplemented by hand-searching reference lists and searches on six National Health Technology Assessment Agency websites. Studies were included if they: investigated populations that were dependent on non-prescription opioids and were receiving opioid agonist or maintenance therapy; compared any pharmacological maintenance intervention with any other maintenance regimen (including placebo or no treatment); and were health-economic models of any type.

Results: A total of 18 unique models were included. These used a range of modelling approaches, including Markov models (n = 4), decision tree with Monte Carlo simulations (n = 3), decision analysis (n = 3), dynamic transmission models (n = 3), decision tree (n = 1), cohort simulation (n = 1), Bayesian (n = 1), and Monte Carlo simulations (n = 2). Time horizons ranged from 6 months to lifetime. The most common evaluation was cost-utility analysis reporting cost per quality-adjusted life-year (n = 11), followed by cost-effectiveness analysis (n = 4), budget-impact analysis/cost comparison (n = 2) and cost-benefit analysis (n = 1). Most studies took the healthcare provider's perspective. Only a few models included some wider societal costs, such as productivity loss or costs of drug-related crime, disorder and antisocial behaviour. Costs to individuals and impacts on family and social networks were not included in any model.

Conclusion: A relatively small number of studies of varying quality were found. Strengths and weaknesses relating to model structure, inputs and approach were identified across all the studies. There was no indication of a single standard emerging as a preferred approach. Most studies omitted societal costs, an important issue since the implications of drug abuse extend widely beyond healthcare services. Nevertheless, elements from previous models could together form a framework for future economic evaluations in opioid agonist therapy including all relevant costs and outcomes. This could more adequately support decision-making and policy development for treatment of non-prescription opioid dependence.

Keywords: Systematic review, Non-prescription opioid dependence, Opioid agonist maintenance therapy, Economic evaluation

*Correspondence: will.dunlop@mundipharma.com
[2] Mundipharma International Ltd, Cambridge Science Park, Milton Road, Cambridge CB4 0GW, UK
Full list of author information is available at the end of the article

Background

Physical and psychological dependence can occur with any opioid drug, but the non-prescription or 'street' use of heroin presents the greatest problems to society [1]. In 2010, the global prevalence of opioid use was estimated at 0.6–0.8% of the population aged 15–64 years (between 26.4 and 36.0 million opioid users), of which approximately half, or between 13 and 21 million, were using heroin [2].

Illicit non-prescription opioid dependence is associated with major medical, personal and social problems, including increased risk of infection with human immunodeficiency virus (HIV) or hepatitis C virus (HCV), increased risk of death due to suicide, overdose or violence, decreased quality of life, high rates of psychiatric co-morbidity, and involvement in criminal activity [3, 4].

It was estimated in 2008 that there are approximately 16 million injecting drug users (IDU) worldwide and that 3 million (18.9%) of them were living with HIV. Global prevalence of HCV infection among injecting drug users in 2010 was 46.7%, meaning that some 7.4 million injecting drug users worldwide are infected with HCV and 2.3 million injecting drug users are infected with hepatitis B [2].

In 2010, illicit drug use was found to be associated with between 99,000 and 253,000 deaths globally, with drug-related deaths accounting for between 0.5 and 1.3% of all-cause mortality among those aged 15–64 years [2].

Heroin addiction also has significant economic costs to society, resulting from the association between crime and opioid dependence. Many opioid-dependent individuals become involved in crime to support their drug use, but crime may also provide the money and the contacts to buy drugs [1]. Based on a review, the average heroin user is likely to engage in criminal activity for 40–60% of the time they are not incarcerated or not in treatment [5].

Other societal impacts result from the psychopharmacological effects of the drug, which may result in mistakes at work, lost productivity or unemployment [6]. Personal relationships may suffer or parental capacity may be hampered. Evidence from the United Kingdom (UK) shows neglect among children is correlated strongly with parental heroin use, and in the United States of America (US) parental problem drug use is one of the commonest reasons for children entering the care system [7].

The economic and social costs of Class A drug use were estimated to be £15.4 billion in 2003–2004 in England and Wales [6], with opioid and/or crack use accounting for 99%. Health and social care costs accounted for £557 million, implying that the majority of the costs are borne outside of health and social care provision.

Effective treatment for opioid dependence is available but is likely to be long-term or even life-long. Options include psychosocial/behavioural assistance, and pharmacological interventions including opioid agonist therapy. The most commonly used medications for opioid substitution include the opioid agonist methadone, and buprenorphine (with/without naloxone), a partial agonist/antagonist combination; less commonly used treatments include naltrexone, morphine sulphate, naloxone, diamorphine, and medical use of heroin [8].

Recent Cochrane reviews, as well as additional studies of maintenance treatment options, have consistently found opioid agonist therapy to be clinically effective and more cost-effective than no drug therapy in opiate-dependent users [1], and have found no major differences in rates of mortality or illicit drug use achieved with these treatments [9].

In financially constrained health systems with finite resources, increasing emphasis is being placed on the ability to demonstrate that healthcare interventions are not only effective, but also cost-effective. Economic evaluations, which use modelling techniques to consider the comparative clinical effects, patient values and cost of care of alternative options, are used by payers and healthcare policymakers to inform the decision-making process.

The emphasis when conducting an economic evaluation is on including all relevant evidence on costs and outcomes. Given the significant impacts on society, the economic framework in economic evaluations of non-prescription opioid dependence should include not only the direct medical costs associated with treatment and preventive interventions, but also costs borne by other areas of society such as social welfare services and the criminal justice system, and indirect costs associated with lost productivity [4].

In order to explore the ways in which previous modelling studies have approached this issue, we undertook a systematic review of published model-based economic evaluations of opioid agonist therapy in treating opioid dependence, including modelling of long-term costs and outcomes and budget impact modelling. The aim was to identify any 'best practice' methods for modelling approaches and the costs and outcomes considered, which could be used to guide and inform future health economic models in this area. To our knowledge, this is the first systematic review to examine the modelling approaches that have been applied in opioid agonist therapy for non-prescription opioid dependence.

Methods

Search strategy

Search strategies and searches of published literature were designed and performed by an experienced medical librarian. The searches were conducted on 17–18 March 2015 in eight electronic databases: Medline (OvidSP); Medline

In-Process Citations and Daily Updates (OvidSP); Embase (OvidSP); the Cochrane Library (Wiley); the Cochrane Database of Systematic Reviews (CDSR) (Wiley); the Database of Abstracts of Reviews of Effects (DARE) (Wiley); the Health Technology Assessment (HTA) Database (Wiley); and the National Health Service Economic Evaluation Database (NHS EED) (Wiley). The databases were searched from the beginning of the database to the date of the search. No date or language limits were applied.

Search terms appropriate for each database were used for the disorder (non-prescription opioid dependence), interventions (any pharmacological maintenance regimen) and study type (health economic studies of any type). The detailed search strategies are presented in Additional file 1.

These searches were supplemented by hand searching of the reference lists of review papers.

In addition, general title searches were conducted, also on 17–18 March 2015, on the websites of HTA agencies in six countries. Health technology assessment (HTA) involves the systematic evaluation of properties, effects and/or impacts of health technologies and interventions. It covers both the direct, intended consequences of technologies and interventions as well as their indirect, unintended consequences, and the HTA approach is used to inform policy and decision-making in health care, especially on how best to allocate limited funds to health interventions and technologies. The assessment is conducted by interdisciplinary groups using explicit analytical frameworks, drawing on clinical, epidemiological, health economic and other information and methodologies. The six HTA agencies selected below are well established and with clearly defined processes and references cases for economic models and were therefore included in this search.

- Australia: Pharmaceutical Benefits Advisory Committee (PBAC);
- Canada: Canadian Agency for Drugs and Technologies in Health (CADTH);
- England and Wales: National Institute for Health and Clinical Excellence (NICE);
- Germany: Gemeinsamer Bundesausschuss (G-BA); Institute for Quality and Efficiency in Heath Care (IQWIG);
- Scotland: Scottish Medicines Consortium (SMC);
- Sweden: Tandvards-och lakemedelsformansverket (TLV); Swedish Council on Health Technology Assessment (SBU).

These additional searches were intended to identify any additional published or unpublished material missed by the electronic database searches.

Inclusion and exclusion criteria

The inclusion and exclusion criteria used to select studies for the review are shown in Table 1. Each publication had to fulfil all the inclusion criteria and none of the exclusion criteria to be selected for inclusion in the review. Unless specifically stated otherwise, it was assumed that drug abuse pertained to illicit use of opioids.

Study selection

Citations identified by the searches were initially screened for eligibility against the inclusion and exclusion criteria using the title and (where present) the abstract and keywords. Each citation was classified as 'include', 'exclude' or 'unsure'. Full text copies were obtained for publications categorised as 'include' or 'unsure' at the initial screen.

The full-text publications were then screened against the inclusion and exclusion criteria by two independent researchers. Any disagreements were resolved by discussion and consensus. Publications that met all the inclusion criteria and none of the exclusion criteria after full-text review were selected for inclusion in the review. The reason for exclusion was recorded for all studies excluded after full-text review. Excluded publications are listed in Additional file 2.

Information on the modelling approach, perspective, time horizon, comparators and form of evaluation was extracted from each of the included studies and tabulated. Additionally, data were extracted on the type of model used and the range of inputs for costs and outcomes. Data extracted on cost inputs were aimed at addressing the question of what types of costs were used i.e. direct or wider societal and indirect costs, the evidence sources for these types of costs and where gaps may exist in the evidence sources. Data on utility weights for health states in cost-utility analyses were aimed at understanding what values were available, what methods had been used and what gaps might exist.

Economic appraisal checklist

The model-based economic evaluations were assessed using an adapted form of the checklist for economic evaluations developed by the University of Glasgow [10]. The checklist consists of twelve questions in total, of which nine relate to the economic evaluation itself while the remaining questions address the applicability of results to the local population. Therefore, only the nine questions relating to the quality of the economic evaluation were used in the present analysis. Each of the included studies was graded on each of the questions as 'yes', 'no' or 'can't tell' by one researcher, and the results tabulated.

Table 1 Inclusion and exclusion criteria

Parameter	Criteria
Population	People who are dependent on non-prescription opioids and who are receiving opioid agonist therapy or maintenance therapy for opioid dependency
Intervention	Pharmacological maintenance therapy, monotherapy or combination Morphine/morphine sulphate/diacetylmorphine/diamorphine (DIA) Buprenorphine (BUP) Methadone (METH) Codeine, dihydrocodeine Naloxone, naltrexone (NAL) Buprenorphine/naloxone (BUP/NAL) Note naloxone may be used in combination with other treatments (morphine + naloxone) The following operational definition will be employed for "maintenance" treatment: the treatment approach does not include a reduction or cessation of one of the above treatments as part of the approach
Comparators	Any comparator regime used in maintenance therapy (including no therapy or placebo)
Outcomes	Health economic models (any type including Markov, dynamic, Monte-Carlo, simulations, decision-trees etc)
Study types	Cost-effectiveness (CEA), cost-utility (CUA), cost-minimisation (CMA), cost-benefit (CBA), budget impact (BIM), cost-consequence (CC)
Language	English language abstracts
Timeframe	Last 20 years (1995–2015)
Exclusions	Studies indexed as case reports, case series, editorials and letters English language title and abstracts only Economic studies that do not employ modelling techniques (studies describing extrapolation of data beyond the primary clinical evidence time horizon were considered to include modelling techniques. Studies based only on cost and outcomes during the course of a trial were excluded)

Results

Search results and study selection

A total of 2666 citations were identified in the electronic literature searches, which decreased to 2149 after removal of duplicates. Hand searching of reference lists and review of HTA websites retrieved a further 14 citations, making a total of 2163 citations. After initial screening, 63 of these progressed to full-text review.

After review of the full text, 45 publications were excluded for the following reasons: non-model or trial-based analysis (n = 18); non-model-based cost analysis (n = 12); review articles (n = 10); HTA reports that did not contain new information of relevance to the review (n = 3); and outdated references, defined as pre-dating 1995 (n = 2). The reference lists of the review articles were hand searched for new references. Three of the HTA reports cited models that had already been captured by the searches and selection process. The outdated references were considered too old to be relevant or useful compared with current treatment programmes. This was in line with the HTA publication by Connock et al. [1], which excluded the same references for the same reason.

A total of 18 unique models were included in the review. Figure 1 shows a preferred reporting items for systematic reviews and meta-analyses (PRISMA) flow diagram for the study screening and selection process.

Summary of included studies

Twelve of the included models were reported in full-text publications [11–22]. Four were HTA evaluations [1, 23–25]. Of the four HTA reports, two were economic models supporting NICE technology appraisal for naloxone, methadone and buprenorphine in maintenance treatment of opioid dependence, one was the Schering-Plough manufacturer's submission to the NICE technology assessment (cited in Connock et al. [1]), and one was the SMC advice document based on the manufacturer's submission by Schering-Plough for suboxone. The remaining two models were published only as abstracts [26–28].

Table 2 summarises the characteristics of the 18 included models.

Interventions and populations considered

The interventions evaluated were established treatments in opioid dependence, including methadone maintenance treatment, buprenorphine maintenance treatment, medical heroin prescription, and buprenorphine combined with naloxone. Two US studies investigated the effect of expanding existing methadone maintenance treatment programmes. Studies compared between active treatments (for example, methadone maintenance treatment versus buprenorphine maintenance treatment), or between active treatment and no treatment or placebo (Table 2).

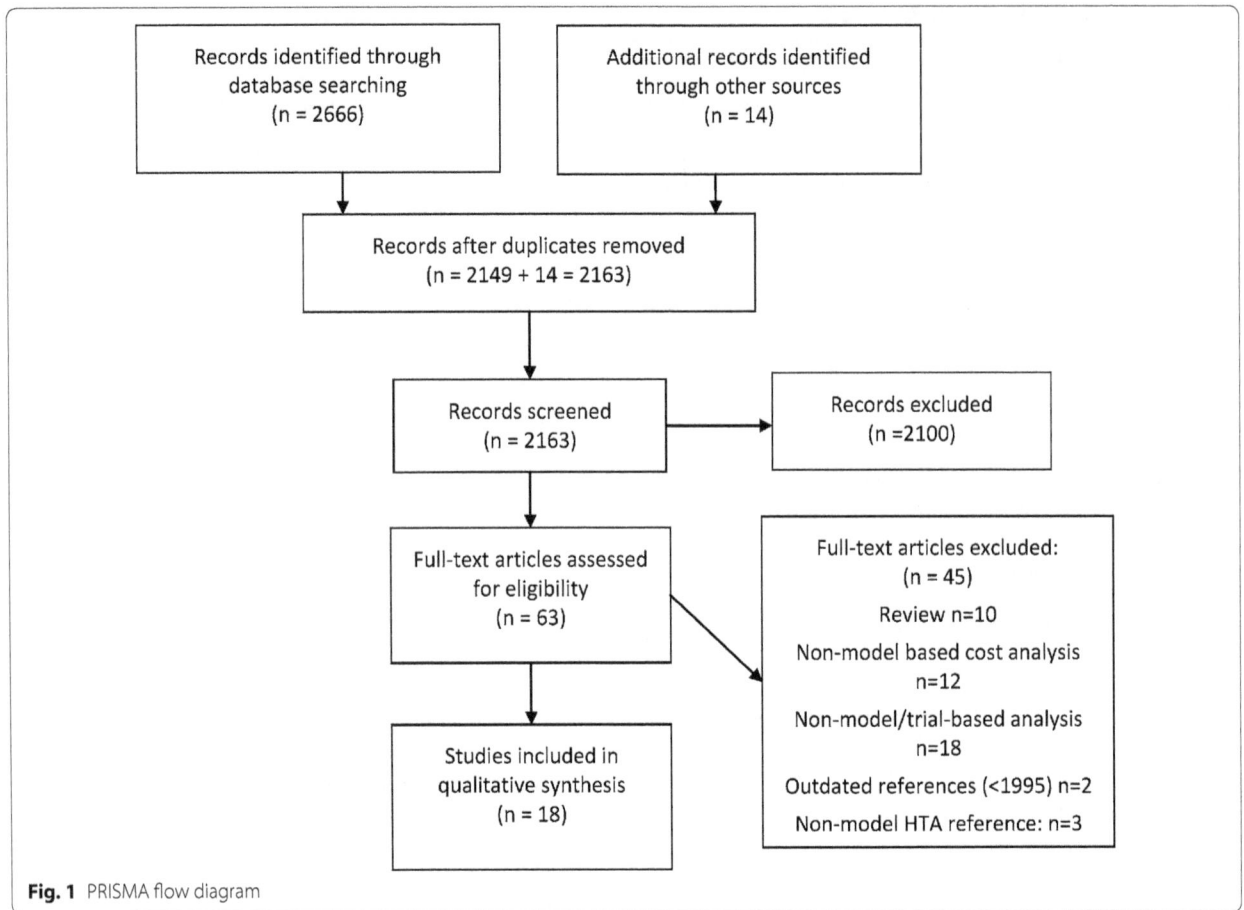

Fig. 1 PRISMA flow diagram

Three of the models did not report their baseline population. Of those studies that did report the baseline population, most used a hypothetical cohort of opioid-dependent patients (Table 2).

Evaluation type

Figure 2 summarises the evaluation types, time horizons and modelling approaches in graphical form. The most common form of evaluation was a cost-utility analysis reporting the cost per quality-adjusted life-year (QALY) gained, followed by cost-effectiveness analysis reporting cost per life-year gained/saved. No other type of evaluation was used in more than one study (Table 2; Fig. 2).

Cost-utility evaluation was employed in 11/18 studies, and cost-effectiveness evaluation in 4/18 studies. The remaining three studies included a cost-benefit evaluation, a budget impact analysis, and a cost comparison (one study each).

Assessing studies using an economic appraisal checklist

The results of the economic appraisal checklist are shown in Fig. 3 and Additional file 3. The two abstracts are included for completeness, but the limited space available in an abstract is likely to have restricted their ability to report full information on the models and the assessment should therefore be interpreted with caution. Of the 16 studies reported in journals or HTA reports, more than half (9/16) scored 'Yes' on at least seven of the nine questions on the checklist, and almost all (14/16) scored 'Yes' on at least five of the nine questions. Only five studies scored 'Yes' on all nine questions (Fig. 3).

Country and perspective

The most commonly modelled countries were the US and the UK (Table 2). Eleven of the models were Canadian or US-based and one of the ten US studies did not explicitly report its perspective. Six US studies were from the perspective of the healthcare provider, and three from a societal perspective. The study based in Canada took a societal perspective by including costs associated with crime and considering the proportion of patients in employment [14].

Four studies used a UK National Health Service (NHS) perspective. Of these, three also included a societal perspective as a secondary analysis, although one of these

Table 2 Summary of characteristics of included studies

Journal-based publications

Study/references	Cost year/currency	Country	Form of the evaluation	Perspective taken	Treatments evaluated	Model population	Time horizon	Study design[a]	Outcome measure	Societal costs	Health states
Barnett [11]	1996 (US $)	US	CEA	US Healthcare provider	METH versus Drug-free treatment	Hypothetical cohort of 1000 25 year old heroin users	Life-time	Markov	Cost/LYG	No	NR
Barnett [12]	1998 (US $)	US	CUA	US Healthcare provider	BMT versus MMT	Hypothetical cohort	10 years	Dynamic model	QALY	No	9 states based on HIV status (uninfected, asymptomatic HIV +ve, AIDS) and drug user status (IDU not on tx, IDU on tx, non-user)
Masson [13]	NR (US $)	US	CEA	US Healthcare provider	MMT versus Enriched Detox	Based on 179 patients in a RCT	10 years	Markov	LYG (base case) QALY (SA)	No	Alive and dead
Negrin [15]	NR/(Euro (€))	Spain	CEA	Drug Treatment centres	3 MMT programmes (high, medium, low intensity)	Based on 586 patients in drug tx centre	1 year	Bayesian	CEAC & CEAPF	NR	NR
Schackman [16]	2010 (US $)	US	CUA	Societal	Office-based BUP/NAL versus no treatment	Hypothetical cohort of stable patients on treatment for 6 months	24 months	Cohort simulation	Cost/QALY	Patient costs	In tx off drugs, Off tx off drugs, In tx on drugs, Off tx on drugs
Sheerin [17]	1999/2000 (NZ $)	New Zealand	CEA	New Zealand Healthcare	MMT	Hypothetical cohort of 1000 IDU	Lifetime	Markov	Cost/LYS	No	HCV + ve, no HCV, Chronic HCV, HCC, Compensated LC, Decompensated LC, Liver transplant, Death
Stephen [18]	2011 (US $)	US	CUA	Societal	MMT versus theoretical course of Deep Brain stimulation	NR	6 months	Decision analytical	QALY	Yes (productivity losses, crime costs)	NA (decision tree)

Table 2 continued

Study/references	Cost year/currency	Country	Form of the evaluation	Perspective taken	Treatments evaluated	Model population	Time horizon	Study design[a]	Outcome measure	Societal costs	Health states
Tran [19]	2009 (US $)	Vietnam	CUA	Vietnamese Health Service	MMT versus non-MMT	Based on 370 drug users from a cohort study	1 year (5% discounting)	Decision tree	Case of HIV averted QALY of MMT versus non-MMT	No	NA (decision tree)
Zaric [20]	1998 (US $)	US	CUA	US Healthcare provider	Expanding MMT programme (HIV prevalence rate of 5% & 40% versus 15% baseline)	Hypothetical cohort	10 years	Dynamic model	Cost/QALY & cost/LYG	No	10 states based on HIV status (uninfected, asymptomatic HIV +ve, AIDS) and drug user status (IDU not on tx, IDU on tx, non-user) and AID death
Zaric [21]	1998 (US $)	US	CUA	US Healthcare provider	Expanding MMT programme (HIV prevalence rates of 5,10,20, 40%)	Hypothetical cohort	10 years	Dynamic model	QALY and LYG	No	10 states based on HIV status (uninfected, asymptomatic HIV +ve, AIDS) and drug user status (IDU not on tx, IDU on tx, non-user) and AID death
Zarkin [22]	2001 (US $)	US	CBA	Societal	METH	Hypothetical cohort of 1 million adult patients	Lifetime	Monte Carlo simulation model	Cost/benefit ratio	Yes (productivity losses, crime costs)	Heroin non user & not in tx, Heroin user and not in tx, In tx, Incarcerated heroin user, Incarcerated non-user
Miller [14]	NR/(Canadian $)	Canada	Cost Comparison	Societal	MHPP versus non-MHPP	≥20 years old with > 5 year history of injecting heroin, to inject heroin at least daily, and to have previously failed MMT	5 years	Monte Carlo simulation model	Total cost over 5 years	Yes (criminal activity costs)	NA

Table 2 continued

Study/references	Cost year/currency	Country	Form of the evaluation	Perspective taken	Treatments evaluated	Model population	Time horizon	Study design[a]	Outcome measure	Societal costs	Health states
HTA-sourced models											
Adi [23]	2004 (GBP £)	UK	CUA	NHS & Societal	NTX versus standard psychosocial care	Hypothetical cohort	1 year	Decision tree with Monte Carlo simulations	QALY	Yes, in a secondary analysis	NA (decision tree)
Connock [1]	2004 (GBP £)	UK	CUA	NHS & Societal	MMT versus BMT versus Placebo	Hypothetical cohort	1 year	Decision tree with Monte Carlo simulations	QALY	Yes, in a secondary analysis	NA (decision tree)
Schering-Plough [24]	2004 (GBP £)	UK	CUA	NHS & PSS	Maintenance versus no drug tx, BUP versus no tx, BUP versus METH	NR	1 year'	Decision tree with Monte Carlo simulations	QALY	NR	NA (decision tree)
SMC [25]	NR/(GBP £)	UK	CUA	NHS & Societal	BUP/NAL versus METH, BUP or no treatment	NR	1 year	Decision analytical	QALY	NR	NR
Abstracts only											
Clay [26, 27]	NR/(US $)	US	BIM	US Healthcare provider	BUP/NAL film versus BUP/NAL tablets	Patients initiating treatment for opioid dependence	5 years	Markov model	Cost impact comparing 100% on BUP/NAL film versus 100% on BUP/NAL	No	NR
Fowler [28]	NR/US ($)	US	CUA	NR	MMT versus BMT	Hypothetical cohort of opioid-dependent pregnant women	NR	Decision analytical model	QALY	NR	NR

AIDS acquired immunodeficiency syndrome, *BIM* budget impact model, *BMT* buprenorphine maintenance treatment, *BUP* buprenorphine, *BUP/NAL* buprenorphine–naloxone combination, *CBA* cost-benefit analysis, *CEA* cost effectiveness analysis, *CEAC* cost-effectiveness acceptability curve, *CEAPF* cost-effectiveness frontier, *CUA* cost utility analysis, *HCC* Hepatocellular carcinoma, *HCV* hepatitis C virus, *HIV* human immunodeficiency virus, *HTA* health technology assessment, *IDU* injecting drug user, *LC* Liver Cirrhosis, *LYG* life-year gained, *MCBR* marginal cost-benefit ratio, *METH* methadone, *MHPP* Medical Heroin Prescription Program, *MMT* methadone maintenance treatment, *NA* not applicable, *NAL* naltrexone, *NHS* National Health Service, *NR* not reported, *NTX* extended release naltrexone, *NZ* New Zealand, *outpx* outpatient, *PSS* Personal & Social services, *QALY* quality-adjusted life-year, *RCT* randomised controlled trial, *SA* sensitivity analysis, *SMC* Scottish Medicines Consortium, *tx* treatment, *UK* United Kingdom, *US* United States of America

[a] Design as described by authors

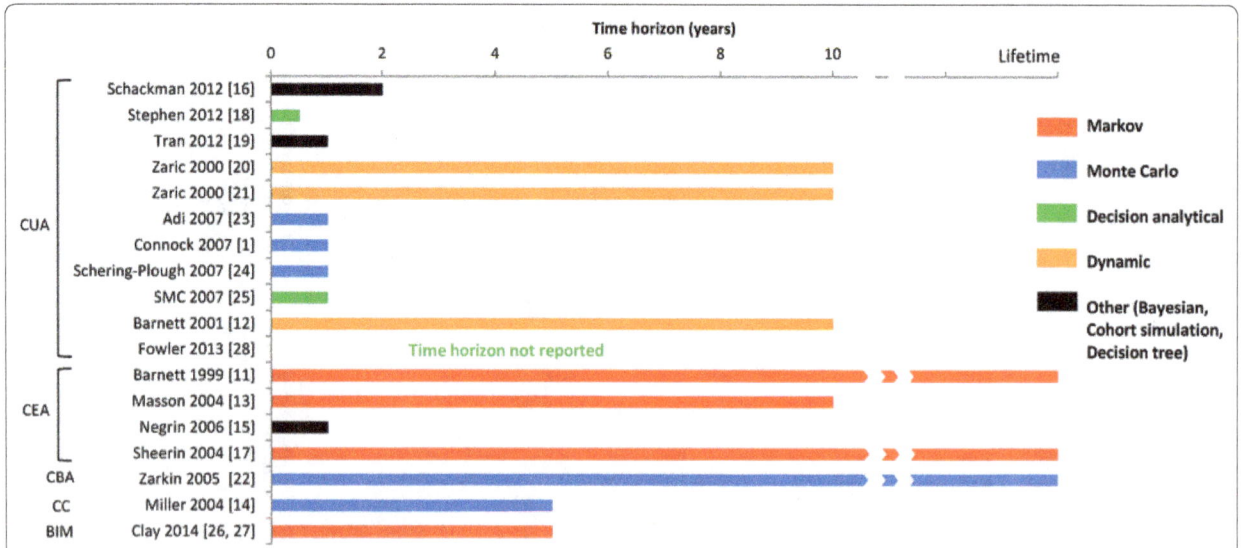

Fig. 2 Modelling approaches, time horizons and evaluation types used in the included models. *BIM* budget impact, *CBA* cost-benefit analysis, *CC* cost comparison, *CEA* cost-effectiveness analysis, *CUA* cost-utility analysis

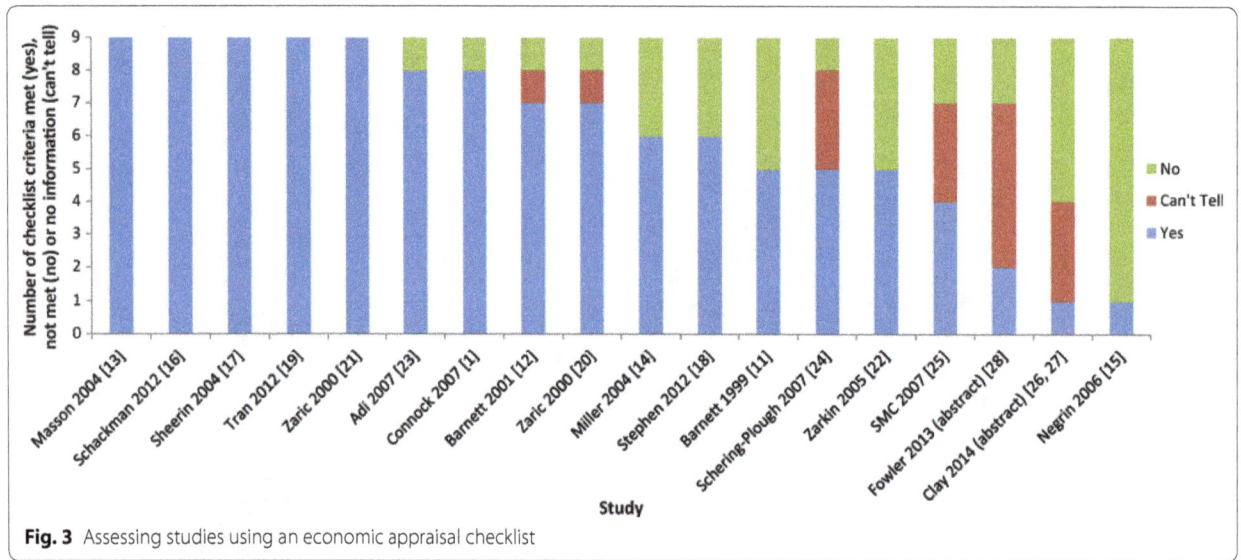

Fig. 3 Assessing studies using an economic appraisal checklist

reported no details of the societal perspective analysis. All four UK models were HTA reports.

Of the three remaining models, one was from the perspective of Spanish drug treatment centres, one from the perspective of the New Zealand healthcare system, and one from the perspective of the Vietnamese healthcare system.

Studies conducted from a societal perspective included costs borne outside the healthcare system, such as out-of-pocket costs incurred by patients, effects on employment and productivity, and the impact of criminal activity on the criminal justice system and on victims of crime.

Time horizons

The time horizons varied widely, ranging from 6 months to a lifetime. Seven studies had short time horizons (6 months to a year), seven had time horizons of 2–10 years, and three models had a lifetime horizon. One abstract did not report the time horizon used (Table 2; Fig. 2).

Modelling approaches

The 18 models used a range of different modelling approaches reported by authors. There did not seem to be any single approach that emerged as a preferred standard.

The most commonly used approaches were Markov modelling, which was used by four of the included models, and decision tree modelling with Monte Carlo simulations, which was used by three models.

Two further models used Monte Carlo simulations. Of the remaining nine, three were decision-analytical models, three were dynamic transmission models using epidemiological data on HIV prevalence, one used a decision tree, one used cohort simulation, and one used a Bayesian approach (Table 2; Fig. 2).

Decision-analysis trees are simple forms of health economic models that aim to represent clinical pathways over time and allows synthesis of evidence to estimate costs and effectiveness. These models are best suited to modelling acute conditions or short-term interventions. However, decision-analysis trees are generally too simple to be used for the modelling of situations where there are multiple alternative actions (for example, treatment pathways, drug options) that are encountered in complex or chronic conditions (such as long-term management of addiction) or in cases where events may be repeated (such as treatment cycles).

Markov models are particularly suited to modelling repeated events and/or progression of disease. In Markov models, there are a finite set of health states (for example, in treatment, illicit drug user, non-user not on treatment) and individuals move between these health states over a discrete time period, known as a Markov cycle and according to a set of transition probabilities (describing the probability of moving from one health state to another). By attaching costs and outcomes to the health states, and running the model over a number of cycles, the long term costs and outcomes for hypothetical cohorts can be estimated. In reality, the transitions/probabilities may vary based on individual patient treatment history, and Monte Carlo simulations may be used. These simulations use repeated random calculations to obtain a distribution of a particular outcome and take account of different treatment histories or varying transition probabilities.

Outcomes measures and data sources

The data used in the models for outcomes and resource use were mainly derived from published literature, clinical trials, meta-analyses or indirect comparisons. The budget impact analysis used a health claims database (Table 2).

For those studies that reported details of the clinical outcomes used as model inputs, the choice of outcomes used depended on the scope of the economic evaluations.

In all cases outcomes associated with maintenance treatment were either based on impacts on mortality, retention in the maintenance programme or successful detoxification and cessation of the maintenance treatment (Additional file 4). Other clinical outcomes/clinical effectiveness outcomes used were related to whether an individual was taking illicit drugs while on maintenance treatment, or while off treatment. Five economic evaluations considered the impact of needle-sharing and sexual behaviour of IDU on the spread of HIV, acquired immunodeficiency syndrome (AIDS) and HCV disease [12, 17, 19–21].

The impact of disease and treatment on quality of life is an important indicator of outcomes. When this is combined with clinical outcomes such as life-years gained, QALYs can be calculated. This outcome measure is recommended by HTA authorities [29–32]. The results of this review highlight the lack of evidence in this area of modelling. Additional file 5 summarises the sources of utility data used in the models reviewed. While utility weights are reported for HIV, AIDS and HCV, these are not specific to individuals with heroin abuse. Of the 11 studies which used a cost-utility approach and QALYs, four economic evaluations derived utility weights from a UK panel study which used general population members to make valuations of given health states using a standard gamble method (an approach recommended by NICE). One economic evaluation used mapping of a generic psychometric scale to QALY-based estimates [19]. For the remaining studies, assumptions were made based on plausible estimates in other diseases.

Costs included in the economic evaluations are summarised in Additional file 6. These included direct medical costs, which comprised all consumption of resources resulting from maintenance treatment (such as drug costs, healthcare resources); and direct non-medical costs such as staff costs, capital and building costs. The far-reaching consequences of heroin use, namely wider societal costs such as the costs of crime, employment, and support services have been included in only a limited number of studies. Only one study included costs to patients such as transport costs and their time spent travelling to and from treatment centres. The studies that included societal costs in the primary analysis varied widely in the type of costs they included; Schackman et al. [16] included only patient costs (travel, visit time and transport costs), Miller et al. [14] included the costs of criminal activity; Zarkin et al. [22] included criminal costs and productivity; and Stephen et al. [18] included criminal costs and productivity costs for both victim and crime perpetrator. A further two studies included societal costs as part of an additional analysis: for both, the costs included were criminal justice service costs [1, 23]. One further study mentioned an additional analysis including societal costs but reported no details [25].

Figure 4 summarises the outcome measures used in the studies and whether societal costs were included in the primary analysis. Only four studies included societal costs in the primary analysis [14, 16, 18, 22]. The most commonly used outcome measure was the QALY.

Sensitivity analyses

A range of different types of sensitivity analyses have been reported in existing models in order to test the robustness of results. Deterministic and probabilistic analyses have been used.

In general, the results from the models did not vary significantly for the parameters tested in the various forms of sensitivity analyses, and ICERs usually remained within cost-effectiveness thresholds. However, the parameters which did impact on the results included treatment completion rates, health-related quality of life, and costs associated with criminal justice services.

Discussion

Opioid dependence is typically a chronic condition with a dynamic and variable course. Individuals may have periods of illicit drug use interspersed with periods of treatment and periods of abstinence, and outcomes vary greatly from one individual to another. Opioid dependence also has complex effects on wider society, for example on the criminal justice system and victims of crime, so economic models should aim to capture these aspects in order to reflect the decision-making framework.

To our knowledge, this systematic review is the first to evaluate economic modelling studies conducted in opioid agonist therapy for non-prescription opioid dependence.

Several different modelling approaches have been reported, each with its own strengths and limitations. Decision-tree models typically accepted by HTA bodies are simple to construct and useful where short time horizons are appropriate and the estimation of outcomes is straightforward, but they do not easily capture time dependency or recurrent events in chronic or complex diseases such as heroin addiction. However, decision-tree models can be adapted to better reflect aspects of time dependency and/or longer term outcomes. An example of this is incorporation of Monte Carlo simulations, as was done in two of the HTA models reported [1, 23].

Other approaches that overcome the issues associated with modelling long-term or chronic conditions with discrete health states include cohort models or Markov models. In this type of model, patients are in one of a number of finite health states, which are mutually exclusive and represent clinically and economically important events. Movements between health states are determined by transition probabilities. Decision-tree models, cohort models and Markov models are favoured by HTA agencies for their simplicity of construction and analysis. However, the transition probability of moving from one disease state to another is independent of the patient's disease history, and there is a fixed cycle time before a patient is eligible to move into a new state. These are potentially important limitations in opioid dependence, as transitions are affected by individual patient characteristics, previous behaviour and treatment history [22]. Ways to address these limitations within the Markov/cohort framework include using additional health states to account for disease history (as long as the number of states does not become too cumbersome), or the transition probabilities can be made time-dependent [1].

Patient-level simulation models such as dynamic models and Monte Carlo simulations can also be used to capture stochastic variation in outcomes between individuals, and can take account of heterogeneity in factors such as demographic characteristics and previous history. Their main deficiency is lack of transparency with regard to data inputs and how they are combined within the model, coupled with the prolonged time taken to run sensitivity analyses [1].

Dynamic models, used by three studies identified in this review [12, 20, 21] to evaluate population effects associated with needle sharing, allow internal feedback loops and time delays that permit the modelling of health changes across entire populations or systems. They are well established in the study of infectious disease transmission through populations [1].

Four studies identified in this review used Monte Carlo simulation [1, 22–24], and a further study used it for the sensitivity analyses [14]. However, these types of models are known to produce different results from those of static models, and the direction of the results may be unpredictable compared with models such as decision trees or Markov models. Comparisons of results between dynamic models and static models cannot easily be made. As a result, dynamic models may not be accepted by HTA assessment groups, as noted in a systematic review and economic evaluation of methadone and buprenorphine for the management of opioid dependence in 2007 [1].

A limitation of our review is that it did not include health economic models based solely on data from the duration of a randomised controlled trial, i.e. those that did not extrapolate beyond the trial duration. Whilst this does represent another possible modelling approach, the short duration of such trials means it is unlikely to be suitable for modelling a chronic condition such as non-prescription opioid dependence.

● Societal costs included in the primary analysis

● Societal costs not included in the primary analysis but included in a secondary analysis

● Societal costs not included

● No information on whether societal costs were included

Study/ Reference	Outcome measure				
	QALY	LYG	Cost/LYG	Cost/QALY	Other*
Barnett (1999) [11]			●		
Barnett (2001) [12]	●				
Masson (2004) [13]	●	●			
Negrin (2006) [15]					●
Schackman (2012) [16]				●	
Sheerin (2004) [17]			●		
Stephen (2012) [18]	●				
Tran (2012) [19]	●				●
Zaric (2000) [20]			●	●	
Zaric (2000) [21]	●	●			
Zarkin (2005) [22]					●
Miller (2004) [14]					●
Adi (2007) [23]	●				
Connock (2007) [1]	●				
Schering Plough (2007) [24]	●				
SMC (2007)** [25]	●				
Clay (2014) [26,27]					●
Fowler (2013) [28]	●				

*Other includes: Cost Impact comparing 100% on buprenorphine-naloxone combination film vs. 100% on buprenorphine-naloxone combination (Clay 2014); Total cost over 5 years (Miller 2004); Cost/ benefit ratio (Zarkin 2005); Case of HIV averted (Tran 2012); Cost-effectiveness acceptability curve and cost-effectiveness frontier (Negrin 2006)

**Secondary analysis including societal costs is mentioned, but no details presented

Fig. 4 Overview of outcomes and costs considered. *HIV* human immunodeficiency virus, *LYG* life-years gained, *QALY* quality-adjusted life-years

Model parameters such as time horizons were reflected in the modelling approach. Time horizons in decision analytical models ranged from 6 months to 1 year while cohort/simulation models ranged from 5 years to a lifetime. Modelling guidelines [30] recommend that the time horizon of a model should be long enough to capture all important differences in costs or outcomes between two or more treatments or between treatment and no treatment. Both models used in NICE HTA appraisals were 1 year in length [1, 23]. As opioid dependence may require long-term or life-long treatment [4], longer time horizons are likely to be more appropriate for models of opioid dependence, so that a realistic picture of lifetime costs and benefits of treatment can be adequately presented.

The model inputs reflected the perspective taken. Costs included in the economic evaluations were mainly those relating to healthcare service costs associated with opioid agonist therapy, including costs to primary care services and hospital services. Wider societal costs, such as costs of drug-related crime, disorder and antisocial behaviour, and loss of productivity in the workplace, were included in some form in only a few of the models. Impacts on family and social networks have not been included in any model. Costs to the individual patient, such as out-of-pocket costs, the costs related to premature death, drug-related illness and the loss of earnings through criminality/imprisonment, sickness, temporary or permanent unemployment and reduced educational attainment are also not routinely included in economic models. This may be because these types of costs are not ordinarily included in economic evaluations of healthcare interventions, so comparability with other interventions would be hampered if they were included. Indeed, HTA groups around the world have varying guidelines regarding costs to be included in a reference case for economic evaluations. In Sweden and The Netherlands, all relevant direct and indirect costs and revenues for treatment and ill health, irrespective of the payee, should be considered [29, 32]; in Norway, unrelated medical and non-medical costs should not be included [31]; in the UK a broader perspective on costs (beyond the NHS and Personal Social Services) may only be considered in exceptional circumstances [30]; while in Australia, PBAC mainly considers the costs of providing health care resources but may also consider costs and cost offsets of non-health care resources, although these might not be as influential in decision making as health care resources [33]. In the treatment of drug addiction, consistent omission of wider costs and benefits in the reported models means that the impact of effective maintenance treatments will not be fully captured; this will under-estimate the benefit of maintenance treatment to society. For example, reducing

the spread of HIV will benefit non-drug users who will avoid HIV infection [11, 12] and is an important societal impact of maintenance treatment. In the US, total lifetime treatment cost for HIV based on new diagnoses in 2009 was estimated to be $16.6 billion [34].

The most common form of evaluation was cost-utility analysis, with an outcome measure of the number of QALYs gained. This may reflect the preference of HTA agencies for this type of analysis as it incorporates the value placed on health effects by society [30, 33]. However, there are limited data sources available for utility weights for substance abuse. Including the impact on quality of life is important because substance abuse is associated with significant co-morbidities and personal and social impacts, all of which should be considered when estimating the benefit of maintenance treatment. Thus, QALY weights should take account of reductions in health due to the disease of addiction itself and the impact of treatment on quality of life. In this review, only one source was available where the standard gamble method was used with members of the general public to obtain QALY weights for health states in substance abuse [16]. Choice-based preference measures to capture the value of health-related quality of life impacts are recommended by HTA groups such as NICE in the UK [30], PBAC in Australia [33] and HTA groups in European countries such as Norway [31], The Netherlands [29] and Sweden [32]. However, with addiction therapies and services the question could be asked about whose values should be used. Members of the public valuing vignettes developed by patients may be skewed by moral judgements, so perhaps people who have recovered from drug addiction might be the best-informed group.

Conclusions

This systematic review identified 18 economic modelling studies in non-prescription opioid dependence reporting a range of modelling approaches. There appears to be no single standard emerging as the preferred approach and there are a number of advantages and disadvantages to the different modelling approaches, some of which can be overcome using advanced modelling techniques. These factors, together with acceptability to HTA agencies, need to be considered when selecting a model structure for economic evaluation of a new therapy indicated for the maintenance treatment of non-prescription opioid dependence.

The most common evaluation type was cost-utility analysis reporting the cost per QALY gained (11/18 models), reflecting the preference of HTA agencies for this form of evaluation, although the data on utility weights are limited. Typical outcomes include mortality and treatment retention. However, wider societal costs such as the cost of crime (expenditure by the criminal justice system in dealing with crimes committed, and cost consequences for the victims of crime), productivity, employment impacts, transmission of HIV and HCV and costs of treatment borne by patients (for example, transportation costs and value of time spent receiving treatment) are not typically included in health economic modelling. Given the wide ranging impact of illicit opioid abuse on the workplace, the healthcare system, and in the communities, including these non-typical costs may help present a more complete story of the economic burden.

This review identified some key elements that could form a standard framework and guide for future models, such as:

- Selecting a modelling approach that is able to capture the complexities of opioid use, allow for transitions to be affected by past behaviour and include transmission of HIV and other drug-related infectious diseases;
- Selecting a time horizon that is long enough to capture the impact of treatment and disease on patients in this chronic condition;
- Inclusion of societal consequences associated with heroin use that also have important economic consequences;
- Capturing the impact of disease and treatment-related health-related quality of life/utility specific to this patient population through appropriately sourced and valued health states.

The range of modelling approaches found in the literature could not easily be compared in terms of quality but the evidence does indicate that there is currently no single standard emerging as the preferred approach. Indeed, a number of the methodological approaches taken in different modelling studies could be used together to begin to build a framework for future models in this disease area. Furthermore, some of the disadvantages of current model structures could be overcome by using more advanced modelling techniques or choosing a different model approach. We propose that to develop a future model for the pharmacoeconomic evaluation of opioid agonist interventions, researchers should first identify the most robust model currently available, replicate the model, and then extend that model in terms of the range of inputs described above. Such a model should be applicable to a range of scenarios, e.g. intervention versus no intervention, comparison between interventions, changes over time, societal impact. Providing access to the model and the associated model code to the health care community could stimulate future dialogue and

make it easier to recognise the strengths and weakness of different modelling approaches.

Abbreviations

AIDS: acquired immunodeficiency syndrome; CADTH: Canadian Agency for Drugs and Technologies in Health; DARE: Database of Abstracts of Reviews of Effects; DBS: deep brain stimulation; G-BA: Gemeinsamer Bundesausschuss; HCV: hepatitis C virus; HIV: human immunodeficiency virus; HTA: health technology assessment; IDU: injecting drug users; IQWIG: Institute for Quality and Efficiency in Heath Care; NHS: National Health Service; NHS EED: National Health Service Economic Evaluation Database; NICE: National Institute for Health and Clinical Excellence; PBAC: Pharmaceutical Benefits Advisory Committee; QALY: quality-adjusted life-year; SBU: Swedish Council on Health Technology Assessment; SMC: Scottish Medicines Consortium; TLV: Tandvards-och lakemedelsformansverket; US: United States of America; UK: United Kingdom.

Authors' contributions

MC carried out the review of the literature and drafted the manuscript. JK reviewed the manuscript, revised it critically for intellectual content, and was also involved in the interpretation and cross-checking of selected original sources. WD was involved in the planning of the manuscript at all stages, reviewed the manuscript and revised it critically for intellectual content, and was also involved in the interpretation and cross-checking of selected original sources. SL reviewed the manuscript, revised it critically for intellectual content, and was also involved in the interpretation and cross-checking of selected original sources. AW reviewed the manuscript and revised it critically for intellectual content. All searches, reviewing and data extraction were performed by PHMR without influence from Mundipharma. All authors read and approved the final manuscript.

Author details

[1] PHMR Ltd, London, UK. [2] Mundipharma International Ltd, Cambridge Science Park, Milton Road, Cambridge CB4 0GW, UK. [3] University of Glasgow, Glasgow, UK.

Acknowledgements

The authors thank Carole Nadin and Jo Whelan for editorial assistance on behalf of PHMR Ltd, and Dave Fox (PHMR Ltd, Newcastle) for conducting the literature searches. This piece of work, including preparation of the manuscript, was funded by Mundipharma International, which was involved in: study design; collection, analysis and interpretation of data; writing of the manuscript; and decision to submit the manuscript for publication. Two Mundipharma employees (JK and WD) were authors of the paper under ICJME criteria.

Competing interests

JK and WD are employees of Mundipharma International. MC and SL are employees of PHMR, which was contracted by Mundipharma International to undertake this research. AW contribution was voluntary and without payment.

References

1. Connock M, Juarez-Garcia A, Jowett S, Frew E, Liu Z, Taylor RJ, et al. Methadone and buprenorphine for the management of opioid dependence: a systematic review and economic evaluation. Health Technol Assess. 2007;11:1–171.
2. United Nations World Drug Report. Recent statistics and trend analysis of illicit drug market. 2012. https://www.unodc.org/documents/data-and-analysis/WDR2012/WDR_2012_Chapter1.pdf. Accessed 23 Jun 2015.
3. Ross J, Teesson M, Darke S, Lynskey M, Ali R, Ritter A, et al. The characteristics of heroin users entering treatment: findings from the Australian treatment outcome study (ATOS). Drug Alcohol Rev. 2005;24:411–8.
4. World Health Organization. Guidelines for the psychosocially assisted pharmacological treatment of opioid dependence. 2009. http://www.who.int/substance_abuse/publications/opioid_dependence_guidelines.pdf. Accessed 28 May 2015.

5. Doran C. Economic evaluation of interventions for illicit opioid depend-
    ence: a review of evidence. 2007. http://www.who.int/substance_abuse/
    activities/economic_evaluation_interventions.pdf. Accessed 18 Nov
    2015.
6. BMA Board of Science. Drugs of dependence (full report). Chapter 3—the
    burden of illicit drug use. 2013. http://bma.org.uk/news-views-analysis/
    in-depth-drugs-of-dependence/full-report. Accessed 26 Jun 2015.
7. Barnard M, McKeganey N. The impact of parental problem drug use on
    children: what is the problem and what can be done to help? Addiction.
    2004;99:552–9.
8. Soyka M. New developments in the management of opioid dependence:
    focus on sublingual buprenorphine-naloxone. Subst Abuse Rehabil.
    2015;6:1–14.
9. Institute for Clinical and Economic Review. Management of patients
    with opioid dependence: a review of clinical, delivery system, and policy
    options 2014. https://icer-review.org/wpcontent/uploads/2016/01/
    CEPAC-Opioid-Dependence-Final-Report-For-Posting-July-211. Accessed
    28 May 2015.
10. University of Glasgow, Department of General Practice. Critical appraisal
    checklist for economic evaluations. 2015. http://www.gla.ac.uk/media/
    media_64048_en.pdf Accessed 3 Jun 2015.
11. Barnett PG. The cost-effectiveness of methadone maintenance as a
    health care intervention. Addiction. 1999;94:479–88.
12. Barnett PG, Zaric GS, Brandeau ML. The cost-effectiveness of buprenor-
    phine maintenance therapy for opiate addiction in the United States.
    Addiction. 2001;96:1267–78.
13. Masson CL, Barnett PG, Sees KL, Delucchi KL, Rosen A, Wong W, et al. Cost
    and cost-effectiveness of standard methadone maintenance treatment
    compared to enriched 180-day methadone detoxification. Addiction.
    2004;99:718–26.
14. Miller CL, Schechter MT, Wood E, Spittal PM, Li K, Laliberte N, et al. The
    potential health and economic impact of implementing a medically
    prescribed heroin program among Canadian injection drug users. Int J
    Drug Policy. 2004;15:259–63.
15. Negrin MA, Vazquez-Polo FJ. Bayesian cost-effectiveness analysis with
    two measures of effectiveness: the cost-effectiveness acceptability plane.
    Health Econ. 2006;15:363–72.
16. Schackman BR, Leff JA, Polsky D, Moore BA, Fiellin DA. Cost-effectiveness
    of long-term outpatient buprenorphine-naloxone treatment for opioid
    dependence in primary care. J Gen Intern Med. 2012;27:669–76.
17. Sheerin IG, Green FT, Sellman JD. What is the cost-effectiveness of hepa-
    titis C treatment for injecting drug users on methadone maintenance in
    New Zealand? Drug Alcohol Rev. 2004;23:261–72.
18. Stephen JH, Halpern CH, Barrios CJ, Balmuri U, Pisapia JM, Wolf JA, et al.
    Deep brain stimulation compared with methadone maintenance for
    the treatment of heroin dependence: a threshold and cost-effectiveness
    analysis. Addiction. 2012;107:624–34.
19. Tran BX, Ohinmaa A, Duong AT, Nguyen LT, Vu PX, Mills S, et al. The cost-
    effectiveness and budget impact of Vietnam's methadone maintenance
    treatment programme in HIV prevention and treatment among injection
    drug users. Glob Public Health. 2012;7:1080–94.
20. Zaric GS, Barnett PG, Brandeau ML. HIV transmission and the cost-
    effectiveness of methadone maintenance. Am J Public Health.
    2000;90:1100–11.
21. Zaric GS, Brandeau ML, Barnett PG. Methadone maintenance and HIV
    prevention: a cost-effectiveness analysis. Manag Sci. 2000;46:1013–31.
22. Zarkin GA, Dunlap LJ, Hicks KA, Mamo D. Benefits and costs of metha-
    done treatment: results from a lifetime simulation model. Health Econ.
    2005;14:1133–50.
23. Adi Y, Juarez-Garcia A, Wang D, Jowett S, Frew E, Day E, et al. Oral naltrex-
    one as a treatment for relapse prevention in formerly opioid-dependent
    drug users: a systematic review and economic evaluation. Health Technol
    Assess. 2007;11:1–85.
24. Schering-Plough. Manufacturer's submission. Cited in Connock et al.
    Health Technol Assess. 2007;11:1–171, iii–iv.
25. Scottish Medicines Consortium. Buprenorphine/naloxone 2 mg/0.5 mg,
    8/2 mg sublingual tablet (Suboxone). No. 355/07. 2007. https://www.
    scottishmedicines.org.uk/files/buprenorphine_naloxone_sublingual_tab-
    let__Suboxone__355-07_.pdf. Accessed 3 Jun 2015.
26. Clay E, Kharitonova E, Ruby J, Aballea S, Zah V. Medicaid population
    budget impact analysis of buprenorphine/naloxone film and tablet
    formulation. Value Health. 2014;17:A212.
27. Clay E, Khemiri A, Ruby J, Aballea S, Zah V. A studies-based private insur-
    ance budget impact analysis of buprenorphine/naloxone film and tablet
    formulations. Value Health. 2014;17:A213.
28. Fowler J, Emerson J, Allen A, Dilley S, Gideonse N, Rieckmann T, et al.
    Buprenorphine vs methadone for maintenance of opioid addiction
    during pregnancy: a cost-effectiveness analysis. Am J Obstet Gynecol.
    2013;208((1 SUPPL.)):S65–6.
29. College voor zorgverzekeringen, Diemen. Guidelines for pharmacoeco-
    nomic research, updated version. 2006. http://www.ispor.org/PEguide-
    lines/source/HTAGuidelinesNLupdated2006.pdf. Accessed 27 Jul 2015.
30. National Institute for Health and Care Excellence. Process and methods
    guides: guide to the methods of technology appraisal. 2013. http://www.
    nice.org.uk/article/PMG9/chapter/Foreword. Accessed 4 Mar 2015.
31. Norwegian Medicines Agency (NOMA). Guidelines on how to conduct
    pharmacoeconomic analyses. 2012. http://www.ispor.org/PEguidelines/
    source/Norwegian_guidelines2012.pdf. Accessed 27 Jul 2015.
32. Pharmaceutical Benefits Board, Sweden. General guidelines for economic
    evaluations from the Pharmaceutical Benefits Board (LFNAR 2003:2).
    2003. http://www.ispor.org/PEguidelines/source/Guidelines_in_Sweden.
    pdf. Accessed 27 Jul 2015.
33. Pharmaceutical Benefits Advisory Committee (PBAC). Guidelines for pre-
    paring submissions to the Pharmaceutical Benefits Advisory Committee
    (Version 4.3). 2008. http://www.pbac.pbs.gov.au/content/information/
    archived-versions/pbac-guidelines-v4.3-2008.pdf. Accessed 21 Jul 2015.
34. Centers for Disease Control. HIV cost-effectiveness. 2013. http://www.cdc.
    gov/hiv/prevention/ongoing/costeffectiveness/. Accessed 18 Nov 2015.

7

Emergency department use and hospitalizations among homeless adults with substance dependence and mental disorders

Adrienne Cheung[1], Julian M Somers[2], Akm Moniruzzaman[2], Michelle Patterson[2], Charles J Frankish[3], Michael Krausz[3,4] and Anita Palepu[1]*

Abstract

Background: Homelessness, substance use, and mental disorders each have been associated with higher rates of emergency department (ED) use and hospitalization. We sought to understand the correlation between ED use, hospital admission, and substance dependence among homeless individuals with concurrent mental illness who participated in a 'Housing First' (HF) intervention trial.

Methods: The Vancouver At Home study consisted of two randomized controlled trials addressing homeless individuals with mental disorders who have "high" or "moderate" levels of need. Substance dependence was determined at baseline prior to randomization, using the Mini International Neuropsychiatric Interview diagnostic tool, version 6.0. To assess health service use, we reviewed the number of ED visits and the number of hospital admissions based on administrative data for six urban hospitals. Negative binomial regression modeling was used to test the independent association between substance dependence and health service use (ED use and hospitalization), adjusting for HF intervention, age, gender, ethnicity, education, duration of lifetime homelessness, mental disorders, chronic health conditions, and other variables that were selected a priori to be potentially associated with use of ED services and hospital admission.

Results: Of the 497 homeless adults with mental disorders who were recruited, we included 381 participants in our analyses who had at least 1 year of follow-up and had a personal health number that could be linked to administrative health data. Of this group, 59% (n = 223) met criteria for substance dependence. We found no independent association between substance dependence and ED visits or hospital admissions [rate ratio (RR) = 0.85; 95% CI 0.62–1.17 and RR = 1.21; 95% CI 0.83–1.77, respectively]. The most responsible diagnoses (defined as the diagnosis that accounts for the length of stay) for hospital admissions were schizo-affective disorder, schizophrenia-related disorder, or bipolar affective disorder; collectively reported in 48% (n = 263) of admissions. Fifteen percent (n = 84) of hospital admissions listed substance dependence as the most responsible diagnosis.

Conclusions: Substance dependence was not independently associated with ED use or hospital admission among homeless adults with mental disorders participating in an HF trial. Hospital admissions among this cohort were primarily associated with severe mental disorders.

Trial registration: ISRCTN57595077 and ISRCTN66721740

*Correspondence: apalepu@hivnet.ubc.ca
[1] Department of Medicine, Centre for Health Evaluation and Outcome Sciences, University of British Columbia, 588B-1081 Burrard Street, Vancouver, BC V6Z 1Y6, Canada
Full list of author information is available at the end of the article

Keywords: Emergency department use, Hospital admission, Substance dependence, Homelessness, At Home study, Mental disorders

Background

Homelessness is associated with a number of health and policy challenges in urban settings around the world. A significant proportion of individuals struggling with homelessness also suffer from substance dependence and other concurrent mental illnesses [1, 2]. A higher prevalence of these disorders has been observed among homeless populations in Canada, the United States, Europe, and Australia [3, 4]. In Toronto, Canada, lifetime diagnosis of mental illness and substance use or dependence has been recorded as high as 67 and 68%, respectively, among users of homeless shelters [1]. In the Hotel Study, which included 297 adults living in single-room occupancy hotels in Vancouver, the lifetime prevalence of mental illness and substance dependence was 98 and 85%, respectively [5].

Homelessness, substance use, and mental disorders each have been associated with higher rates of emergency department (ED) use, hospitalization, and involvement with other publicly-funded services in the United States and Canada [6–10]. One survey of 2,500 adults who were homeless in the United States found that less stable housing, history of psychiatric hospitalization, and substance abuse were associated with repeated use of ED services (defined as four or more visits in the previous year) [10]. Tsai et al. reported similar findings in comparing homeless to housed persons accessing Veterans Affairs EDs in the U.S. Homeless veterans had four times the odds of using the ED as housed veterans, and they were also more likely to have been diagnosed with a substance use disorder or schizophrenia in the preceding year [11]. Another study, examining discharge data from New York City hospitals, found that patients who were homeless stayed in the hospital, on average, 4.1 days (36%) longer than a comparison group [12]. Using the same sample as the present study, Palepu et al. found that daily substance use was associated with more severe mental health symptoms [2], which could lead to increased health care utilization. It follows that interventions addressing substance use and mental disorders among the homeless may reduce downstream health care expenditures.

Housing First (HF) is a low-barrier intervention designed to target the most vulnerable among the homeless, including those with severe mental illness experiencing chronic homelessness [7, 13]. HF provides immediate access to subsidized housing with supports and does not impose prerequisites of abstinence from substance use or adherence to medication for mental disorders. The model prioritizes consumer choice and an individual's rights to appropriate housing, with the proposition that helping to meet immediate needs will enable the patients to address addiction and other psychiatric conditions. In addition to the housing component, different methods of support and treatment are offered to support recovery in a more effective way [13, 14]. These services have multiple goals, including the reduction of unnecessary hospitalizations and ED visits. We found that the assertive community treatment intervention of HF was associated with a reduction in ED visits [15].

Positive outcomes have been observed with HF in homeless adults with concurrent disorders, including greater residential stability and greater perception of choice among participants [16–18]. A number of studies have reported reductions in health service use and health care costs with HF interventions, including reductions in ED visits, hospitalizations, and length of hospital stay [7, 19–21]. Contrary to these findings, however, Hwang et al. found no difference in health service use between a group of supportive housing program participants and a control group in a study conducted in Toronto [21]. Another study, following a cohort of applicants to a supportive housing program in the United States, also failed to find reductions in health care use over time; this retrospective cohort study showed no significant difference in utilization rates of ambulance services and the ED before and after the intervention, and no difference was detected between the intervention group and a wait-list control group [22]. Although promising results have been published regarding the effectiveness of HF, some controversy remains as to its effect on participants' use of health services.

In spite of the documented higher prevalence of substance use among the homeless, evidence is lacking on the effect of substance dependence on various outcomes, such as health service use for this group [23–25]. The objective of this study was to examine whether substance dependence at baseline predicted health service use at 2-year follow-up among participants assigned to HF or to treatment as usual (TAU), using data from the Vancouver At Home (VAH) study. We were also interested in whether or not substance dependence altered the effect of HF on ED use and hospitalization. We hypothesized that persons who were homeless and met criteria for substance dependence would have significantly higher levels of ED use and hospital admission at 2-year follow-up compared to persons without substance dependence.

Methods

The detailed methods for the At Home/Chez Soi collaboration and the VAH study have been previously described [13, 14]. Essentially, At Home/Chez Soi is a pragmatic, multisite randomized controlled trial (RCT) assessing the effectiveness of a complex housing and support intervention in five Canadian cities. The VAH study includes additional measures, a site-specific intervention, and has a particular focus on substance use. In this manuscript, we report findings from the VAH study using survey data from participants recruited between October 2009 and June 2011, and administrative data on ED use and hospitalization spanning April 2007–September 2012. The VAH study is comprised of two RCTs examining the effectiveness of HF interventions among homeless adults with mental disorders who were differentiated based on their assessed levels of need (high vs. moderate). We pooled data from the two trials (ISRCTN57595077 and ISRCTN66721740) to examine the relationship between substance dependence and ED use and hospitalization [14]. Institutional Research Ethics Board approval was received from Simon Fraser University and the University of British Columbia.

Participants were recruited through referrals from a range of community agencies including shelters, drop-in centers, homeless outreach teams, mental health teams, inpatient hospital wards, and criminal justice programs [13, 14]. Individuals were eligible if they were age 19 years or older, met criteria for a current mental disorder on the Mini International Neuropsychiatric Interview (MINI) 6.0 [26], with or without concurrent substance dependence, and were either absolutely homeless or precariously housed.

Initial screening with referring service providers was conducted over the telephone [14]. This was followed by a face-to-face screening interview with the potential participant, where trained interviewers determined eligibility, explained study procedures, and obtained informed consent. A total of 800 individuals were screened for eligibility. Approximately 100 individuals did not meet eligibility criteria in the telephone screen. Another 200 were excluded through the baseline interview procedure due to ineligibility (n = 94), the inability to be contacted for baseline interview (n = 100), declining to participate (n = 3), or an incomplete interview (n = 3).

Once participants were enrolled, interviewers administered a baseline questionnaire, which consisted of detailed questions regarding sociodemographic characteristics, symptoms of mental disorders, substance use, physical health, and service involvement [14]. Participants received an honorarium of $35 upon completing the baseline interview. Participants were identified as high needs (HN) if they had a score of 62 or lower on the Multnomah Community Ability Scale [27], met criteria for current psychotic disorder or a (hypo)manic episode on the MINI, and had at least one of the following: two or more hospitalizations for mental illness in any one of the last 5 years, substance dependence in the past month, or legal involvement in the past year [13, 14]. All other included participants were designated as moderate needs (MN).

A detailed description of the intervention arms has been published previously [14]. Briefly, HN participants were randomized to one of three intervention arms: (1) HF with assertive community treatment (HF-ACT), where participants were given a choice of up to three market rentals and had to fulfill the commitments of their lease and check in with an ACT team member on a weekly basis with a client/staff ratio of 9:1; (2) HF in a congregate housing unit (HF-CONG) with onsite support; or (3) HF with treatment as usual (HN-TAU), which provided no additional housing or support aside from what was available in the community. MN participants were randomized to one of two intervention arms: (1) HF with intensive case management (HF-ICM), where participants were given a choice of up to three market rentals and connected to existing community services through case managers and a client/staff ratio of 16:1; or (2) MN-TAU.

Randomization was computer-generated at a national data center using an adaptive randomization procedure. This allowed for sequential allocation of participants immediately after enrollment, without affecting the predictability of future assignments. Blinding of participants was impossible, and blinding of interviewers was not feasible as interviewers were required to obtain data on participants' housing status. Interviewers met with participants at 3-month intervals over the 2-year follow-up period. Participants were asked to provide consent to access administrative hospital data through their provincial personal health numbers.

Variables of interest

Our primary outcome was health service use, defined as the number of ED visits and hospitalizations during the observation period. Both ED use and hospital admissions were captured through the administrative data. This administrative data included information related to ED visits (such as number and type of ED visits, mode of arrival, name of hospital, chief complaint, discharge diagnosis, and disposition) and hospitalizations (such as number of hospital admissions, name of hospital, most responsible diagnosis) from April 2007 to September 2012 at six urban hospitals in the Vancouver Coastal Health Authority.

Our primary independent variable, substance dependence (yes/no), was identified at baseline using the MINI

6.0. Self-reported frequency of substance use over the past month was captured using the Maudsley Addiction Profile at baseline and every 6 months thereafter up to 24 months [28]. Drug use frequency was dichotomized to compare daily substance use versus nondaily use (less than daily or none) [2]. HF intervention was the combination of the three housing intervention arms (HF-ACT, HF-CONG, HF-ICM), and TAU was comprised of the two TAU arms (HN and MN). Mental health symptoms and severity were collected through the Colorado Symptom Index (CSI) [29, 30]. Sociodemographic information (including gender, self-reported race/ethnicity, marital status, highest educational attainment, and monthly income) was collected at baseline.

For mental disorders, the severe cluster included at least one current psychotic disorder, mood disorder with psychotic features, and (hypo)manic episode, as identified through the MINI [26]. The less-severe cluster included at least one current major depressive episode, panic disorder, or post-traumatic stress disorder. Based on a list of 31 chronic health conditions, participants were also asked to report any conditions that were expected to last or already had lasted at least 6 months. Chronic health conditions listed in the survey tool were adapted from the Canadian Community Health Survey [31] and the National Population Health Survey [32]. Positivity for blood-borne infectious diseases was obtained by self-report. Participants were asked three questions pertaining to access to care that we included in our analyses: (1) do you have a regular medical doctor? (2) Is there a place you go when you are sick or need advice about your health? (If answered yes, named a hospital ED); (3) in the past 6 months, was there ever a time when you felt that you needed health care but you didn't receive it?

Statistical analysis

We pooled data from the two trials for the analyses. We used descriptive statistics to characterize the sample (mean and SD for continuous variables, and proportion for categorical variables). We compared variables between groups using parametric (Student's t-test or one-way ANOVA for continuous variables) and nonparametric (Pearson's Chi square test for categorical variables) tests, as appropriate. We estimated the rate of ED visits and hospitalizations by dividing the total number of occurrences (visits or admissions) by the total follow-up time (person-years). We fit separate models for the number of ED visits and the number of hospitalizations. We used negative binomial regression (NBR) analysis to estimate the association between each outcome variable and the primary independent variable (substance dependence). We chose NBR due to over-dispersion, the count nature of outcome data, and better goodness of fit

statistics compared to Poisson regression. Post randomization period (exposure time) was estimated from the differences between time 0 (date of randomization) and time 1 (date of death or administrative data cutoff date, September, 2012), which varied across individuals (range 1.1–2 years). We used this exposure time (using the log transformation) as an offset variable in the regression analysis to adjust for these variations across individuals.

We examined the effects of substance dependence on health care use in both bivariate and multivariable settings. For the multivariable regression models, we included variables that were selected a priori to be potentially associated with ED visits and hospital admission [HF intervention (combined HF-ACT, HF-ICM, HF-CONG), need-level (HN vs. MN), employment, age, gender, ethnicity, education, age at first homelessness, mental disorders, chronic health conditions (3 or more), blood-borne infectious disease, prior health care utilization, having a regular doctor, and where one goes when sick]. In the model-building process, we chose all variables that were significant in bivariate models ($p \leq 0.05$). In addition, we forced several demographic variables and substance dependence into the multivariable models, regardless of significance in bivariate models. We tested the interaction term between HF intervention and substance dependence, but did not include it in the final model due to nonsignificance ($p > 0.05$). We also conducted two sub-analyses fitting NBR models: one for the association of daily substance use and ED use and hospitalization using a similar set of covariates; and another model examining the association of substance dependence on psychiatric hospitalization. All reported p values were two-sided. Rate ratios (RRs) obtained from the NBR models were reported as effect sizes. The missing values for covariates that ranged from zero to 2% were excluded from the analysis. IBM SPSS statistics (version 19.0, August 2010) and STATA 12 (StataCorp. 2011) were used to conduct these analyses.

Results

The eligible sample consisted of 381 participants who had at least 1 year of follow-up, provided consent to access administrative health data, and had a personal health number that could be used to access those data. There were no significant differences in the characteristics of the eligible sample compared to the total sample (Table 1). Among the eligible sample, 59% (n = 223) met criteria for substance dependence, and 29% (n = 110) reported daily substance use. Twenty-eight percent (n = 105) of the sample was female, and 16% (n = 62) identified as Aboriginal. Seventy percent (n = 266) of participants reported having at least three or more chronic health conditions, and 32% (n = 121) reported

Table 1 Characteristics of "At Home" participants by Housing First allocation status

Variable	Entire sample (N = 497) n (%)/mean (SD)	Eligible sample (n = 381) n (%)/mean (SD)	Housing First-yes (n = 250) n (%)/mean (SD)	Housing First-no (n = 131) n (%)/mean (SD)	p value[a]
Housing First interventions	297 (60)	250 (66)			
Substance dependence	288 (58)	223 (59)	150 (60)	73 (56)	0.421
Daily substance use	143 (29)	110 (29)	78 (31)	32 (25)	0.172
Need level (high)	297 (59)	223 (59)			
Age at randomization (in years)	40.8 (11.0)	40.6 (10.9)	40.6 (10.8)	40.6 (11.1)	0.968
Age of first homelessness (in years)	30.3 (13.3)	29.9 (13.4)	29.5 (12.9)	30.5 (14.2)	0.477
Female gender	134 (27)	105 (28)	65 (26)	40 (31)	0.313
Aboriginals	77 (16)	62 (16)	45 (18)	17 (13)	0.119
White	280 (56)	206 (54)	139 (56)	67 (51)	
Other	140 (28)	113 (30)	66 (26)	47 (36)	
Education (incomplete high school)	280 (57)	214 (57)	147 (60)	67 (51)	0.118
Single/never married	343 (70)	254 (67)	168 (68)	86 (66)	0.755
Income ($800 CDN or more)[b] in past month	257 (52)	201 (54)	138 (56)	63 (49)	0.180
Lifetime duration of homelessness (in months)	60.2 (70.3)	56.8 (62.2)	60.6 (66.4)	49.5 (52.7)	0.099
Longest episode of homelessness (in months)	30.9 (40.1)	29.7 (38.8)	31.1 (40.2)	27.2 (36.0)	0.353
Less severe cluster of mental disorders	264 (53)	201 (59)	130 (52)	71 (54)	0.683
Severe cluster of mental disorders	363 (73)	272 (71)	180 (72)	92 (70)	0.716
Multiple mental disorders (≥3)	114 (25)	88 (23)	61 (24)	27 (21)	0.405
Suicidality (high)	87 (17)	68 (18)	44 (18)	24 (18)	0.861
Mental health severity/CSI score (per unit)	37.2 (12.5)	37.3 (12.6)	36.6 (12.8)	38.7 (12.2)	0.116
Chronic health conditions (≥3)	344 (69)	266 (70)	172 (69)	94 (72)	0.551
Blood-borne infectious disease (HIV, hepatitis B or C)	157 (32)	121 (32)	83 (33)	38 (29)	0.416
Have a regular medical doctor	320 (65)	257 (67)	170 (68)	87 (67)	0.831
Place to go when you are sick	395 (81)	302 (81)	202 (82)	100 (78)	0.396
Needed health care, but didn't receive it	209 (43)	156 (42)	97 (40)	59 (46)	0.239
ED visit before randomization (last year)		4.1 (7.0)	4.2 (7.1)	4.0 (6.8)	0.778
Hospital admissions before randomization (last year)		0.9 (1.5)	0.9 (1.5)	0.9 (1.5)	0.805

[a] P values based on comparisons of characteristics between HF-yes participants and HF-no participants in the eligible sample (n = 381).

[b] Dichotomized based on median value.

having a blood-borne infectious disease (HIV, hepatitis B, or hepatitis C). Most participants (67%) reported having a regular medical doctor. The average follow-up time was 1.94 years (SD 0.15 years, range 1.1–2 years). Tables 2 and 3 present the participant characteristics by ED and hospital admission rate (per person, per year).

The 381 participants incurred a total of 3,086 ED visits during the 2-year study period. The average number of ED visits was 4.2 per person, per year (Table 2). Less than one-quarter (23%) had no visits and one individual accumulated 176 ED visits. The multivariable NBR model (Table 4) showed no significant association between substance dependence and ED visits [adjusted incidence rate ratio (ARR) = 0.85; 95% CI 0.62–1.17]. The HF intervention was associated with a reduction in subsequent ED visits (ARR = 0.74; 95% CI 0.55–1.00). We found that having an ED visit in the year prior to randomization (ARR = 1.11; 95% CI 1.08–1.14) and reporting the ED as

a place to go when sick (ARR = 1.45; 95% CI 1.01–2.09) were associated with higher rates of ED use. There were no significant interactions between substance dependence and the HF intervention on ED visits (p = 0.50) or between substance dependence and ACT on ED visits (p = 0.45).

Participants in the eligible sample incurred a total of 550 hospital admissions during the 2-year follow-up period. The average number of admissions was 0.8 per person, per year (Table 3). The maximum number of admissions per person was 15. Sixty-one percent (n = 336) of admissions occurred during the first year post randomization. Psychiatric hospital admissions comprised 81% of the total hospitalizations (443/550) and were incurred by 137 homeless persons. The most responsible diagnosis for hospital admission was schizoaffective or schizophrenia-related disorder in 233 admissions (42%), followed by bipolar affective disorder

Table 2 ED visit during the post randomization period, by "At Home" participant characteristics (n = 381)

Variable	# of ER visits	Total person-years (PYs)	ED rate (per person, per year)
Overall	3,086	738.2	4.2
Housing First interventions	1,925	482.8	4.0
Treatment as usual	1,161	255.4	4.6
Substance dependence			
Yes	1,784	430.9	4.1
No	1,302	307.3	4.2
Daily substance use			
Yes	921	213.3	4.3
No	2,165	524.9	4.1
Need level			
High	2,038	430.6	4.7
Moderate	1,048	307.6	3.4
Male	2,127	529.5	4.0
Female	947	202.7	4.7
Aboriginals	672	119.7	5.6
White	1,794	398.5	4.5
Other	620	219.0	2.8
Incomplete high school	2,008	416.5	4.8
High school or higher	1,062	315.7	3.4
Single/never married	2,225	493.2	4.5
Other	796	239.0	3.3
Income ($800 CDN or more) in past month			
Yes	1,660	387.0	4.3
No	1,413	339.5	4.2
Less severe cluster of mental disorders			
Yes	1,605	390.1	4.1
No	1,481	348.1	4.3
Severe cluster of mental disorders			
Yes	2,369	527.5	4.5
No	717	210.7	3.4
Multiple mental disorders (≥3)			
Yes	826	171.3	4.8
No	2,260	566.9	4.0
Suicidality (high)			
Yes	592	132.5	4.5
No	2,494	605.7	4.1
Chronic health conditions (≥3)			
Yes	2,426	516.6	4.7
No	660	221.6	3.0
Blood-borne infectious disease (HIV, hepatitis B or C)			
Yes	941	235.6	4.0
No	2,143	498.6	4.3
Have a regular medical doctor			
Yes	2,204	497.6	4.4
No	882	240.6	3.7
Place to go when you are sick			
Yes	2,757	595.2	4.6
No	328	143.0	2.3

Table 2 continued

Variable	# of ER visits	Total person-years (PYs)	ED rate (per person, per year)
Needed health care, but didn't receive it			
Yes	1,568	321.3	4.9
No	1,518	416.9	3.6

in 30 admissions (6%). These diagnoses collectively accounted for 48% (n = 263) of hospital admissions, while 15% (n = 84) of admissions were attributable to substance use. As shown in Table 5, substance dependence was not independently associated with hospital admissions (ARR = 1.21; 95% CI 0.83–1.77). Higher rates of hospital admission were associated with having a hospital admission in the year prior to randomization (ARR = 1.33; 95% CI 1.19–1.49) and having a mental disorder in the severe cluster (ARR = 1.76; 95% CI 1.09–2.86). There was no significant interaction between substance dependence and the HF intervention on hospital admissions (p = 0.60).

We did not find an association between daily substance use and health service use in the sub-analysis, when we fit separate models for the number of ED visits and the number of hospitalizations (data not shown). We also did not find a significant association between substance dependence and psychiatric hospitalization (ARR 1.14; 95% CI 0.73–1.80).

Discussion

We found no association between substance dependence and health service use in the form of ED visits and hospitalizations. Daily substance use also was not associated with ED use or hospital admission in these models. Two studies also found no association between substance use and health service involvement [9, 33]. The first examined 2,974 homeless persons in the United States and did not find an association between alcohol and drug abuse with ED use or hospitalization [9]. The second study in Toronto also found no association between having an alcohol and drug problem with frequent ED visits (4.7 visits/year) [33]. In contrast, many studies have shown that homelessness, substance use, and mental disorders are all independently associated with higher rates of ED use and hospitalization [6–10, 22, 34, 35]. HF has been linked to increased residential stability and reductions in these health services in a number of studies [7, 19–21, 24, 25, 36], while others have found no significant association [21, 22]. Differences in these findings may be due to differences in the homeless samples in terms of the higher burden of medical and psychiatric comorbidities, severity of substance use, and health care systems in

different jurisdictions. We found a reduction in ED visits among HF participants compared to the TAU group but did not detect a difference in hospitalizations, which is consistent with a finding previously reported among VAH high-needs participants in the HF-ACT arm that has been discussed elsewhere [15].

It is notable that our observed average rate of ED use was high, at 4.2 visits per year. This is in contrast to a recent study of 1,189 homeless adults who were followed for 4 years in Toronto [33]. Those researchers measured average ED visits per year at ~2, and they defined high utilizers as 4.7 visits per year, which corresponded to the top 10 percentile. Interestingly, the average ED visits among these frequent ED users was 12.1 per person-year. Unlike other studies of homeless persons, our criteria for study inclusion stipulated that they had to have a mental disorder, and 71% were classified as having severe cluster of mental disorders, including psychosis, mood disorder with psychotic features, and hypomanic or manic episode. Furthermore, 70% of our sample had at least three or more chronic health conditions, which is similar to a study of frequent ED use (>4 visits per year) among homeless veterans within the Veterans Affair health care system that found an association between the high burden of chronic medical and psychiatric diagnoses and frequent ED use [37]. Many other studies report lower annual rates of ED use among persons who are homeless, and those who had ≥4 ED visits annually are defined as frequent users [22, 38, 39]. In contrast, D'Amore et al. recorded an average ED visit rate of 6.2 per homeless person per year at one ED in New York City. This sample was similar to ours, with a high prevalence of mental health disorders and substance use [40].

In this study, we found no significant interaction between substance dependence and HF vs. TAU intervention on ED visits and hospitalization. Few studies have examined the effect of HF interventions in homeless populations with substance dependence [23]. It is reasonable to suspect that outcomes of HF may differ among this subgroup from the general homeless population, and further investigation is warranted considering the high prevalence of addiction among chronically homeless and mentally ill adults [16, 41]. Edens et al. examined health service costs in a population of active substance users,

Table 3 Acute hospital admissions during the post randomization period among "At Home" participants (n = 381)

Variable	Hospital admissions (N)	Total person-years (PYs)	Hospitalization rate (per person, per year)
Overall	550	721.9	0.8
Housing First interventions	367	471.6	0.8
Treatment as usual	183	250.3	0.7
Substance dependence			
Yes	338	421.2	0.8
No	212	300.7	0.7
Daily substance use			
Yes	124	207.9	0.6
No	426	514.0	0.8
Need level			
High	366	420.2	0.9
Moderate	184	301.7	0.6
Male	390	518.8	0.8
Female	157	197.1	0.8
Aboriginals	79	116.2	0.7
White	299	389.9	0.8
Other	172	215.8	0.8
Incomplete high school	355	407.1	0.9
High school or higher	195	308.8	0.6
Single/never married	410	482.0	0.9
Other	138	234.0	0.6
Income ($800 CDN or more) in past month			
Yes	319	377.9	0.8
No	229	332.6	0.7
Less severe cluster of mental disorders			
Yes	227	381.0	0.6
No	323	340.9	1.0
Severe cluster of mental disorders			
Yes	465	516.0	0.9
No	85	205.9	0.4
Multiple mental disorders (≥3)			
Yes	118	167.8	0.7
No	432	554.1	0.8
Suicidality (high)			
Yes	106	129.1	0.8
No	444	592.8	0.8
Chronic health conditions (≥3)			
Yes	352	506.6	0.7
No	198	215.3	0.9
Blood-borne infectious disease (HIV, hepatitis B or C)			
Yes	167	231.8	0.7
No	383	486.2	0.8
Have a regular medical doctor			
Yes	324	484.0	0.7
No	226	236.0	1.0
Place to go when you are sick			
Yes	460	570.8	0.8
No	88	140.7	0.6

Table 3 continued

Variable	Hospital admissions (N)	Total person-years (PYs)	Hospitalization rate (per person, per year)
Needed health care, but didn't receive it			
Yes	198	299.5	0.7
No	335	406.1	0.8

Table 4 Negative binomial regression analysis to estimate the effect of substance dependence on ED visits during the post randomization period among "At Home" participants (n = 381)

Variable	Unadjusted RR (95% CI)	p value	Adjusted RR (95% CI)
Substance dependence (yes vs. no)	0.99 (0.73, 1.34)	0.953	0.85 (0.62, 1.17)
Housing First interventions (yes vs. no)	0.89 (0.65, 1.22)	0.468	0.74 (0.55, 1.00)
Need level (high vs. moderate)	1.37 (1.02, 1.86)	0.039	1.11 (0.79, 1.56)
Age at randomization (per year)	0.99 (0.98, 1.01)	0.265	1.00 (0.98, 1.02)
Age of first homelessness	1.00 (0.99, 1.01)	0.900	0.99 (0.97, 1.00)
Female gender	1.13 (0.81, 1.58)	0.459	1.03 (0.75, 1.70)
Aboriginals	1.94 (1.23, 3.05)	0.004	1.32 (0.95, 1.84)
White	1.60 (1.14, 2.24)	0.006	1.05 (0.65, 1.76)
Other	Reference		
Education (incomplete high school)	0.71 (0.53, 0.96)	0.027	0.78 (0.58, 1.05)
Single/never married	1.33 (0.97, 1.83)	0.080	
Income ($800 CDN or more) in past month	1.05 (0.78, 1.41)	0.762	
ER visit before randomization (last year)	1.12 (1.09, 1.15)	<0.001	1.11 (1.08, 1.14)
Less severe cluster of mental disorders	0.97 (0.72, 1.31)	0.861	0.98 (0.73, 1.32)
Severe cluster of mental disorders	1.28 (0.92, 1.78)	0.141	1.32 (0.91, 1.92)
Chronic health conditions (≥ 3)	1.56 (1.12, 2.16)	0.007	1.13 (0.79, 1.63)
Blood-borne infectious disease (HIV, hepatitis B or C)	0.93 (0.68, 1.29)	0.678	1.28 (0.92, 1.79)
Have a regular medical doctor	1.20 (0.87, 1.65)	0.264	1.06 (0.77, 1.46)
Place to go when you are sick	2.06 (1.41, 3.00)	<0.001	1.45 (1.01, 2.09)
Needed health care, but didn't receive it	1.36 (1.01, 1.84)	0.046	0.93 (0.69, 1.27)

and Larimer et al. analyzed overall costs (including jail, ED, inpatient and outpatient contacts, emergency medical service calls, and transports) in chronically homeless adults with severe alcohol addiction. Both studies involved a low-barrier housing intervention similar to HF, and both studies found a reduction in costs when participants were stably housed [24, 25]. Martinez examined placement in permanent supportive housing and found that stable housing significantly reduced the percentage of residents with an ED visit, the average number of ED visits per person, and the total number of ED visits among homeless adults with substance use and mental disorders [36]. Our results support this existing research showing that HF can be equally effective in persons with and without substance dependence in reducing ED visits.

Of note, hospital admissions in this study were associated with the severe cluster of mental disorders, which accounted for 48% of hospital admissions in the follow-up period. Contrary to general perception, disorders attributed to substance use accounted for a relatively small proportion of hospital admissions (15%). Substance dependence also was not a driver for ED visits. In a study of New York City hospital discharge data, Salit et al. reported that 80.6% of hospital admissions among homeless adults involved either a principal or secondary diagnosis of substance use or mental illness, but did not report what proportion of admissions were attributed to substance use and mental illness independently [12]. It also may be that these results reflect the high level of stigma towards substance users among health professionals [42].

Hospitalization among homeless adults in Toronto was also recently examined [43], and 921 hospitalizations were incurred during the 4-year follow-up, of which 548 (59.5%) were medical or surgical and 373 (40.5%) were psychiatric. We observed 550 hospital admissions during the 2-year follow-up period and found a higher average yearly hospital admission rate (medical, surgical, and psychiatric combined) of 0.72 vs. 0.26 in their study. This

Table 5 Negative binomial regression analysis to estimate the effect of substance dependence on acute hospital admissions during the post randomization period among "At Home" participants (n = 381)

Variable	Unadjusted RR (95% CI)	p value	Adjusted RR (95% CI)
Substance dependence (yes vs. no)	1.15 (0.81, 1.65)	0.433	1.21 (0.83, 1.77)
Housing first interventions (yes vs. no)	1.08 (0.75, 1.56)	0.682	0.65 (0.25, 1.72)
Need level (high vs. moderate)	1.42 (0.99, 2.03)	0.056	0.88 (0.58, 1.35)
Age at randomization (per year)	0.98 (0.97, 1.00)	0.044	0.99 (0.97, 1.01)
Age of first homelessness	1.00 (0.98, 1.01)	0.475	1.00 (0.98, 1.02)
Female gender	1.04 (0.70, 1.54)	0.844	1.05 (0.71, 1.55)
Aboriginals	0.83 (0.48, 1.44)	0.508	0.89 (0.51, 1.53)
White	0.97 (0.65, 1.45)	0.897	1.06 (0.73, 1.56)
Other	Reference		Reference
Education (incomplete high school)	1.35 (0.95, 1.93)	0.095	1.27 (0.88, 1.83)
Single/never married	1.42 (0.97, 2.08)	0.070	
Income ($800 CDN or more) in past month	1.23 (0.87, 1.75)	0.247	
Hospital admissions before randomization (last year)	1.34 (1.20, 1.50)	<0.001	1.33 (1.19, 1.49)
Less severe cluster of mental disorders	0.65 (0.46, 0.92)	0.015	0.76 (0.53, 1.10)
Severe cluster of mental disorders	2.12 (1.42, 3.17)	<0.001	1.76 (1.09, 2.86)
Chronic health conditions (≥3)	0.75 (0.51, 1.09)	0.127	0.99 (0.67, 1.46)
Blood-borne infectious disease (HIV, hepatitis B or C)	0.92 (0.63, 1.35)	0.682	
Have a regular medical doctor	0.70 (0.48, 1.01)	0.053	0.78 (0.54, 1.12)
Place to go when you are sick	1.28 (0.81, 2.01)	0.284	
Needed health care, but didn't receive it	0.81 (0.57, 1.16)	0.260	

is likely attributable to differences in the sample characteristics, where VAH had many more persons with severe mental disorders and did not include homeless families with children (who tend not to use as much health services). The Toronto researchers also found that a large proportion of the psychiatric admissions were for schizophrenia and other psychotic disorders and noted that some hospitalizations may be difficult to avoid [43].

These findings may be relevant to policymakers wishing to reduce health care expenditures among this population. Increasing availability and access to mental health services may reduce costly acute health service use more so than targeting substance dependence alone. One tertiary intervention that included a residential treatment program for persons with severe substance dependence and concurrent mental illness (of whom half were homeless at intake) found a reduction in substance use and psychopathology symptoms among those who completed the follow-up assessment at 6 months [44].

Several limitations should be considered when interpreting our results. The HF-CONG location was a few blocks away from a hospital, which may have influenced the frequency of ED use. It should be noted that given the high burden of mental disorders and chronic health conditions in this population, the provision of regular care

may have identified the need for ED and hospital admissions, and the use of such services may have been appropriate. We would expect the use of these health services to decline with longer time in HF. We did not examine the effect of substance dependence within each HF intervention arm on ED visits and hospitalizations, given that the interaction term of substance dependence by HF was nonsignificant. Participants may also have been inclined to under-report substance use due to stigma and/or the fear of losing their housing/services. Access to administrative data provided a more accurate portrayal of health service use than self-reported measures; however, our analyses were based on incomplete data from the VAH study sample because some participants did not provide consent to access data, could not be linked to the database, or had less than 1 year of follow-up. Further, we were able to acquire data on ED visits and hospital admissions from six urban hospitals, but may have missed visits to other hospitals in British Columbia or outside of the province. Finally, the effect sizes observed in our multivariable analyses were generally small.

This study contributes to the body of evidence examining HF interventions in a homeless population with high rates of substance use and mental disorders, an area in which research is lacking. We analyzed data collected from an RCT as a longitudinal cohort with controls. This is an improvement on much of the previous research that has been based on cross-sectional or observational designs without controls. We were also able to achieve exceptionally high rates of follow-up among our participants.

Conclusions

We found no significant association between substance dependence and health service use in the form of ED visits and hospital admissions. Hospital admissions in the VAH cohort were mainly associated with severe mental disorder diagnoses rather than substance use disorders, suggesting that exploring interventions to better optimize management of these categories of mental disorders may be key to reducing hospitalization, but may prove to be challenging among persons who are homeless with concurrent disorders. It is likely that any such intervention will need to be comprehensive and integrate both housing and social support in the long term.

Abbreviations

HF: Housing First; ED: emergency department; VAH: Vancouver At Home; ACT: assertive community treatment; ICM: intensive case management; CONG: congregate; AU: treatment as usual.

Authors' contributions

AC and AP made substantial contributions to study conception and design and the interpretation of data; MP made substantial contributions to the acquisition and interpretation of data; AM made substantial contributions to the analyses and interpretation of data; JS, JF, and MK made substantial contributions to the analyses and interpretation of data. All authors were involved in drafting the manuscript or revising it critically for important intellectual content; gave final approval of the version to be published; and agreed to be accountable for all aspects of the work in ensuring that questions related to the accuracy or integrity of any part of the work were appropriately investigated and resolved. All authors read and approved the final manuscript.

Author details

[1] Department of Medicine, Centre for Health Evaluation and Outcome Sciences, University of British Columbia, 588B-1081 Burrard Street, Vancouver, BC V6Z 1Y6, Canada. [2] Faculty of Health Sciences, Simon Fraser University, Vancouver, Canada. [3] School of Population and Public Health, Vancouver, Canada. [4] Department of Psychiatry, University of British Columbia, Vancouver, Canada.

Acknowledgements

This research was supported by a Grant to Simon Fraser University, made possible through a financial contribution from Health Canada to the Mental Health Commission of Canada. The authors gratefully acknowledge the study participants and the support of colleagues and collaborators on this project. An abstract of these results was presented at the International Conference on Urban Health, March 6, 2014, in Manchester, England.

Compliance with ethical guidelines

Competing interests

The authors declare that they have no competing interests.

Appendix

See Table 6.

Table 6 Correlation between baseline substance dependence and daily substance use at each follow-up visit in the eligible sample (n = 381)

	All N (%)	SD-No N (%)	SD-Yes N (%)	p value
Daily substance use at baseline (n = 379)[a]	110 (29)	27 (17)	83 (37)	<0.001
Daily substance use at 6-month visit (n = 346)	93 (27)	24 (17)	69 (34)	<0.001
Daily substance use at 12-month visit (n = 357)	106 (30)	23 (16)	83 (39)	<0.001
Daily substance use at 18-month visit (n = 341)	89 (26)	24 (17)	65 (32)	0.003
Daily substance use at 24-month visit (n = 319)	75 (23)	21 (16)	54 (28)	0.014

[a] Participants with valid response to the questions related to daily substance use at each follow-up visit are presented in the parentheses. The remaining participants had either declined response or did not complete the interview.

References

1. Goering P, Tolomiczenko G, Sheldon T, Boydell K, Wasylenki D (2002) Characteristics of persons who are homeless for the first time. Psychiatr Serv 53(11):1472–1474
2. Palepu A, Patterson M, Strehlau V, Moniruzzamen A, Tan de Bibiana J, Frankish J et al (2013) Daily substance use and mental health symptoms among a cohort of homeless adults in Vancouver, British Columbia. J Urban Health 90(4):740–746
3. Madianos MG, Chondraki P, Papadimitriou GN (2013) Prevalence of psychiatric disorders among homeless people in Athens area: a cross-sectional study. Soc Psychiatry Psychiatr Epidemiol 48(8):1225–1234
4. Fazel S, Khosla V, Doll H, Geddes J (2008) The prevalence of mental disorders among the homeless in western countries: systematic review and meta-regression analysis. PLoS Med 5(12):e225
5. Vila-Rodriguez F, Panenka WJ, Lang DJ, Thornton AE, Vertinsky T, Wong H et al (2013) The hotel study: multimorbidity in a community sample living in marginal housing. Am J Psychiatry 170(12):1413–1422
6. Chartier M, Carrico AW, Weiser SD, Kushel MB, Riley ED (2012) Specific psychiatric correlates of acute care utilization among unstably housed HIV-positive adults. AIDS Care 24(12):1514–1518
7. Culhane DP, Metraux S, Hadley T (2002) Public service reductions associated with placement of homeless persons with severe mental illness in supportive housing. Hous Policy Debate 13:107–162
8. Kim TW, Kertesz SG, Horton NJ, Tibbetts N, Samet JH (2006) Episodic homelessness and health care utilization in a prospective cohort of HIV-infected persons with alcohol problems. BMC Health Serv Res 6:19
9. Kushel MB, Vittinghoff E, Haas JS (2001) Factors associated with the health care utilization of homeless persons. JAMA 285(2):200–206
10. Kushel MB, Perry S, Bangsberg D, Clark R, Moss AR (2002) Emergency department use among the homeless and marginally housed: results from a community-based study. Am J Public Health 92(5):778–784
11. Tsai J, Doran KM, Rosenheck RA (2013) When health insurance is not a factor: national comparison of homeless and nonhomeless US veterans who use Veterans Affairs Emergency Departments. Am J Public Health 103(Suppl 2):S225–S231
12. Salit SA, Kuhn EM, Hartz AJ, Vu JM, Mosso AL (1998) Hospitalization costs associated with homelessness in New York City. N Engl J Med 338(24):1734–1740
13. Goering PN, Streiner DL, Adair C, Aubry T, Barker J, Distasio J et al (2011) The At Home/Chez Soi trial protocol: a pragmatic, multi-site, randomised controlled trial of a Housing First intervention for homeless individuals with mental illness in five Canadian cities. BMJ Open 1(2):e000323

14. Somers JM, Patterson ML, Moniruzzaman A, Currie L, Rezansoff SN, Palepu A et al (2013) Vancouver At Home: pragmatic randomized trials investigating Housing First for homeless and mentally ill adults. Trials 14:365

15. Russolillo A, Patterson M, McCandless L, Moniruzzaman A, Somers J (2014) Emergency department utilisation among formerly homeless adults with mental disorders after one year of Housing First interventions: a randomised controlled trial. Int J Hous Policy 14(1):79–97

16. Palepu A, Patterson ML, Moniruzzaman A, Frankish CJ, Somers J (2013) Housing first improves residential stability in homeless adults with concurrent substance dependence and mental disorders. Am J Public Health 103(Suppl 2):e30–e36

17. Tsemberis S, Gulcur L, Nakae M (2004) Housing First, consumer choice, and harm reduction for homeless individuals with a dual diagnosis. Am J Public Health 94(4):651–656

18. Tsai J, Mares AS, Rosenheck RA (2010) A multi-site comparison of supported housing for chronically homeless adults: "Housing first" versus "residential treatment first". Psychol Serv 7(4):219–232

19. Sadowski LS, Kee RA, VanderWeele TJ, Buchanan D (2009) Effect of a housing and case management program on emergency department visits and hospitalizations among chronically ill homeless adults: a randomized trial. JAMA 301(17):1771–1778

20. Srebnik D, Connor T, Sylla L (2013) A pilot study of the impact of housing first-supported housing for intensive users of medical hospitalization and sobering services. Am J Public Health 103(2):316–321

21. Hwang SW, Gogosis E, Chambers C, Dunn JR, Hoch JS, Aubry T (2011) Health status, quality of life, residential stability, substance use, and health care utilization among adults applying to a supportive housing program. J Urban Health 88(6):1076–1090

22. Kessell ER, Bhatia R, Bamberger JD, Kushel MB (2006) Public health care utilization in a cohort of homeless adult applicants to a supportive housing program. J Urban Health 83(5):860–873

23. Kertesz SG, Crouch K, Milby JB, Cusimano RE, Schumacher JE (2009) Housing first for homeless persons with active addiction: are we overreaching? Milbank Q 87(2):495–534

24. Larimer ME, Malone DK, Garner MD, Atkins DC, Burlingham B, Lonczak HS et al (2009) Health care and public service use and costs before and after provision of housing for chronically homeless persons with severe alcohol problems. JAMA 301(13):1349–1357

25. Edens EL, Mares AS, Rosenheck RA (2011) Chronically homeless women report high rates of substance use problems equivalent to chronically homeless men. Womens Health Issues 21(5):383–389

26. Sheehan DV, Lecrubier Y, Sheehan KH, Amorim P, Janavs J, Weiller E et al (1998) The Mini-International Neuropsychiatric Interview (M.I.N.I.): the development and validation of a structured diagnostic psychiatric interview for DSM-IV and ICD-10. J Clin Psychiatry 59(Suppl 20):22–33 (quiz 34–57)

27. Barker S, Barron N, McFarland BH, Bigelow DA, Carnahan T (1994) A community ability scale for chronically mentally ill consumers: part II. Applications. Commun Ment Health J 30(5):459–472

28. Marsden J, Gossop M, Stewart D, Best D, Farrell M, Lehmann P et al (1998) The Maudsley Addiction Profile (MAP): a brief instrument for assessing treatment outcome. Addiction 93(12):1857–1867

29. Shern DL, Wilson NZ, Coen AS, Patrick DC, Foster M, Bartsch DA et al (1994) Client outcomes II: longitudinal client data from the Colorado treatment outcome study. Milbank Q 72(1):123–148

30. Conrad KJ, Yagelka JR, Matters MD, Rich AR, Williams V, Buchanan M (2001) Reliability and validity of a modified Colorado Symptom Index in a national homeless sample. Ment Health Serv Res 3(3):141–153

31. Canadian Community Health Survey (2010) http://www23.statcan.gc.ca/imdb/p2SV.pl?Function=getSurvey&SurvId=3226&SurvVer=1&InstaId=15282&InstaVer=7&SDDS=3226&lang=en&db=imdb&adm=8&dis=2. Accessed 15 May 2015

32. National Population Health Survey, Canada (1998–1999) http://www23.statcan.gc.ca/imdb/p2SV.pl?Function=getSurvey&SDDS=5004&lang=en&db=imdb&adm=8&dis=2. Accessed 15 May 15 2015

33. Chambers C, Chiu S, Katic M, Kiss A, Redelmeier DA, Levinson W et al (2013) High utilizers of emergency health services in a population-based cohort of homeless adults. Am J Public Health 103(Suppl 2):S302–S310

34. Hwang SW, Chambers C, Chiu S, Katic M, Kiss A, Redelmeier DA et al (2013) A comprehensive assessment of health care utilization among homeless adults under a system of universal health insurance. Am J Public Health 103(Suppl 2):S294–S301

35. Thakarar K, Morgan JR, Gaeta JM, Hohl C, Drainoni ML (2015) Predictors of frequent emergency room visits among a homeless population. PLoS One 10(4):e0124552

36. Martinez TE, Burt MR (2006) Impact of permanent supportive housing on the use of acute care health services by homeless adults. Psychiatr Serv 57(7):992–999

37. Tsai J, Rosenheck RA (2013) Risk factors for ED use among homeless veterans. Am J Emerg Med 31(5):855–858

38. Ku BS, Scott KC, Kertesz SG, Pitts SR (2010) Factors associated with use of urban emergency departments by the U.S. homeless population. Public Health Rep 125(3):398–405

39. Mandelberg JH, Kuhn RE, Kohn MA (2000) Epidemiologic analysis of an urban, public emergency department's frequent users. Acad Emerg Med 7(6):637–646

40. D'Amore J, Hung O, Chiang W, Goldfrank L (2001) The epidemiology of the homeless population and its impact on an urban emergency department. Acad Emerg Med 8(11):1051–1055

41. Glasser I, Zywiak WH (2003) Homelessness and substance misuse: a tale of two cities. Subst Use Misuse 38(3–6):551–576

42. van Boekel LC, Brouwers EP, van Weeghel J, Garretsen HF (2013) Stigma among health professionals towards patients with substance use disorders and its consequences for healthcare delivery: systematic review. Drug Alcohol Depend 131(1–2):23–35

43. Chambers C, Katic M, Chiu S, Redelmeier DA, Levinson W, Kiss A et al (2013) Predictors of medical or surgical and psychiatric hospitalizations among a population-based cohort of homeless adults. Am J Public Health 103(Suppl 2):S380–S388

44. Schutz C, Linden IA, Torchalla I, Li K, Al-Desouki M, Krausz M (2013) The Burnaby treatment center for mental health and addiction, a novel integrated treatment program for patients with addiction and concurrent disorders: results from a program evaluation. BMC Health Serv Res 13:288

8

VA residential substance use disorder treatment program providers' perceptions of facilitators and barriers to performance on pre-admission processes

Laura S. Ellerbe[1], Luisa Manfredi[1*], Shalini Gupta[1], Tyler E. Phelps[1], Thomas R. Bowe[1], Anna D. Rubinsky[2], Jennifer L. Burden[3] and Alex H. S. Harris[1]

Abstract

Background: In the U.S. Department of Veterans Affairs (VA), residential treatment programs are an important part of the continuum of care for patients with a substance use disorder (SUD). However, a limited number of program-specific measures to identify quality gaps in SUD residential programs exist. This study aimed to: (1) Develop metrics for two pre-admission processes: *Wait Time* and *Engagement While Waiting*, and (2) Interview program management and staff about program structures and processes that may contribute to performance on these metrics. The first aim sought to supplement the VA's existing facility-level performance metrics with SUD program-level metrics in order to identify high-value targets for quality improvement. The second aim recognized that not all key processes are reflected in the administrative data, and even when they are, new insight may be gained from viewing these data in the context of day-to-day clinical practice.

Methods: VA administrative data from fiscal year 2012 were used to calculate pre-admission metrics for 97 programs (63 SUD Residential Rehabilitation Treatment Programs (SUD RRTPs); 34 Mental Health Residential Rehabilitation Treatment Programs (MH RRTPs) with a SUD track). Interviews were then conducted with management and front-line staff to learn what factors may have contributed to high or low performance, relative to the national average for their program type. We hypothesized that speaking directly to residential program staff may reveal innovative practices, areas for improvement, and factors that may explain system-wide variability in performance.

Results: Average wait time for admission was 16 days (SUD RRTPs: 17 days; MH RRTPs with a SUD track: 11 days), with 60% of Veterans waiting longer than 7 days. For these Veterans, engagement while waiting occurred in an average of 54% of the waiting weeks (range 3–100% across programs). Fifty-nine interviews representing 44 programs revealed factors perceived to potentially impact performance in these domains. Efficient screening processes, effective patient flow, and available beds were perceived to facilitate shorter wait times, while lack of beds, poor staffing levels, and lengths of stay of existing patients were thought to lengthen wait times. Accessible outpatient services, strong patient outreach, and strong encouragement of pre-admission outpatient treatment emerged as facilitators of engagement while waiting; poor staffing levels, socioeconomic barriers, and low patient motivation were viewed as barriers.

Conclusions: Metrics for pre-admission processes can be helpful for monitoring residential SUD treatment programs. Interviewing program management and staff about drivers of performance metrics can play a complementary role by

---

*Correspondence: Luisa.Manfredi@va.gov
[1] Center for Innovation to Implementation, Department of Veterans Affairs (VA) Palo Alto Health Care System, 795 Willow Road (MPD-152), Menlo Park, CA 94025, USA
Full list of author information is available at the end of the article

identifying innovative and other strong practices, as well as high-value targets for quality improvement. Key facilitators of high-performing facilities may offer programs with lower performance useful strategies to improve specific pre-admission processes.

Keywords: Substance use disorders, Residential treatment, Standards of care, Quality measurement, Quality improvement

Background

In the United States Department of Veterans Affairs (VA), residential rehabilitation treatment programs are an integral part of the continuum of care for patients with a mental health or substance use disorder (SUD) [1]. Research on the effectiveness of residential treatment for substance use disorders is mixed but overall suggests that it fills a particular niche and is a valuable option for some types of patients [2]. Veterans with SUD who need specialized, 24/7 structure and support may seek treatment in one of the VA's 63 SUD Residential Rehabilitation Treatment Programs (SUD RRTPs) or 34 Mental Health Residential Rehabilitation Treatment Programs (MH RRTPs) with a SUD track. Each of the 97 programs offers recovery-oriented, patient-centered care, including evidence-based individual, and group psychotherapy and pharmacotherapy, to address SUD, co-occurring mental health conditions and other severe psychosocial concerns such as homelessness and unemployment.

Despite their place in the continuum of care, residential programs are resource-intensive and costly, with associated health care costs (including indirect costs) estimated to be roughly $210 million for VA in FY 2014, posing a fiscal challenge for a capitated healthcare system with competing demands [3]. Patient demand for SUD RRTPs, in particular, has increased steadily, with a 10.7% increase in admissions from FY 2012 to FY 2014 [4].

In order to reduce undesirable variability in quality of care across VA residential SUD treatment programs, core standards and practices for these programs have been codified in two VA handbooks, the Uniform Mental Health Services Handbook (revised in 2008) and the MH RRTP Handbook (published in 2010) [1, 5]. These handbooks outline requirements to ensure that Veterans have access to comprehensive, evidence-based SUD and other mental health services. For example, all residential programs are required to provide or arrange pre-admission treatment and case management to Veterans waiting for admission [1, 5].

VA Mental Health Services and the VA Office of Mental Health Operations have made adhering to these standard requirements for care delivery, managing costs, and improving outcomes their highest priority. Recognizing the need for a mechanism to routinely monitor the performance of all mental health services, including those provided in residential treatment programs, the Office of Mental Health Operations developed the Mental Health Information System (MHIS) [6]. The MHIS is an informatics dashboard comprised of dozens of metrics, including 15 metrics assessing access to and the quality of SUD treatment. However, only two metrics focus specifically on *residential* SUD treatment: (a) an access measure—the proportion of patients with a SUD diagnosis that receive care in a residential SUD treatment program, and (b) average length of stay in a residential SUD treatment program among patients admitted. While these measures are useful, VA would benefit from a comprehensive suite of measures to monitor other important structures, processes and outcomes of residential SUD treatment programs.

Therefore, we sought to develop metrics using electronic health records data for VA residential SUD treatment programs in three key domains: pre-admission (e.g., wait time, engagement while waiting), in-treatment (e.g., use of addiction pharmacotherapy), and post-discharge (e.g., outpatient SUD follow-up, readmission, subsequent detoxification episodes). After calculating the metrics for all programs, we interviewed residential SUD treatment program management and front-line staff. This enabled us to validate that the metric data corresponded with their day-to-day experience, and to learn their impressions regarding the facilitators and/or challenges that may have impacted their program's performance on metrics for which the program was substantially higher or lower than the VA national average. In this paper, we focus on the *Pre-Admission* domain and the corresponding qualitative data which describe factors that may explain observed variability, in order to learn about potential innovative practices, and identify possible areas for improvement.

Methods
Study population
National data collected by the VA Northeast Program Evaluation Center (NEPEC) were used to identify 97 VA residential SUD treatment programs (63 SUD RRTPs; 34 MH RRTPs with a SUD track). Patients receiving treatment from these programs were then located in VA electronic health records data using combinations of station and specialty treatment (bed section) codes.

Developing and calculating metrics

Quality measures prioritized for metric development were chosen in collaboration with our operational partners in VA Mental Health Services (MHS) and the Office of Mental Health Operations (OMHO). The selected metrics include SUD-specific versions of other Mental Health Information System (MHIS) metrics, and processes of care emphasized in program evaluation reports [e.g., OIG (Department of Veterans Affairs (VA) Office of the Inspector General (OIG)), 2009 and 2011] [7, 8]. These new metrics capture critical aspects of pre-admission processes, in-treatment processes and practices, and post-discharge follow-up.

Two *pre-admission* processes are the focus of this paper—wait time (two metrics) and engagement while waiting for admission (three metrics). Descriptions of how these metrics were operationalized are presented in Table 1. If the percent of admissions with a pre-admissions screening visit was less than 25% for a program then wait time and engagement metrics were not calculated since the screening visit (stop code 596) marked the start of the clock for those metrics. Since these wait time and engagement while waiting data metrics rely on the use of the 596 stop code, non-use or low use of the code would render it difficult or impossible to calculate and meaningfully interpret a program's performance. While 25% is admittedly arbitrary, the threshold was chosen with consultation from our operational partners. For programs without valid metric data, participants were interviewed about factors that impacted their program's low screening rates, as well as typical wait time and engagement while waiting.

Metrics data from FY 2012 were linked to the VA Program Evaluation and Resource Center's FY 2012 *Drug and Alcohol Program Survey* (*DAPS*) and NEPEC's *MH RRTP Annual Survey* for FY 2012 to create individualized program profile reports. Each report summarized the program's performance on the *Pre-Admission* metrics compared to the national average for similar VA residential SUD treatment programs (i.e., SUD RRTPs or MH RRTPs with a SUD track). See Table 1. The research team then reviewed each report in order to highlight metrics in which the program was a high or low performer compared to the national average and in reference to program-level distributions. This information was used to tailor specific questions in the interview protocol.

Study population and recruitment

Program managers from the 97 programs were identified using *DAPS* and NEPEC databases and invited to participate in a telephone interview to discuss their program. First, a flyer describing the study was e-mailed to potential participants. If no response was received, a follow-up e-mail was sent a week later which featured select performance data for their program, highlighting both an area of success and an area for improvement (if applicable). A week later, a follow-up telephone call was made to the potential participant to answer any questions about the study. If the point-of-contact could not be reached, a telephone message was left and a subsequent follow-up call was made. To supplement initial recruitment efforts, research staff announced the study on VA-wide SUD representative calls and sent the recruitment flyer to several national VA e-mail groups. At scheduled telephone interviews, participants provided informed consent and were asked permission for interviews to be audiotaped. If the person declined to be audiotaped, then notes were taken. At the end of the interview, participants were asked to recommend front-line staff from their program who might be interested in participating in the study to provide additional perspectives. Interviews were conducted from March 2014 to August 2014. The study protocol was approved by the Stanford University Institutional Review Board.

Interview content

The interview guide was developed by an interdisciplinary project team with input and feedback from our VA operational partners. It consisted of reviewing a "snapshot" of the program (e.g., occupancy rate), followed by questions about the program's clinical processes (e.g., screening) and metric performance within the pre-admission, in-treatment, and post-discharge domains. We used a unique data collection technique which combined a semi-structured telephone interview (60–75 min) with Microsoft Lync computer screen-sharing. This method allowed the interviewer to walk the participant, point by point, through the individualized profile report that included their program's performance relative to the national average for each metric. Participants were asked if the metric data seemed realistic given their knowledge of the program, and what factors may have contributed to their program's high or low performance on specific metrics. For example, high performers were asked if there is anything they would like to share with other programs on how they achieved success on the metric, whereas low performers were asked if there were barriers and/or resource needs that impacted their performance.

Qualitative analysis

The interviews were transcribed, cleaned for quality control, and imported into the qualitative data analysis software, ATLAS.ti (Version 7.5.7) [9]. A coding scheme that utilized typical coding techniques for qualitative data [10] was developed to identify common facilitators and barriers described by the participants. The coding scheme included 11 primary codes corresponding to

Table 1 Pre-admission metric definitions and national averages for SUD RRTPs and MH RRTPs with a SUD track

Metric	Definition	SUD RRTPs* Data (SD)	MH RRTPs with a SUD track* Data (SD)
Wait time			
Mean days from screen to admission (based on patient-level wait times from 42 SUD RRTPs and 19 MH RRTPs with a SUD track)	Time (days) between screen and admission, averaged at the program level, for Veterans screened with a 596 stop code** and admitted to a residential SUD treatment program	17 days (35.46)	11 days (34.49)
Percent of admissions with >7 day wait (for SUD RRTPs, based on 1047 out of 4550 Veterans, and for MH RRTPs with a SUD track, based on 676 out of 1780 Veterans)	Percent of Veterans admitted to a residential SUD treatment program who waited >7 days after screening to enter the program	23%	38%
Engagement while waiting			
Percent of weeks with any outpatient SUD or MH contact (based on patient-level number of waiting weeks)	Among Veterans who waited >7 days between screening and admission to residential SUD treatment, percent of weeks while waiting in which Veterans received at least one outpatient SUD or MH contact	55% (.336)	47% (.389)
Percent of weeks with any outpatient SUD contact only (based on patient-level number of waiting weeks)	Among Veterans who waited >7 days between screening and admission, percent of weeks while waiting in which Veterans received at least one outpatient SUD contact	39% (.355)	24% (.343)
Percent of weeks with any outpatient MH contact only (based on patient-level number of waiting weeks)	Among Veterans who waited >7 days between screening and admission, percent of weeks while waiting in which Veterans received at least one outpatient MH contact	31% (.31)	35% (.34)

Data are from fiscal year (FY) 2012

SUD substance use disorder, *RRTP* Residential Rehabilitation Treatment Program, *MH* mental health, *SD* standard deviation

* Includes programs with less than 10 admissions

** The 596 clinic stop code was activated in FY 2009 and indicates RRTP Admission Screening Services. Per the VHA Handbook 1162.02, this code must be used to document a screening for residential treatment. Any outpatient SUD or MH contact is defined in this paper as any SUD or MH outpatient care (e.g., psychotherapy, group or individual therapy, case management, or phone contact)

the sections of the interview (e.g., Pre-admission) and two thematic codes (facilitator, barrier). Then, the lead qualitative analyst (LSE) coded each interview according to the 11 primary codes and their section subcodes (e.g., Pre-admission wait time). Next, the lead analyst and two other qualitative analysts (TEP and LM) separately coded quotes in the Pre-admission section based on the thematic codes. The two sets of coded interviews were then merged and queries run separately in ATLAS. ti to extract facilitators and barriers for each pre-admission metric. Lastly, qualitative analysts reviewed the output, *individually* developed lists of barrier themes and facilitator themes, and met to resolve discrepancies and jointly arrive at a consensus of the major facilitator themes, major barrier themes, and their illustrative text components.

Results

The total number of admissions in FY12 for all programs combined was 14,281 (10,425 admissions to SUD RRTPs; 3856 admissions to MH RRTPs with a SUD track). Among all programs combined, there were 6330 patients with a pre-admission screening (4550 patients in SUD RRTPs; 1780 patients in MH RRTPs with a SUD track). The wait time and engagement while waiting metrics were not calculated if the percentage of patients with a pre-admission screening visit was less than 25%. Roughly a third of the programs (36 out of 97), failed to meet this threshold and, therefore are not included in the summary statistics presented here. In 27 programs, less than 25% of patients had a pre-admission screening visit. For 9 programs, there were no pre-admission screening data.

Program performance for wait time and engagement while waiting

During FY 2012, the average number of days that a Veteran waited from pre-admission screening to admission into a residential SUD treatment program ("average wait time") was 17 days for SUD RRTPs (see Table 1), 11 days for MH RRTPs with a SUD track (see Table 1), and 16 days for all programs combined. A total of 60% of Veterans in all programs waited longer than 7 days to be admitted. These Veterans had at least one SUD or mental health contact outpatient encounter during 54% of the weeks while they were waiting (SUD RRTPs: 55%; MH RRTPs with a SUD track: 47%). SUD or mental health contact was defined as psychotherapy, group or individual therapy, case management, or phone contact in a SUD or MH clinic.

Variation in program performance

Program performance on the pre-admission metrics varied greatly: 0–100% of patients waited longer than 7 days to be admitted, and weeks waiting with at least one SUD or mental health contact (i.e., SUD or mental health outpatient encounter/appointment) ranged from 0 to 100% (0–100% SUD contact only, and 0–94% mental health contact only).

Interview response rate

A total of 59 interviews were conducted, representing 63 participants (36 female; 27 male) from 44 unique treatment programs (35 SUD RRTPs and 9 MH RRTPs with a SUD track; facility-level response rate of 45%). The interviewees were from 17 of the 21 VA networks and included four joint interviews (i.e., two program staff interviewed together). The majority of providers either had some type of social work degree (40%) or a PhD (35%). MDs and some type of nursing degree each comprised 5%. Program management comprised 37 providers (20 female; 17 male). Similar to the overall providers interviewed, the majority of program management either had some type of social work degree (41%) or a PhD (41%). Four participants declined to be audio-taped but agreed that notes could be taken during the interview. In these cases, an electronic copy of the notes was then uploaded into ATLAS.ti.

Wait time facilitators

Participants at 11 programs with high performance on either of the two *Wait Time* metrics were asked if they had advice for other programs that may struggle with longer wait times. In response, program staff described process and structural factors that may have contributed to shorter wait times. Several interrelated key facilitators were identified and are described below, with supporting quotations listed in Table 2.

Wait time facilitator 1: efficient screening processes

Many participants described ways in which they optimized efficiency in their screening and assessment processes, which in turn may have contributed to shorter wait times for Veterans waiting to enter the program. Among the strategies employed by programs were (a) keeping the number of assessments or screening appointments per patient to a minimum, and (b) flexibility in scheduling screening appointments or other processes to accommodate more timely screenings.

Wait time facilitator 2: effective patient flow

The residential treatment program process includes waiting for admission, going through the process of being admitted, working through the components of the program, and the discharge process. In some cases, these processes overlap. Effectively managing patient flow, whether at an individual, team, or facility level, appeared to be

Table 2 Interview participants' perceptions of key facilitators of pre-admission metric performance

Metric	Facilitator	Supporting quotations
I. Wait time	1. Efficient screening processes	"…we don't schedule face-to-face screens. So there's no time in between like when we get the consult and then we close the consult, we're not setting up another additional evaluation meeting with the Veteran that they have to come here which would potentially delay their admission, as far as I know." "So as we get referrals throughout the day—whether it's 9:00 or 2 p.m.—we'll get the referral and we'll do the screening that day. Prior to the Lean Thinking initiative, we would have one time a day where we would meet at like 11 a.m. But if you get the referral at noon then you gotta wait all the way till 11 a.m. the next day."
	2. Effective patient flow	"We meet daily for a staffing meeting for 15 minutes to decide, to talk about who's coming, who's going, what the plan for the people who are here are, how people are doing in treatment, and that's when we discuss who's on the list and how we can get them in." "…one of the things that we did was add a fourth day and open up the possibility of doing two admissions on 1 day when our census is low. So we're trying to be a little bit more flexible, a little more accommodating and we've also sort of decreased the requirements for being admitted to the program. So we used to have a hard line that they had to have a TB test, for example, prior to admission. Now we can do a test on the day of admission and if they have symptoms, isolate them…"
	3. Available beds	"Okay, we actually had about 120 beds for the Domiciliary which makes us a very large Domiciliary. And that's a good size for the community and what our needs are. And so generally, it was a fairly short period of time that someone needed to wait to come in." "And then what's great about the SA side is that it's a 45-day program so we can turn around beds a little bit easier."
II. Engagement while waiting	1. Accessible outpatient services	"…we open all of our groups up to anybody that is interested in participating. We try to individualize that care to the Veteran. So we will let them look at our group schedule and if there's one or two groups that they can make during the week then we go ahead and invite them in until they get into the inpatient part of the program…And they have some evening groups too that are available like 3 days a week, I believe, 4 days a week, which I think helps." "There may be a wait to get into a residential bed, but we'll get you screened quickly and what we do in the interim then if we don't have a residential bed available, we have an early recovery group, we have individual options for some people and sometimes we'll even have them do a little bit of our IOP program until a bed opens. So they should be getting services pretty quickly."
	2. Strong patient outreach	"And we work really hard at calling them if they don't show up and just really an intensive outreach process. I think because it seems the nature of the population is that they easily disappear, so we work really hard to try not to let that happen."
	3. Strong encouragement of pre-admission outpatient treatment	"So, anyone on the list, we tell them if you're coming to outpatient, you're staying involved and we can see that you're maintaining and motivated and someone doesn't show, well, we're going to come to outpatient and say, 'Hey somebody didn't show' or 'Someone left AMA.' And so, it gives you a better chance of getting into the program quicker and the fact that we're all on the same floor, I think that, you know, they can check in with us on a daily basis even if they want to." "Well, I think that one of the things is that we tell people it's an expectation. So, when we screen them, and say our wait is like two and a half weeks at this point or something, we tell them a couple of things, that we're really requiring you to do outpatient unless there's really some legitimate reason, like you live too far away or whatever, to not come." "But when the patients are screened, they automatically are enrolled or scheduled for, number one, a pre-treatment group that we call "Preparation Group," that meets twice a week and that's done in the outpatient clinic."

integral in efforts at keeping program wait times below the national average. Key facilitators included: (a) regularly-scheduled meetings to review patient status to make sure they are not unnecessarily stalled between processes and (b) flexible admissions processes and requirements.

Wait time facilitator 3: available beds

The availability of beds was another factor that was commonly attributed to lower wait times. How long a Veteran waits to enter the program may be reflected, in part by the sheer number of beds that a residential treatment program has available at any given time. Several

participants described how their program's high capacity may have positively influenced their program's performance on the wait time metrics.

Wait time barriers

Participants at 14 programs with low performance on either of the two *Wait Time* metrics reported the following reasons and challenges. See Table 3.

Wait time barrier 1: lack of beds

Many participants indicated that the lack of available beds impacted how long Veterans waited to enter their

Table 3 Interview participants' perceptions of key barriers affecting pre-admission metric performance

Metric	Barrier	Supporting quotations
I. Wait time	1. Lack of beds	"Well, we only have 20 beds and we're serving four hospitals…We have 20 beds for a lot of people." "…there were two medical centers in the X area up until 2011…Basically the substance abuse program was consolidated here at the X Hospital in X. So prior to that, the SUD program was actually out at a separate VA medical center and we had more beds there and little to no waitlist. So ever since the move here and the consolidation, we actually lost a significant number of beds and ever since then basically wait time has been an ongoing issue."
	2. Poor staffing levels	"…we had only one psychiatrist who was doing the work so we had to keep our census at half…" "We were pretty well staffed and then we had a kind of an exodus of social workers and all at once. Then we had to rehire, and that took a long time. And then at that same time, we just kept getting more and more referrals, more and more applications."
	3. Length of stay	"The other side of it could be that our length of stay is too long. We are working on that and have revamped our program to have an eight-week option, as well as a longer option. So, we're trying to address that part of it." "In addition to a variable length of stay for folks, I mean, one of the things that we struggled with was if people needed more time than we're able to extend them; if we extend them, it creates a longer wait for people on that admissions list."
II. Engagement while waiting	1. Poor staffing levels	"I think even adding the X CBOCs, there's 12 of them up north; only this month have they gotten CBT SUD groups in all the rural areas. So, you can imagine our continuity of care fallouts because they were sending guys out, you know, to the boondocks with no SUD providers available even by CBT." "A lot of our people would be seeing people in CBOCs, and I would very much doubt if those people are stop coding, you know, for SUD. We have a single social worker or whatever trying to cope. And then in this medical center, our SUD is way understaffed. So, they don't give a lot of outpatient contact to anybody. So, it's very hard to get in." "We've talked about having a waiting for treatment group. But that has been something that staffing-wise we have not been able to pull off."
	2. Socioeconomic barriers	"Well, right now, out in one of the X CBOCs, the bus station is actually like five or six miles away, the closest bus stop to the CBOC. So, you couldn't even take a bus to get to the CBOCs…" "I think for a lot of these people who are more indigent, or they don't have cars. Or, if they even have cars, they might not have what they call gas money to get to the place. I think they tend to no-show a lot, or they don't' have a way of getting in to treatment."
	3. Low patient motivation	"Sometimes it's motivation as well. I mean sometimes they're using hard, they're drinking hard or whatever. They're just not that motivated to get up and come into a weekly group. They'll show up for their admission appointment because at that point they're like 'Okay I'm ready to dry out and get serious.' But up until that point, they're continuing to party and use." "We don't have a group, because we tried to do a group for people waiting and nobody showed up. So we do offer individual visits and rarely—I'd say less than 10% of the people waiting take advantage of that."

program in FY 2012. Key factors affecting bed availability were high demand and reduction of bed availability.

Wait time barrier 2: poor staffing levels
Participants indicated that staff shortages (psychiatrists, social workers) at the residential programs hindered their ability to admit patients more quickly and having fewer staff at the smaller Community Based Outpatient Clinics (CBOCs) delayed important processes such as medical clearances.

Wait time barrier 3: length of stay
Several participants acknowledged that program length or extending a Veteran's length of stay after program completion when warranted can unintentionally lead to some Veterans waiting longer to enter the program.

The programs in which we interviewed program management and front-line staff were more likely to be low performers on the 7-day wait metric. However, among these programs in which patients waited longer than 7 days to be admitted, they were more likely to be high performers with respect to the proportion of waiting weeks with at least one SUD/mental health outpatient encounter (these data exclude programs with less than 25% pre-admission screening, for which these metrics were not calculated).

Engagement while waiting facilitators

Participants at 17 programs with high performance on any of the three *Engagement While Waiting* metrics were asked if there were particular aspects of their pre-admission processes that may have facilitated the provision of outpatient SUD and/or MH treatment while Veterans were waiting to enter the program. Several interrelated key factors were identified and are described below, with supporting quotations listed in Table 2.

Engagement while waiting facilitator 1: accessible outpatient services

Programs that were successful at engaging Veterans pre-admission leveraged their ability to offer and connect Veterans to SUD and mental health outpatient services within and/or outside the VA. In addition, some participants emphasized to Veterans the importance of staying connected to their outpatient providers if they were already accessing VA outpatient services. Fourteen of the 17 programs with high performance on this metric tried to engage Veterans waiting for admission in treatment groups such as pre-existing groups within the VA residential treatment program and VA intensive outpatient programs. Eight of the 17 high performing sites offered Veterans the opportunity to attend an established pre-admission group.

Engagement while waiting facilitator 2: strong patient outreach

In general, participants described a variety of motivational and outreach strategies believed to be instrumental in successfully engaging Veterans in treatment activities while waiting for admission. Program staff commonly reached out to and followed up with Veterans by telephone (e.g., daily, weekly, biweekly).

Engagement while waiting facilitator 3: strong encouragement of pre-admission outpatient treatment

Strongly encouraging pre-admission group participation was perceived to have a favorable impact on the degree to which Veterans engaged in treatment activities prior to admission. One participant illustrated how the staff incentivized Veterans to attend outpatient treatment by letting them know that pre-admission group participation would "improve their chance of getting into the program quicker" (Table 2).

Engagement while waiting barriers

Participants at 14 programs with low performance on any of the three *Engagement While Waiting* metrics, relative to the national average for their program type, were asked about barriers they faced in facilitating pre-admission engagement. The most commonly-cited barriers are described below, with corresponding supporting quotations listed in Table 3.

Engagement while waiting barrier 1: poor staffing levels

One of the primary obstacles voiced by participants was staffing constraints, which can make it difficult for program staff to provide optimal access to outpatient treatment.

Engagement while waiting barrier 2: socioeconomic barriers

Participants also noted that due to socioeconomic factors, Veterans themselves find it difficult to access outpatient treatment even when it is available. The most common socioeconomic barriers voiced by participants were (a) geographic location/driving distance to outpatient treatment, (b) lack of public transportation, and (c) financial constraints, such as lacking money to buy gas.

Engagement while waiting barrier 3: low patient motivation

Fewer participants perceived that Veterans themselves may hinder their own opportunities to engage in treatment. In other words, some Veterans do not avail themselves of outpatient services.

Discussion

This study aimed to: (1) Develop metrics for two pre-admission processes: *Wait Time* and *Engagement While Waiting*, and (2) Interview program management and staff about program structures and processes that may contribute to performance on these metrics. The first aim sought to close a gap in the VA's existing performance metrics in order to identify high-value targets for quality improvement. The second aim recognized that not all key processes are reflected in the administrative data, and even when they are, new insight may be gained from viewing these data in the context of day-to-day clinical practice. We hypothesized that speaking directly to residential program staff may reveal innovative practices, areas for improvement, and factors that may explain system-wide variability in performance.

In this project, we learned that program-level performance on the pre-admission metrics was highly variable. Across programs, 0–100% of Veterans waited longer than 7 days to be admitted (average: 60%). For these Veterans, at least one SUD or mental health contact occurred in

3–100% of the waiting weeks (average: 54%). This degree of clinical variability is consistent with previous studies and evaluative reports of SUD treatment in VA SUD RRTPs [11, 12].

We found that program management and staff shared common perceptions of the structures and processes that may have contributed to their program's high or low performance on the pre-admission metrics. This information can be useful for designing interventions to improve access to residential SUD treatment and reduce system-wide variability. Efficient screening processes and effective patient flow are processes that theoretically could be implemented across programs to help reduce wait times if there is good communication among all levels of staff. The availability of beds which emerged as a key determinant (barrier and facilitator) of wait times is structural, more static and largely dependent upon factors external to the program (e.g., facility/VA budget).

Given resource constraints, it may be tempting to concentrate efforts on other processes such as efficient screening and effective patient flow to reduce wait times, rather than increasing number of beds. However, systems can only become so efficient and resources spent on efficiency may take away resources from more beds. In addition, effective patient flow often depends upon sufficient staffing within the program itself and its ancillary components, which can be costly depending on the program's needs. When staffing levels are suboptimal, this can potentially impact how quickly Veterans can be admitted to and discharged from the program. Most of the interview comments related to staffing levels were general in nature, although some respondents mentioned specific staffing needs. As noted in Table 3, one respondent indicated that with only one psychiatrist doing the work, they were compelled to reduce their census by half. Another program lacked sufficient social workers, particularly during a time of increased referrals and applications, which staff perceived as potentially affecting wait time. Therefore, it is important to advocate for more beds and sufficient staffing along with low-cost, effective processes that may also ease wait times. It is also worth noting that although programs in which we interviewed staff were more likely to be low performers on the 7-day wait metric, among the low performers, they were more likely to be high performers with respect to the proportion of waiting weeks with at least one SUD/mental health outpatient encounter. This finding is heartening in that it appears that programs are seeking to provide outpatient care during this critical window of time despite difficult circumstances.

We found that successfully engaging Veterans in outpatient treatment while they wait appears to depend heavily on efforts by staff, at the individual provider, program,

and facility level. Overall, good internal and inter-facility communication appears vital to providing Veterans with timely access to residential treatment, and may also have positive ripple effects (e.g., engaging Veterans pre-admission may lead to fewer "no shows" to group treatment activities).

Poor staffing levels and socioeconomic barriers (e.g., lack of transportation) which were often perceived to be beyond the staff's control may be difficult to surmount as they are dependent on sufficient financial resources at the medical center. Yet, they are important to address as they potentially affect quality of care. As noted in Table 3, one respondent indicated that there had been a shortage of SUD providers in the Community Based Outpatient Clinics (CBOCs) "up north" and "no SUD providers available even by CBT" in rural areas, which impacted the type of outpatient care available to Veterans waiting for admission to the program. Another respondent mentioned that their program has only one social worker and that their medical facility is "way understaffed" in terms of SUD providers. Staffing costs will invariably depend on the type of staff required per site as well as the particular needs of the program.

Some programs however, showed resiliency and creativity in the face of these challenges. For instance, several programs were in the midst of advocating for transportation "workarounds" or creating their own (e.g., asking other Veterans if they were willing to give others a ride). Another program had not yet set up a group for Veterans who are waiting, but found peer support specialists to be particularly helpful in the interim. Others cited strategies (e.g., telemental health for patients in rural areas) that their program would benefit from having.

While some patients who do not engage in outpatient treatment may truly lack motivation, it is possible that some factors perceived as low motivation (e.g., failing to show up for a group or individual session while waiting), may stem from things beyond their control. Veterans struggling with issues such as transportation/housing may not be able to avail themselves of outpatient care, and for some, these factors may have been the driving force for seeking residential care in the first place. As such, these Veterans would also be precluded from an improved chance of getting into a residential program if they are incentivized to attend outpatient treatment—a strategy previously indicated by one provider as facilitating engagement while waiting. Any unintended consequences like this deserve attention to ensure equitability in access to services.

The potential value of these pre-admission metrics is significant given that they provide VA leadership, as well as program management and staff, with a way to easily monitor the access, quality, and efficiency of residential

SUD treatment programs. In response to an identified need to rapidly develop metrics for monitoring access to residential treatment, MHS and OMHO built upon the initial metrics developed by this study and implemented wait time metrics for the residential programs in October of 2014. These metrics continue to be refined with quarterly updates provided to the field and are part of a broader set of metrics that have been developed to understand access to residential treatment. By operationalizing this wait time metric, residential SUD treatment staff can view their program's performance over time and identify opportunities for implementation and quality improvement efforts. It has been a critical component to ensuring a clear understanding of residential access and guiding strategic planning efforts at the regional and local level to improve access. Further, MHS and OMHO are working towards refinement and implementation of the remaining metrics. The initial data provided by this study serves as baseline data and a point of comparison as new metrics are implemented.

The identification of common perceived facilitators and barriers offer opportunities for clinical leadership and health services researchers to craft interventions to improve timely access to services and disseminate "best practices" to the field. Although some of the identified "best practices" may appear to simply be the expected standard of care, the responses from interview participants reflect how a Veteran's quality of care is critically tied to the consistent execution of these tasks. In addition, the support, cooperation, and communication among program staff and facility-wide appeared to play a vital role.

We recognize some limitations of this study. We did not interview peripheral VA staff members (e.g., outpatient personnel who conduct pre-admissions screenings) that are located at another site/campus within the facility, nor did we interview Veterans. In addition, less than half of the VA's residential SUD programs were represented in the interviews, so our findings may not be generalizable to all VA residential SUD programs or to residential SUD programs outside the VA system. Moreover, there was substantially less representation from MH RRTPs with a SUD track (20%), compared to SUD RRTPs (80%). While we believe that provider interviews can be a beneficial component of quality improvement, we did not evaluate the effect of conveying what we learned back to our stakeholders. The next step would be to assess the potential value of interviewing program management and front-line staff while developing performance metrics. Since this endeavor can be labor-intensive, this reaffirms the need for evaluation. Despite these limitations, this study successfully created new metrics to monitor performance and identify areas for improvement, as well

as an inventory of potential solutions informed by residential program management and front-line staff.

Conclusion
Pre-admission process metrics developed in this study have been refined and are proving to be helpful for monitoring residential SUD treatment programs within the VA. Interviewing program management and staff about drivers of performance metrics can play a critical and complementary role by identifying innovative and other strong practices, as well as high-value targets for quality improvement. Key facilitators of pre-admission processes in high-performing facilities may offer programs with lower performance useful strategies to improve the quality of their pre-admission processes.

Abbreviations
VA: United States Department of Veterans Affairs; SUD: substance use disorder; SUD RRTPs: SUD Residential Rehabilitation Treatment Programs; MH RRTPs: Mental Health Residential Rehabilitation Treatment Programs; FY: fiscal year; MHIS: Mental Health Information System; NEPEC: Northeast Program Evaluation Center; MHS: VA Mental Health Services; OMHO: VA Office of Mental Health Operations; OIG: Office of the Inspector General; DAPS: VA Drug and Alcohol Program Survey; CBOCs: Community Based Outpatient Clinics.

Authors' contributions
LSE conducted the majority of the interviews; was the main qualitative analyst; interpreted the qualitative results; and drafted the manuscript. LM was a qualitative analyst, assisting in the analysis and interpretation of the data; contributed to the drafting of the manuscript; and is the corresponding author. SG developed and calculated the majority of the metrics; performed data analysis; and contributed to the design of the program profile report. TB developed and calculated the metrics; performed data analysis; and contributed to the design of the program profile report. TEP contributed to the design of the program profile report; conducted interviews; and was a qualitative analyst, assisting in the analysis and interpretation of the data. ADR developed the metrics and the interview guide; and edited the manuscript. JLB and ASH designed the study; interpreted the quantitative and qualitative results; and edited the manuscript. All authors read and approved the final manuscript.

Author details
[1] Center for Innovation to Implementation, Department of Veterans Affairs (VA) Palo Alto Health Care System, 795 Willow Road (MPD-152), Menlo Park, CA 94025, USA. [2] Department of Medicine, University of California, San Francisco and the San Francisco VA Medical Center, San Francisco, CA, USA. [3] Salem VA Medical Center, Salem, VA, USA.

Acknowledgements
None.
    This work was funded in part by the Department of Veterans Affairs (VA) Quality Enhancement Research Initiative (RRP-12-468) and a VA Research Career Scientist Award to Dr. Harris (RCS-14-232). The views expressed are those of the authors and do not represent the position or policy of the Department of Veterans Affairs or the United States Government.

Competing interests
The authors declare that they have no competing interests.
conducted from March 2014 to August 2014. This research was approved by the Stanford University Institutional Review Board for Human Subject Research and VHA Palo Alto Health Care System Research and Development Committee.

Funding and roles

This study was funded by the United States Department of Veterans Affairs (VA) Quality Enhancement Research Initiative (RRP 12-468) and a VA Research Career Scientist Award to Dr. Harris (RCS-14-232). The funding bodies for this study had no role in the design of the study, nor in collection, analysis, interpretation of data, or in writing the manuscript.

References

1. Department of Veterans Affairs, V.H.A. VHA handbook 1162.02: Mental Health Residential Rehabilitation Treatment Program (MH RRTP). Washington, DC: Author; 2010.
2. Reif S, et al. Residential treatment for individuals with substance use disorders: assessing the evidence. Psychiatr Serv. 2014;65(3):301–12.
3. Department of Veterans Affairs, O.o.I.G.O. Independent review of the FY 2014 detailed accounting submission to the office of national drug control policy. 2015.
4. Department of Veterans Affairs, O.o.I.G.O. Review of the operations and effectiveness of VHA residential substance use treatment programs. 2015.
5. Department of Veterans Affairs, V.H.A. VHA handbook 1160.01: Uniform Mental Health Services in VA Medical Centers and Clinics. Washington, DC: Author; 2008.
6. Trafton JA, et al. VHA mental health information system: applying health information technology to monitor and facilitate implementation of VHA Uniform Mental Health Services Handbook requirements. Med Care. 2013;51(3 Suppl 1):S29–36.
7. Department of Veterans Affairs, O.o.I.G.O. Review of Veterans Health Administration Residential Mental Health Care Facilities. 2009.
8. Department of Veterans Affairs, O.o.I.G.O. A Follow-up review of VHA Mental Health Residential Rehabilitation Treatment Programs (MH RRTP). 2011.
9. ATLAS.ti Scientific Software Development GmbH, Berlin.
10. Miles MB, Huberman AM, Saldana J, editors. Qualitative data analysis: a methods sourcebook. 3rd ed. Thousand Oaks: Sage Publications Inc; 2014.
11. Harris AH, et al. Validation of the treatment identification strategy of the HEDIS addiction quality measures: concordance with medical record review. BMC Health Serv Res. 2011;11:73.
12. Harris AH, et al. Examining the specification validity of the HEDIS quality measures for substance use disorders. J Subst Abuse Treat. 2015;53:16–21.

9

Hazardous drinking among young adults seeking outpatient mental health services

Anna E. Ordóñez[1,3]*, Rachel Ranney[1], Maxine Schwartz[1], Carol A. Mathews[1,4] and Derek D. Satre[1,2]

Abstract

Background: Alcohol use can have a significant negative impact on young adults in mental health treatment. This cross-sectional study examined prevalence and factors associated with hazardous drinking among young adults seeking outpatient mental health services, rate of alcohol use disorders (AUDs), and the relationship between hazardous drinking and other types of substance use.

Methods: Participants were 487 young adults ages 18–25 who completed self-administered computerized screening questions for alcohol and drug use. Alcohol use patterns were assessed and predictors of hazardous drinking (≥5 drinks on one or more occasions in the past year) were identified using logistic regression.

Results: Of the 487 participants, 79.8 % endorsed prior-year alcohol use, 52.3 % reported one or more episodes of hazardous drinking in the prior year and 8.2 % were diagnosed with an AUD. Rates of recent and lifetime alcohol, tobacco and marijuana use were significantly greater in those with prior-year hazardous drinking. In logistic regression, prior-year hazardous drinking was associated with lifetime marijuana use (OR 3.30, p < 0.001; 95 % CI 2.05, 5.28), lifetime tobacco use (OR 1.88, p = 0.004; 95 % CI 1.22, 2.90) and older age (OR 1.18 per year, p < 0.001; 95 % CI 1.08, 1.29).

Conclusions: In an outpatient mental health setting, high rates of hazardous drinking were identified, and drinking was associated with history of other substance use. Results highlight patient characteristics associated with hazardous drinking that mental health providers should be aware of in treating young adults, especially older age and greater use of tobacco and marijuana.

Keywords: Alcohol, Hazardous drinking, Cannabis, Depression, Mental health, Young adults

Background

Substance use disorders, hazardous drinking and mental illness all peak in prevalence in early adulthood, yet few young adults receive appropriate services. For example, the 2011 National Household Survey on Drug Use and Health (NHSDUH) found that the 1-year prevalence of illicit drug or alcohol abuse or dependence increased from 7 % among 12–17 year olds to 19 % for 18–25 year olds, decreasing to 6 % for individuals over 25 [1]. The same report found that adults ages 18–25 had higher rates of mental illness and were less likely to receive treatment in the prior year than older adults.

Alcohol use can adversely impact symptom severity and treatment of co-occurring mental illness [2–5]. Reduced response to antidepressants and increased risk of side effects have been reported with even moderate levels of alcohol use [5]. In the STAR*D depression treatment cohort, individuals with major depressive disorder and co-occurring substance use disorders (including alcohol) had earlier onset of depression, greater severity and functional impairment, and higher rates of suicide attempts and completed suicide [3]. Similarly, while many individuals with anxiety disorders use alcohol for short-term symptom relief, drinking can ultimately make anxiety more severe [2, 4]. These associations highlight the need to assess alcohol and drug use patterns among young adults with mental health problems, in order to understand potential symptom exacerbation and

*Correspondence: anna.ordonez@nih.gov
[3] Office of Clinical Research, National Institute of Mental Health, 6001 Executive Blvd. MSC 9669, Bethesda, MD 20892, USA
Full list of author information is available at the end of the article

medication interaction risks. Assessment could also help to identify which individuals may benefit from psychiatry-based brief interventions to reduce harmful drinking patterns, and who should be referred to specialty care addiction treatment.

Apart from the potential value of brief interventions, screening provides benchmark medical record data at intake to help providers track potential changes in drinking over time. Some studies suggest that screening alone could help to reduce drinking [6, 7]. In the clinician's guide to identifying and treating drinking problems in health care settings, the National Institutes on Alcohol Abuse and Alcoholism (NIAAA) recommends asking how many times in the past year individuals have had 5 or more drinks for men and 4 or more for women [8]. In 2009 Smith et al., reported a sensitivity of 88 % and specificity 67 % of this cutoff in detecting a current (AUD) in a primary care setting [9]. Using the Alcohol Use Disorders Identification Test (AUDIT) as reference, Massey et al. [10] reported 96 % sensitivity and 82 % specificity of screening question to detect harmful drinking in an alert nonpsychotic consult-liaison population. In the present study we used a similar cutoff (5+ drinks for both men and women) drawn from electronic health record intake data in a psychiatry clinic setting to examine prevalence and correlates of hazardous drinking in young adults. The same cutoff was used for both sexes as this was the information available from the data, which was based on a graduated frequency measure that did not adjust quantities based on sex.

Although young adults are at high risk for alcohol-related problems [11], studies evaluating drinking patterns and their association with clinical characteristics are lacking. This study evaluated self-reported alcohol use patterns and the association between prior-year hazardous drinking and potentially relevant patient characteristics, including gender, age, clinician-assigned psychiatric diagnosis, and other substance use in a sample of young adults presenting for initial mental health treatment. We hypothesized that prior-year hazardous drinking would be associated with an AUD diagnosis, with other common psychiatric diagnoses, in particular, anxiety and depression, and with other types of substance use prevalent in this population such as tobacco and marijuana.

Methods
Participants and measures
Study participants were adults ages 18–25 seeking psychiatric services in an outpatient clinic in a university medical center. This clinic provides a range of assessment and treatment services, including medication management and individual and group psychotherapy. The clinic has no formal services for patients primarily seeking

alcohol or drug treatment. Individuals seeking such services are pre-screened by telephone by clinic staff and referred to local specialty care programs.

The sample included all individuals who presented to the clinic for initial evaluation between September 14th, 2005 and June 29th, 2011, were between the ages of 18 and 25 at intake, and completed routine computerized questionnaires, including a self-administered Electronic Health Inventory (EHI) [12], Beck Depression Inventory-II (BDI-II) and a clinical interview. Other than age range and intake dates, there were no exclusion criteria.

The EHI was completed on private computers in the clinic waiting area. It included questions about demographic characteristics, current and past medical history, and patterns of substance use for alcohol, cannabis and tobacco. For each substance, participants were asked if they had ever used that substance during their lifetime. Positive responses prompted questions on duration and frequently of use. Providers received a printed copy of the EHI questionnaire results for use in evaluation of new patients at intake. The University of California, San Francisco Committee on Human Research approved the study, including the examination of de-identified records of patients who had an initial clinic visit during the study time period.

Participants who endorsed any lifetime alcohol or cannabis/marijuana use were asked the timing of most recent use (in years, months or days) prior to intake. Alcohol use questions included usual quantity consumed per occasion (in standard drinks), frequency of use in the past 30 days and number of days in the past year when 1–2, 3–4, 5–7, and ≥8 drinks were consumed on one occasion (graduated frequency method) [13]. Combining the responses of any consumption of 5–7 or ≥8 drinks consumed on one occasion in the past year, hazardous drinking was defined for this analysis as any past-year consumption of 5 or more drinks on one occasion, consistent with the definition used by the NHIS (5+ drinks for both women and men) during the same time period [14]. While NIAAA currently recommends a different cut-off for hazardous drinking in men (5+) and women (4+), data were not available to assess this distinction.

Substance use and psychiatric disorder diagnoses
By chart review, we obtained all assigned Diagnostic and Statistical Manual of Mental Disorder, Fourth Edition Text Revision (DSM-IV-TR) [15] diagnoses listed on each participants' standardized initial intake evaluation form, as assigned and documented by the clinician. Blinded to responses on the EHI, a study research assistant reviewed and coded all listed diagnoses. We coded only definite diagnoses, excluding "rule out" diagnoses.

We coded drug use disorder positive if abuse or dependence was diagnosed for the following drugs: amphetamine, cannabis, opiates, methamphetamine, mushrooms, benzodiazepines, cocaine, stimulants, or if polysubstance abuse was diagnosed. Given the young age of the sample, disorders in remission would still be temporally relatively recent. Therefore, no distinction was made between diagnoses in remission or active. We coded alcohol use disorder (AUD) positive if alcohol abuse or dependence was diagnosed. Likewise, no distinction was made between diagnoses in remission or still active. We coded depressive disorder positive if major depressive disorder, dysthymia, or depression not otherwise specified (NOS) was diagnosed. Similarly, we coded an anxiety disorder if anxiety disorder NOS, generalized anxiety disorder, social anxiety disorder, panic disorder, specific phobia, post-traumatic stress disorder or obsessive compulsive disorder was diagnosed. We coded bipolar disorder positive if bipolar affective disorder (BAD) type I, II or NOS was diagnosed. We coded psychotic disorder positive if schizophrenia, schizoaffective disorder, delusional disorder or psychosis NOS was diagnosed. We coded attention deficit hyperactivity disorder (ADHD) positive if ADHD (inattentive, hyperactive, or combined type) or ADHD NOS was diagnosed. We coded eating disorder positive if anorexia, bulimia or eating disorder NOS was diagnosed.

Analyses

We linked self-reported demographic and substance use data from the EHI to diagnostic data from the chart review to create a single dataset for analysis. We compared differences in alcohol use rates between men and women using the χ^2 test, and differences in BDI-II score and mean quantity of alcohol consumed between women and men using t tests. Similarly, using χ^2 tests for categorical variables and t tests for continuous variable, rates of alcohol, tobacco and marijuana use, as well as rates of specific psychiatric diagnoses at intake were examined by prior-year hazardous drinking. Underage alcohol use was also examined (rate of any hazardous drinking among those ages 18–20 vs. 21–25). Given that participants could be assigned several diagnoses at intake, individual diagnoses were not included in regression models (as they were not independent of each other). Instead, we assessed diagnostic burden as indicated by the number of diagnoses assigned at intake. We used a single logistic regression model to test the association between number of psychiatric diagnoses, any lifetime use of tobacco and cannabis, age, race/ethnicity and gender as potential predictors of participants reporting any hazardous drinking in the prior year. We used STATA version 13 for all analyses.

Results

During the study intake period, 487 new patients between the ages of 18–25 years were admitted. The sample was racially diverse and predominantly female, and included a substantial percentage of students (Table 1).

Lifetime alcohol use was endorsed by 85.4 % of the sample, prior year alcohol use was endorsed by 79.8 %, and 52.3 % reported prior year hazardous drinking. Frequency of hazardous drinking was: 1–5 times a year (22.8 %), 6–11 times a year (11.5 %), about once a month (3.3 %), 2 or 3 times a month (7.0 %), once or twice a week (6.2 %), 3 or 4 times a week (0.8 %), nearly every day (0.5 %). Lifetime marijuana use was endorsed by 66.7 % of participants and prior year marijuana use was endorsed by 48.1 % of the sample. There were no significant gender differences in any of the above rates. AUD diagnoses were present in 8.2 % of the sample, and were twice as prevalent among women (10.3 %) compared to men (4.2 %) ($\chi^2 = 5.2$, p = 0.02). Participants over age 21 (N = 313) endorsed significantly greater prior-year hazardous drinking than those under 21 (N = 174) (58.8 % vs. 41.2 % respectively; $\chi^2 = 14.5$, p < 0.001) (not shown).

Table 1 Demographic characteristics and occupational status of adults ages 18–25 seeking outpatient mental health treatment (N = 487)

Variables	Mean (SD) or %
Gender (%)	
Men	33.9
Women	66.1
Age (mean, SD)	22.2 (±2.3)
Men	21.9 (±2.4)
Women	22.3 (±2.3)
Race (%)	
Asian	15.2
Black	2.5
White	62.6
Other	19.7
Hispanic origin (%)	9.9
Education (%)	
High school grade 7–12	4.6
High school graduate or GED	47.3
Completed technical training	3.2
College graduate	27.8
In or completed graduate training	17.1
Occupational status (%)	
Student	44.8
Employed (full or part-time)	31.7
Unemployed	21.5
Disability	2.0

The most prevalent psychiatric diagnoses at intake were depression (55 %) and anxiety disorders (43.3 %) with no gender differences. BDI-II scores were available for 395 participants. Overall mean BDI-II score was 22.2 (SD = 10.8), indicative of moderate depression, with a significant difference between men (mean = 18.6, SD = 10.8) and women (mean = 24.1, SD = 13.4) (p ≤ 0.001) (not shown).

Overall, rates and frequency of alcohol, tobacco and marijuana use were significantly greater in those who endorsed hazardous drinking in the prior 12 months compared to those who didn't (Table 2). Rates of AUDs were four times greater among those who endorsed hazardous drinking in the prior 12 months, compared to those who didn't (Table 2). Rate of psychotic disorders among those who endorsed prior 12-month hazardous drinking were less frequent compared to those who denied hazardous drinking in the prior 12 months.

There were no significant differences in the rates of other psychiatric disorders among those who did and those who did not endorse hazardous drinking in the prior 12 months.

Logistic regression analysis was used to examine predictors of prior-year hazardous drinking (Table 3). The single model included number of diagnoses at intake, age, gender, race, and any lifetime marijuana or tobacco use. Variables positively associated with prior-year hazardous drinking included lifetime marijuana use (OR 3.30, p < 0.001; 95 % CI 2.05, 5.28), lifetime tobacco use (OR 1.88, p = 0.004; 95 % CI 1.22, 2.90) and older age (OR 1.18 per year, p < 0.001; 95 % CI 1.08; 1.29) (Table 3). Results from sensitivity analyses using prior-year cannabis and smoking measures (which occurred during the same time frame as the hazardous drinking) were similar, and the significance of the measures in predicting prior-year hazardous drinking did not change (not shown).

Table 2 Substance use patterns and psychiatric diagnoses of young adults ages 18–25 seeking outpatient mental health treatment by hazardous drinking status

Variable	Hazardous drinking in the prior 12 months Total N = 487				p value
	No hazardous drinking N = 232 (47.6 %)		≥1 days of hazardous drinking N = 255 (52.3 %)		
	Mean or %	SD	Mean or %	SD	
Alcohol use (%)					
Lifetime	69.4		100		<0.0001
Prior year	59.1		98.8		<0.0001
Prior month	37.9		87.8		<0.0001
Usual quantity of drinks consumed per occasion	0.9	±1.1	3.1	±1.9	<0.0001
Number of days alcohol was consumed in prior 30 days	2.2	±4.5	6.4	±6.5	<0.0001
Tobacco use (%)					
Lifetime	38.8		65.9		<0.0001
Prior year	22.4		51.0		<0.0001
Prior month	21.1		38.8		<0.0001
Marijuana use (%)					
Lifetime	49.6		82.4		<0.0001
Prior year	29.7		64.7		<0.0001
Prior month	16.0		40.0		<0.0001
Psychiatric diagnoses at initial intake (%)					
Depressive disorder	53.9		56.1		0.6261
Anxiety disorder	42.2		44.3		0.6448
Bipolar disorder	11.6		17.3		0.0794
Eating disorders	14.2		11.8		0.4193
Psychotic disorder	16.4		8.24		0.0059
Drug use disorder (excluding tobacco and alcohol)	5.17		9.41		0.0741
Alcohol use disorder	3.02		12.9		0.0001
Attention deficit disorder	7.33		6.67		0.7750
PTSD	6.47		4.31		0.2914
Mean number of diagnoses at initial intake	2.02	±1.1	2.36	±1.3	0.0300

Significant differences appear in italics

Table 3 Factors associated with prior-year hazardous drinking in young adults seeking outpatient psychiatric services (N = 487)

Predictor	OR	p value	95 % CI
Number of psychiatric diagnoses at intake	1.06	0.459	0.90–1.25
Lifetime cannabis use	*3.30*	*<0.001*	*2.05–5.28*
Lifetime tobacco use	*1.88*	*0.004*	*1.22–2.90*
Age in years	*1.18*	*<0.001*	*1.08–1.29*
Female gender	0.98	0.932	0.64–1.50
Race (reference: white)			
Black	0.52	0.372	0.13–2.17
Asian	*0.43*	*0.007*	*0.23–0.80*
Other	1.20	0.470	0.73–2.00

Results are from a single multivariate logistic regression

Significant differences appear in italics

Discussion

This study examined the relationship of prior-year hazardous drinking to patterns of alcohol, tobacco and cannabis use, as well as psychiatry diagnoses, in a young adult outpatient psychiatry sample. In this treatment-seeking sample, cannabis and tobacco use as well as older age were significant predictors of hazardous drinking.

These results highlight the high rates of hazardous drinking in a young adult population seeking mental health treatment, and the need for systematic screening in this group. The levels of prior-year hazardous drinking in our study were approximately twice as high in men (53.3 vs. 23.7 %) and five times higher in women (51.9 vs. 10.3 %) than in individuals of the same age, during the same time frame in the National Health Interview Survey (NHIS) [14]. Our sample also included a substantial proportion of students, we found comparable rates to those seen in college students (approximately 45 % prior-month hazardous drinking) [16]. These rates are also higher than those seen in a study of hazardous drinking among adults with moderate or greater depression symptoms from the same clinic setting [17]. This sample (N = 1183) ranged in age from 18 to 91, with a mean age of 42.2 (SD = 14.7) 47.5 % of men and 32.5 % of women reported prior-year hazardous drinking, compared to 53.3 and 51.9 % for men and women in our young adult sample. In addition, younger age was an independent predictor of hazardous drinking in this larger clinic sample. Thus, the clinical setting, student composition and age of participants may help to explain our findings.

Based on this same previous study in the psychiatry clinic with a mean age of 42.2 [16], the most common primary psychiatric diagnosis assigned to patients following their first visit was major depressive disorder (48.4 %), followed by bipolar disorder (14.8 %), anxiety disorders (11.2 %), depressive disorder not otherwise specified

(7.5 %), mood disorder not otherwise specified (4.3 %), adjustment disorders (4.3 %), schizophrenia (1.2 %), and 9.1 % all other diagnoses combined. For most diagnoses, rates were similar to those in the current sample. The exception is anxiety diagnoses, which were identified at a higher rate in the current sample. A potential explanation for the difference is sample selection (participants scored 10+ on the BDI-II) as well as the way in which diagnoses were identified. The prior study measured only primary diagnoses, while the current young adult study used manual chart review to include all diagnoses assigned by providers.

Although rate of AUD assignment was low relative to the rate of prior-year hazardous drinking, especially among men, any self-reported prior-year hazardous drinking was associated with a fourfold higher rate of an AUD diagnosis. These findings highlight the relevance of hazardous drinking screening among young adults seeking mental health treatment as a component of psychiatric evaluation and treatment [2, 3, 5] and an indicator of a possible AUD. It is noteworthy that in our sample AUD diagnoses were twice as prevalent in woman as in men. This is in contrast to many prior epidemiological studies, including the National Epidemiologic Survey on Alcohol and Related Conditions (NESARC) [18], which found rates of alcohol abuse and dependence to be a little more than double in men compared to women. It is possible that, rather than reflecting actual gender differences in AUD diagnoses, the higher rate of AUD among women in our sample reflects a greater concern from providers regarding problematic drinking in treatment seeking young women than in young men. This pattern has previously been described in a study of the Veterans Health Administration, which found race and gender differences among VA patients with clinically recognized AUDs [19]. That study outlines the importance of validating diagnoses against structured gold-standard clinical assessments to better understand whether providers are over or under-identifying AUDs.

Analyses of the relationship of psychiatric diagnoses to hazardous drinking indicated that, aside from AUDs, no single psychiatric disorder was particularly associated with increased rates of hazardous drinking. The finding of hazardous drinking being associated with lower rates of psychotic disorder diagnosis was not anticipated. There is a large body of data regarding comorbid substance abuse and psychosis. For example, psychosis has been associated with frequent cannabis use in national surveys [20]. Similarly, several studies have described comorbid AUDs in patients with psychosis [21, 22]. It is therefore unexpected that among all diagnoses, hazardous drinking would be negatively associated with psychotic disorder. One possible explanation is that, given that all participants were seeking outpatient mental health treatment, the variability in the sample was more limited than in those seen in other studies.

Study findings have important implications for clinical practice. Screening for hazardous drinking should be conducted with all psychiatric patients, regardless of diagnosis. The finding that any marijuana use was associated with 3.3 fold greater odds of prior-year hazardous drinking is also noteworthy. This finding was consistent with previous literature in college students, which found that those who use both marijuana and alcohol are more likely to experience alcohol and other drug problems, including higher mean number of drinks per occasion [23]. Helping clinicians be aware of the frequency of co-occurring marijuana use with hazardous drinking may represent an additional opportunity to improve identification of alcohol and other drug problems.

Mental health clinics are important settings in which to address hazardous drinking and identify AUDs. Individuals with AUDs are more likely to seek care in mental health settings than in specialized addiction treatment programs [24]. While effective interventions to reduce co-occurring alcohol problems exist, providers in psychiatry clinics often fail to identify warning signs of problematic drinking and overlook opportunities to intervene [25, 26]. Interventions such as motivational interviewing could be important supplements to mental health treatment [27–29]. The Screening, Brief Intervention and Referral to Treatment (SBIRT) model promoted by the U.S. Substance Abuse and Mental Health Services Administration (SAMHSA) [30] is another example of a potential supplement to existing mental health care. SBIRT is a public health-based approach to early intervention for at-risk individuals identified in primary care and other health settings. Implementing these interventions in general psychiatric treatment for young adults, as well as identifying and referring AUDs to specialty addiction treatment when indicated, could help reduce hazardous drinking and improve overall patient care.

Limitations

This study had several limitations. While computerized self-report measures are valid, under-reporting of alcohol and cannabis use by patients would make our prevalence rates conservative. In addition, the clinic that served as the study site routinely referred patients primarily seeking care for alcohol and drug problems to specialty care treatment programs, which may also lead to lower prevalence rates of hazardous drinking in our population compared to some other psychiatric service settings. Similarly, our study used provider-assigned diagnoses and did not systematically assess AUDs using structured interviews, resulting in potential under- and/ or over-estimate of AUD rates and hindering our ability to determine the sensitivity and specificity of prior-year hazardous drinking as a predictor of AUDs. In addition, the lack of distinction between active AUD or substance use disorder diagnoses and those in remission limits the correlation of hazardous drinking in our study to any lifetime AUD or substance use disorder diagnoses. However, the low number of clinician-assigned AUDs in the context of hazardous drinking remains noteworthy. Lastly, using a lower cutoff for hazardous drinking for women than for men (4 drinks per occasion rather than 5), would increase sensitivity of "at risk" drinking in this group, and is often used in population-based and clinical studies. The use of a higher cutoff in this study may make our estimates of hazardous drinking among women conservative.

Conclusions

This study examined the extent of hazardous drinking, alcohol and other substance use patterns, provider-assigned AUDs, and co-occurring psychiatric disorders among young adults in an outpatient psychiatry clinic. Prior-year hazardous drinking rates for both men and women were substantially higher than those found in studies of young adults in the general population. Lifetime marijuana use and tobacco use significantly predicted prior-year hazardous drinking. There was a strong association of prior-year hazardous drinking with a clinician-assigned AUD, even though overall rate of AUD diagnosis was relatively low. Outpatient mental health service settings offer an excellent opportunity for early identification and intervention to reduce alcohol and other substance use among young adults.

Authors' contributions
AEO led the design of the study, conducted analyses and led manuscript drafting. RR and MS conducted data retrieval via chart reviews and assisted in data management. CAM and DDS assisted in study design, interpretation of findings and manuscript drafting. All authors read and approved the final manuscript.

Authors' information
The authors alone are responsible for the content and writing of this paper. Please note, this article was prepared while Anna E. Ordóñez, M.D., M.A.S. was employed at the University of California, San Francisco. The opinions expressed in this article are the author's own and do not reflect the view of the National Institutes of Health, the Department of Health and Human Services, or the United States government.

Author details
[1] Department of Psychiatry and UCSF Weill Institute for Neurosciences, University of California, 401 Parnassus Avenue, San Francisco, CA 94143, USA. [2] Division of Research, Kaiser Permanente Northern California Region, 2000 Broadway, 3rd Floor, Oakland, CA 94612, USA. [3] Office of Clinical Research, National Institute of Mental Health, 6001 Executive Blvd. MSC 9669, Bethesda, MD 20892, USA. [4] Department of Psychiatry, University of Florida, 100 S Newell Drive, Gainesville, FL 32610, USA.

Acknowledgements
This work was supported by NIH grants T32 DA07250 (Principal Investigator: James L. Sorensen, Ph.D., Professor, Department of Psychiatry, University of California, San Francisco), R01 AA020463 (Principal Investigator: Derek D. Satre, Ph.D.) and 2R25 MH060482 (Principal Investigators: Carol A. Mathews, M.D. and Victor Reus, M.D., Professor, Department of Psychiatry, University of California, San Francisco.)

Competing interests
The authors declare that they have no competing interests.

References
1. Substance Abuse and Mental Health Services Administration. Results from the 2010 national survey on drug use and health: summary of national findings, NSDUH series H-44, HHS publication no. (SMA) 11-4658. September 2011. http://archive.samhsa.gov/data/NSDUH/2k10nsduh/2k10results.htm. Accessed 23 June 2016.
2. Brady KT, Tolliver BK, Verduin ML. Alcohol use and anxiety: diagnostic and management issues. Am J Psychiatry. 2007;164(2):217–21 **(quiz 372)**.
3. Davis LL, Frazier E, Husain MM, Warden D, Trivedi M, Fava M, Cassano P, McGrath PJ, Balasubramani GK, Wisniewski SR, et al. Substance use disorder comorbidity in major depressive disorder: a confirmatory analysis of the STAR*D cohort. Am J Addict. 2006;15(4):278–85.
4. Kushner MG, Abrams K, Borchardt C. The relationship between anxiety disorders and alcohol use disorders: a review of major perspectives and findings. Clin Psychol Rev. 2000;20(2):149–71.
5. Worthington J, Fava M, Agustin C, Alpert J, Nierenberg AA, Pava JA, Rosenbaum JF. Consumption of alcohol, nicotine, and caffeine among depressed outpatients. Relationship with response to treatment. Psychosomatics. 1996;37(6):518–22.
6. McCambridge J, Day M. Randomized controlled trial of the effects of completing the Alcohol Use Disorders Identification Test questionnaire on self-reported hazardous drinking. Addiction. 2008;103(2):241–8.
7. McCambridge J, Bendtsen M, Karlsson N, White IR, Nilsen P, Bendtsen P. Alcohol assessment and feedback by email for university students: main findings from a randomised controlled trial. Br J Psychiatry J Ment Sci. 2013;203(5):334–40.
8. National Institute on Alcohol Abuse and Alcoholism. Helping patients who drink too much: a clinician's guide, updated 2005 edition. 2005. http://pubs.niaaa.nih.gov/publications/Practitioner/CliniciansGuide2005/clinicians_guide.htm. Updated January 2007. Accessed 6 June 2016.
9. Smith PC, Schmidt SM, Allensworth-Davies D, Saitz R. Primary care validation of a single-question alcohol screening test. J Gen Intern Med. 2009;24(7):783–8.
10. Massey SH, Norris L, Lausin M, Nwaneri C, Lieberman DZ. Identifying harmful drinking using a single screening question in a psychiatric consultation-liaison population. Psychosomatics. 2011;52(4):362–6.
11. Naimi TS, Brewer RD, Mokdad A, Denny C, Serdula MK, Marks JS. Binge drinking among US adults. JAMA. 2003;289(1):70–5.
12. Satre DD, Wolfe W, Eisendrath S, Weisner C. Computerized screening for alcohol and drug use among adults seeking outpatient psychiatric services. Psychiatr Serv. 2008;59(4):441–4.
13. Stahre M, Naimi T, Brewer R, Holt J. Measuring average alcohol consumption: the impact of including binge drinks in quantity-frequency calculations. Addiction. 2006;101(12):1711–8.
14. Schoenborn CA, Adams PF, Peregoy JA. Health behaviors of adults: United States, 2008–2010. Vital Health Stat. 2013;10(257):1–184.
15. American Psychiatric Association: Diagnostic and statistical manual of mental disorders, 4th ed., text rev. edn. Washington, DC: American Psychiatric Association; 2000.
16. Hingson RW. Focus on: college drinking and related problems: magnitude and prevention of college drinking and related problems. Alcohol Res Health. 2010;33(1–2):45–54.
17. Satre DD, Chi FW, Eisendrath S, Weisner C. Subdiagnostic alcohol use by depressed men and women seeking outpatient psychiatric services: consumption patterns and motivation to reduce drinking. Alcohol Clin Exp Res. 2011;35(4):695–702.
18. Goldstein RB, Dawson DA, Chou SP, Grant BF. Sex differences in prevalence and comorbidity of alcohol and drug use disorders: results from wave 2 of the National Epidemiologic Survey on Alcohol and Related Conditions. J Stud Alcohol Drugs. 2012;73(6):938–50.
19. Williams EC, Gupta S, Rubinsky AD, Jones-Webb R, Bensley KM, Young JP, Hagedorn H, Gifford E, Harris AH. Racial/ethnic differences in the prevalence of clinically recognized alcohol use disorders among patients from the U.S. Veterans Health Administration. Alcohol Clin Exp Res. 2016;40(2):359–66.
20. Davis GP, Compton MT, Wang S, Levin FR, Blanco C. Association between cannabis use, psychosis, and schizotypal personality disorder: findings from the National Epidemiologic Survey on Alcohol and Related Conditions. Schizophr Res. 2013;151(1–3):197–202.
21. Cassano GB, Pini S, Saettoni M, Rucci P, Dell'Osso L. Occurrence and clinical correlates of psychiatric comorbidity in patients with psychotic disorders. J Clin Psychiatry. 1998;59(2):60–8.
22. Wisdom JP, Manuel JI, Drake RE. Substance use disorder among people with first-episode psychosis: a systematic review of course and treatment. Psychiatr Serv. 2011;62(9):1007–12.
23. Shillington AM, Clapp JD. Heavy alcohol use compared to alcohol and marijuana use: do college students experience a difference in substance use problems? J Drug Educ. 2006;36(1):91–103.
24. Edlund MJ, Booth BM, Han X. Who seeks care where? Utilization of mental health and substance use disorder treatment in two national samples of individuals with alcohol use disorders. J Stud Alcohol Drugs. 2012;73(4):635–46.
25. Satre DD, Leibowitz AS, Mertens JR, Weisner C. Advising depression patients to reduce alcohol and drug use: factors associated with provider intervention in outpatient psychiatry. Am J Addict. 2014;23(6):570–5.
26. Weisner C, Matzger H. Missed opportunities in screening for alcohol problems in medical and mental health services. Alcohol Clin Exp Res. 2003;27(7):1132–41.
27. Babor TF, Higgins-Biddle JC. Alcohol screening and brief intervention: dissemination strategies for medical practice and public health. Addiction. 2000;95(5):677–86.
28. Baker A, Kavanagh DJ, Kay-Lambkin FJ, Hunt SA, Lewin TJ, Carr VJ, McElduff P. Randomized controlled trial of MICBT for co-existing alcohol misuse and depression: outcomes to 36-months. J Subst Abuse Treat. 2014;46(3):281–90.
29. Eberhard S, Nordstrom G, Hoglund P, Ojehagen A. Secondary prevention of hazardous alcohol consumption in psychiatric out-patients: a randomised controlled study. Soc Psychiatry Psychiatr Epidemiol. 2009;44(12):1013–21.
30. Fussell HE, Rieckmann TR, Quick MB. Medicaid reimbursement for screening and brief intervention for substance misuse. Psychiatr Serv. 2011;62(3):306–9.

10

Impact of hepatitis C status on 20-year mortality of patients with substance use disorders

Anthony J. Accurso*, Darius A. Rastegar, Sharon R. Ghazarian and Michael I. Fingerhood

Abstract

Background: The magnitude of the effect of hepatitis C viral infection on survival is still not fully understood. The objective of this study was to determine whether the presence of hepatitis C viral antibodies in 1991 was associated with increased mortality 20 years later within a cohort of patients with substance use disorders. Secondary objectives were to determine other factors that were associated with increased mortality in the cohort.

Methods: A subset of a 1991 study cohort of patients who had presented for detoxification was reexamined 20 years later. The Social Security Death Index was queried to identify which of the original patients had died. Attributes of survivors and non-survivors were compared, with special attention to their hepatitis C status in 1991. The original study and this analysis were conducted in the chemical detoxification unit at Johns Hopkins Bayview (previously Francis Scott Key Hospital), an academic urban hospital. All participants met the criteria for alcohol or opioid dependence at the time of admission in 1991. The primary study outcome was 20-year mortality after initial admission in 1991, with a planned analysis of hepatitis C status.

Results: Twenty years after admission, 362 patients survived and 82 had died. Of the 284 patients who were hepatitis C positive, 228 survived (80 %). Of the 160 patients who were hepatitis C negative, 134 survived (84 %). This absolute risk increase of 4 % was not statistically significant (p = 0.37). Factors associated with increased mortality included male sex, white race, older age, and reported use of alcohol, cocaine, and illicit methadone. Binary logistic regression including hepatitis C status and these other variables yielded an adjusted odds ratio of 0.87 (95 % CI 0.49–1.55); (p = 0.64) for hepatitis C positive 20-year survival.

Conclusions: Hepatitis C positivity was not associated with a statistically significant difference in 20-year survival. The effect of the virus on mortality, if present, is small, relative to the effect of substance use disorders alone.

Keywords: Hepatitis C virus, Chemical dependence, Survival

Background

Hepatitis C has been recognized as the major cause of chronic hepatitis in people who inject drugs since 1992 [1]. Epidemiologic studies have shown the prevalence of hepatitis C infection among drug users to be as high as 85–90 % in a variety of cities worldwide [2–4]. Most individuals who test positive for hepatitis C antibody have circulating hepatitis C virus, but 10–15 % clear the infection on their own [5]. It is estimated that about 50 % of infected individuals progress to chronic liver disease and 20 % progress to cirrhosis [6, 7]. The speed of progression appears multi-factorial, with progression accelerated by concurrent HIV infection and heavy alcohol use [8].

Since 1990, the treatment of hepatitis C has depended on the use of injectable interferon as the backbone of treatment [9, 10]. Related to the need for adherence, significant side effects and the intramuscular route of administration, a relatively small percentage of people who inject drugs have been considered for treatment, let

*Correspondence: antaccurso@gmail.com
Johns Hopkins Bayview Medical Center, 5200 Eastern Ave, Mason F. Lord Bldg, West Tower 5th floor, Baltimore, MD 21224, USA

alone treated. However, recent advances in the treatment of hepatitis C have thrust attention to the consideration of treatment for most individuals with hepatitis C viremia [11–15]. This attention is likely to continue to expand as more treatments without interferon are approved over the next few years.

Along with the expanding pharmacotherapy for hepatitis C, there has come the recommendation for expanded screening for hepatitis C [16–21]. The CDC has advocated for universal screening for hepatitis C for all Americans born between 1945 and 1964. This change in the screening guidelines stems from the fact that chronic hepatitis C infection can now be treated by several highly efficacious therapies [22, 23]. An important factor of these new treatment agents is their cost, ranging from 20 to 80 thousand dollars per treatment attempt [24]. Given the high cost of treatment, many third-party payers currently triage their patients based on the extent of liver disease and the likelihood of death from hepatitis C related illness. Knowledge of the natural history of hepatitis C in patients with substance use disorders can aid in the complex decision of who and when to treat. People who inject drugs have a heavy burden of chronic hepatitis C as a population, due to the viral mode of transmission, and are also known to have a higher risk of early mortality than the general population. The relative contribution of chronic hepatitis C infection in this population, compared to the contribution of other dangers such as overdose, suicide and homicide, is still not fully known [25]. Our study offers a prospective examination of this question.

In 1993, an early report on the prevalence of viral hepatitis C among alcohol and drug users showed the correlation of anti-HCV positivity with elevated liver enzymes in that population [1]. The cohort was found to have a hepatitis C antibody prevalence of 63 % overall, and 86 % for those who reported ever using an illicit drug by injection. The arrival of the twenty-year anniversary of this study prompted us to investigate the 20-year all-cause mortality of the cohort, with specific attention to the presence or absence of anti-HCV positivity in 1991. In this study, we look at mortality of a subset of the original cohort, with a focus on whether or not hepatitis C infection was associated with higher mortality.

Methods

The original study was conducted on the Chemical Dependence Unit at Johns Hopkins Bayview Medical Center (then Francis Scott Key Medical Center), in Baltimore, Maryland, between November 1990 and May 1991. Then and now, the unit has 26 inpatient beds and serves a mostly indigent population in the city of Baltimore. Consecutive admissions were entered into the study. All patients met criteria for substance dependence. Demographic data were recorded and patient history related to substance use disorder, HIV infection, hepatitis and sexually transmitted infections was obtained. On admission to the unit, patients had blood testing which included tests for AST, ALT, hepatitis B surface antigen, hepatitis B surface antibody and rapid plasma regain (RPR) test for syphilis. All patients were offered HIV testing. The presence of hepatitis C antibody (anti-HCV) was determined by a first generation enzyme linked immunosorbent assay (Abbott Laboratories, Abbott Park, Illinois) that detects antibody to the C100-3 antigen. All positive serum samples were retested. Assays for hepatitis B were performed by enzyme immunoassay (Abbott Laboratories). The presence of HIV antibody was determined by an enzyme linked immunosorbent assay (Genetic Systems, Seattle, Washington) and all positive samples were confirmed by Western blot (Dupont Laboratories, Wilmington, Delaware).

Records from January 1991–May 1991 were located and 444 records were obtained. The Social Security Death Index was accessed to determine whether or not patients had died during the 20 years period since the date of admission. Causes of death were not determined. Prior to proceeding, anti-HCV status was chosen as a variable of interest in the data analysis. An initial bivariate analysis was performed on the mortality groups, using Chi-squared or Fisher's Exact tests for categorical variables and independent groups t tests for continuous variables, with significance levels set at $p < 0.05$ using STATA 12.1. Anti-HCV status was then included in a regression analysis with all variables for which the mortality group comparison yielded p values of 0.1 or less. Sex, race, age, history of STD, and histories of alcohol, cocaine and methadone use were found to have p values of 0.1 or less and were therefore included in the analysis. Using SPSS, odds ratios and confidence intervals for each of these variables were obtained. A binary logistic regression was then performed, which generated adjusted odds ratios for each of these variables. Attributes of the anti-HCV positive and anti-HCV negative cohorts were compared, using a Chi squared test in SPSS for categorical variables, and an independent group t test for age. As a final step, a time-to-event plot was created, and the cumulative hazard function was calculated in SPSS, using death dates from the social security death index. This study was approved by the Johns Hopkins Institutional Review Board.

Results

The baseline demographics for the 20-year study cohort are shown in Table 1. There were 288 men and 156 women. The majority were African American (63 %). Of

Table 1 Baseline demographics of cohort analyzed at 20 years

	Number	%
Number of patients	444	
Mean age in 1991	33.7	SD 7.86
Gender		
Male	288	65
Female	156	35
Race		
White	118	19
Black	325	63
Hispanic	1	0.2
History IDU	301	68
Drugs of abuse		
Alcohol	300	68
Cocaine	315	71
Heroin	284	64
Methadone	39	9
Benzodiazepines	80	18
Marijuana	110	25
History of STD	175	39
HCV positive	284	64
HepBSAg positive	14	3
HepBSAb positive	142	32
HIV status		
HIV positive	46	10
HIV negative	149	34
HIV not tested	249	56
RPR positive	29	7

the 444 patients, 284 (63 %) were anti-HCV positive in 1991. A history of cocaine use and heroin use was correlated with anti-HCV positivity in 1991. These results are described in the initial study and the subgroups of the found-records are presented in Table 1 [1].

The results of the query of the Social Security Death Index are presented in Table 2, which compares the attributes of 20-year survivors to non-survivors. After 20 years, 82 of the 444 study participants were found to be deceased (18 %). The remaining patients were presumed to be alive. The mean ages of 20-year survivors and non-survivors in 1991 were 32.8 and 37.9, respectively (p < 0.001). Male patients had higher mortality than female patients, (23 vs. 10 %, p = 0.001) and white patients in the cohort had greater mortality than black patients (30 vs. 14 %, p < 0.001). Alcohol use (21 vs. 13 %, p = 0.05) and illicit methadone use (31 vs. 17 %, p = 0.04) in 1991 were more weakly associated with death at 20 years. Surprisingly, a history of sexually transmitted disease was more common among survivors.

Hepatitis C antibody status from 1991 was compared between 20-year survivors and non-survivors. Patients who were anti-HCV positive in 1991 had a 20 % mortality, while anti-HCV negative patients had a 16 % mortality. This difference was not statistically significant (p = 0.37), and is illustrated in Fig. 1a. These data are then shown in Fig. 1b in comparison with the expected survivorship of the US general population of the same age, using data from the 1993 CDC death table [26]. Hepatitis B surface antigen positivity and hepatitis B surface antibody positivity were also not associated with mortality differences, but sample sizes may have been too small in some cases to provide adequate power for the comparisons. Liver enzymes were recorded in the initial study in three ranges. Those with lower liver enzymes in 1991 had a slightly greater chance of survival, but this too did not reach statistical significance.

The HCV negative and HCV positive cohorts are compared in Table 3, to look for potential confounding variables. HCV positive patients were more likely to have been male, to have used cocaine and to have used illicit methadone. HCV positive patients were also older, on average, although HCV negative patients had a greater distribution of ages, including the youngest and oldest in the study.

Factors associated with decreased 20-year survival are compared in Table 4, and their unadjusted odds ratios are shown. Results of a binary logistic regression are also included, and displayed as adjusted odds ratios. Male sex and a history of illicit methadone use remain statistically significant after regression analysis. Age also remains significant, with the odds of surviving decreasing slightly but significantly for each year of age of the individual at the start of the study. Again, hepatitis C positivity was not significantly associated with survival (OR 0.75, p = 0.29), and the non-significant association further diminished after binary logistic regression (AOR 0.87, p = 0.64).

In a time to event analysis, the survival curves for HCV positive and HCV negative patients were essentially superimposable. The log rank test performed on the curve confirmed that the difference in the curves was not statistically significant (p = 0.410) (Fig. 2).

Discussion

Our current study was remarkable for two findings. The first was the overall increased mortality rate of this cohort of patients with substance use disorders, as compared to that of the general population. The second finding was the lack of a statistical difference in mortality between those who were HCV positive in 1991, and those who were HCV negative at that time.

A query of the 1993 CDC mortality table shows that about 5000 out of 97,000 people aged 30–35 would

Table 2 Mortality at 20 years, by subgroup

Demographic	Alive	Deceased	% deceased, %	P
Totals	362	82	18	
Age mean, years	32.8	37.9		<0.0001
Gender				
M	222	66	23	
F	140	16	10	0.001
Race*				
White	83	35	30	
Black	278	47	14	0.001
Hx IDU				
Yes	244	57	19	
No	118	25	17	0.72
Drugs of abuse				
Alcohol				
Yes	237	63	21	
No	125	19	13	0.05
Cocaine				
Yes	263	52	17	
No	99	30	23	0.1
Heroin				
Yes	233	51	18	
No	129	31	19	0.71
Methadone				
Yes	27	12	31	
No	335	70	17	0.04
Benzodiazepines				
Yes	61	19	24	
No	301	63	17	0.18
Marijuana				
Yes	90	20	18	
No	272	62	19	0.93
Hx STD				
Yes	152	23	13	
No	210	59	22	0.02
Hep C Ab				
Positive	228	56	20	
Negative	134	26	16	0.37
Hep BSAg				
Positive	10	4	29	
Negative	352	78	18	0.32
HepBSab				
Positive	115	27	19	
Negative	247	55	18	0.84
HIV				
Positive	23	7	23	
Negative*	339	74	18	0.46
RPR				
Positive	23	29	56	
Negative	339	415	55	0.75
AST				

Table 2 continued

Demographic	Alive	Deceased	% deceased, %	P
<31	210	39	16	
>31 and <60	86	23	21	0.21
>60	66	20	23	
ALT				
<31	193	39	17	
>31 and <60	91	23	20	0.64
>60	78	20	20	

have been expected to die in 20 years, a death rate of 5.1 % [26]. Our observed death rate in the study population was 18.4 %, indicating that the mortality rate of our cohort of patients with substance use disorders was substantially higher than that of the general US population. Our results are concordant with previous studies showing premature death rates among patients with injection drug use [25]. Of the drugs studied, only illicit methadone use appeared to decrease survival. Cocaine use made hepatitis C positivity more likely, but in concord with prior studies, showed no effect on survival [27].

The presence of the anti-HCV antibody in 1991 did not lead to a statistically significant increase in the 20-year mortality within this cohort. While our study did not have sufficient power to detect a small effect size, ample power was present for moderate or large effect sizes. It is therefore reasonable to conclude that the impact of hepatitis C infection on mortality, if present, was small. This study did not account for morbidity, so it is unknown whether cohort members were living with compensated or decompensated cirrhosis, or experienced other negative effects on their quality of life.

Our comparison of the attributes of the hepatitis C negative and hepatitis C positive cohorts shows that the hepatits C positive patients were more likely to have been male, to be older, and to have used illicit methadone, three factors which we would expect to make them more likely to die, given the data from this study. These attributes of the hepatitis C positive cohort are probably responsible for the diminished association of HCV positivity and mortality after the regression analysis. The fact that hepatitis C positive patients were more likely to have used cocaine likely made little difference in their survival. The fact that illicit use of methadone was associated with decreased survival may have been incidental but may also be related to the medication's potential for respiratory depression and cardiac arrhythmias [28, 29]. Hazard from both of these factors may have been increased in patients using methadone outside of a supervised setting [30, 31].

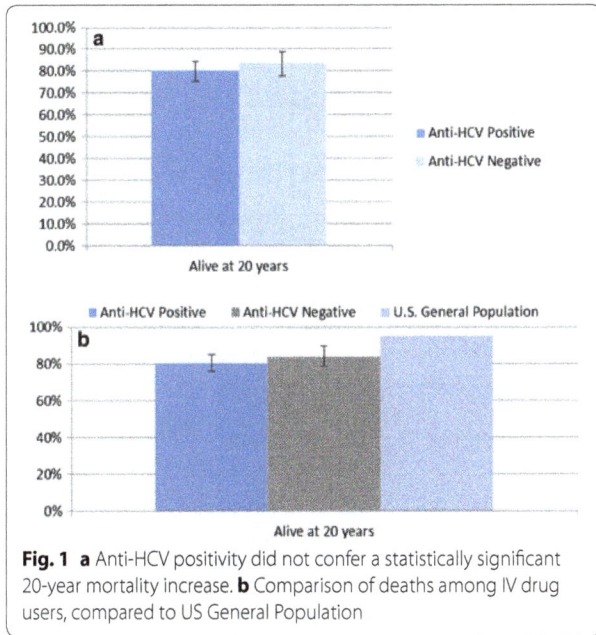

Fig. 1 a Anti-HCV positivity did not confer a statistically significant 20-year mortality increase. **b** Comparison of deaths among IV drug users, compared to US General Population

Table 3 Attributes of hepatitis C negative and positive cohorts

	HCV negative (%)	HCV positive (%)	Total	P value*
Female	70 (0.45)	86 (0.55)	156	0.004
Male	90 (0.31)	198 (0.69)	288	
Nonwhite	123 (0.38)	203 (0.62)	326	0.217
White	37 (0.31)	81 (0.69)	118	
No alcohol	51 (0.35)	93 (0.65)	144	0.851
Alcohol	109 (0.36)	191 (0.64)	300	
No cocaine	66 (0.51)	63 (0.49)	129	<0.001
Cocaine	94 (0.3)	221 (0.7)	315	
No illicit methadone	152 (0.38)	253 (0.62)	405	0.034
Illicit methadone	8 (0.21)	31 (0.79)	39	
Did not report STD History	94 (0.35)	175 (0.65)	269	0.552
Reported STD history	66 (0.38)	109 (0.62)	175	
Mean age (years)	32.48	34.43	N/A	0.028**

* p value computed by Chi-square analysis

** p value computed by independent t test, equal variance not assumed

Previous studies that have examined the mortality of patients with active hepatitis C virus tend to show little impact on mortality early in the disease course. Grady, et al. found 10-year survivals to be similar between seronegative and seropositive patients for the first 10 years, and suggested divergence around 20 years [32]. Gibson et al., similarly only showed increases in liver-related deaths past the 20 year mark, while Grebely et al. show the effect more pronounced only in patients over 50 years of age [33, 34]. Kieland et al. similarly show no change in mortality until three decades out from infection, in patients with an age greater than 50 [35]. Lee et al. documented a substantially greater hepatitis-C associated mortality, although their study did not focus specifically on patients with substance use disorders [36]. Our study serves to validate the emerging trend that hepatitis C positivity among patients with substance use disorders does not manifest a mortality difference for at least the first 20 years, and demonstrates this trend within an urban population in the United States.

The impact of hepatitis C virus specifically on patients with substance use disorders was studied by Evans et al. in San Francisco, CA, in a manner very similar to the one that we employed [37]. Similar to our results, they demonstrated that intravenous drug use itself was a risk factor for higher mortality; hepatitis C positivity only showed a non-significant trend towards higher mortality. Larney et al. studied hepatitis C related mortality among veterans with opioid use disorder and found no difference in overall mortality, although hepatitis C patients were more likely to a have a liver-related cause of death [38]. In an international study of three large national medical systems, Aspinal et al. document that both drug overdose and all-cause liver mortality were important contributors to mortality among patients with hepatitis C infection [39]. Hayashi et al. did a prospective study of patients with intravenous drug use in Vancouver, and did not find any increased liver mortality in the absence of HIV [40]. Several studies do indicate that HIV/HCV co-infection hastens the progression of liver disease [41–43].

Our study had several limitations. Cause of death was unavailable from the social security death index that we queried. As such, we could not make inferences about the frequency of liver-related mortality. At the time of the study in 1991, HCV RNA tests were not yet commonplace, and as such, there was no way to know which of the anti-HCV positive patients in the cohort had experienced spontaneous clearance. It is reasonable to assume that this would have constituted 10–15 % of the group. Another important limitation of this study is the fact that the HIV status of 56 % of the sample is unknown. Of those who were tested, 23 % were positive for HIV, making it a notable comorbidity within the cohort that could have accounted for some of its increased mortality rate as compared to the general population. Our study was also vulnerable to information bias, as it is possible that some of the cohort-members counted in the anti-HCV negative group may have contracted HCV over the 20 year period of the study. Conversely, some members of the anti-HCV positive group may have obtained HCV treatment. It is

Table 4 Regression analysis of hepatitis C viral status and factors associated with decreased 20-year survival

Factor	OR	CI (P value)	AOR	CI (P value)
Hepatitis C antibody (positive)	0.75	0.45–1.27 (0.29)	0.87	0.49–1.55 (0.64)
Sex (male)	0.39	0.22–0.71 (<0.01)	0.51	0.27–0.95 (0.03)
Age	0.93	0.31–0.96 (<0.01)	0.95	0.92–0.98 (<0.01)
Race (white)	0.39	0.24–0.64 (<0.01)	0.51	0.29–0.89 (0.02)
Alcohol use was present	0.58	0.33–1.02 (0.06)	0.76	0.41–1.4 (0.38)
Cocaine use was present	1.47	0.88–2.44 (0.14)	0.99	0.54–1.79 (0.96)
Illicit methadone use was present	0.46	0.22–0.96 (0.04)	0.46	0.21–0.99 (0.05)
History of sexually transmitted disease (true)	1.95	1.15–3.33 (0.01)	1.70	0.95–3.03 (0.07)

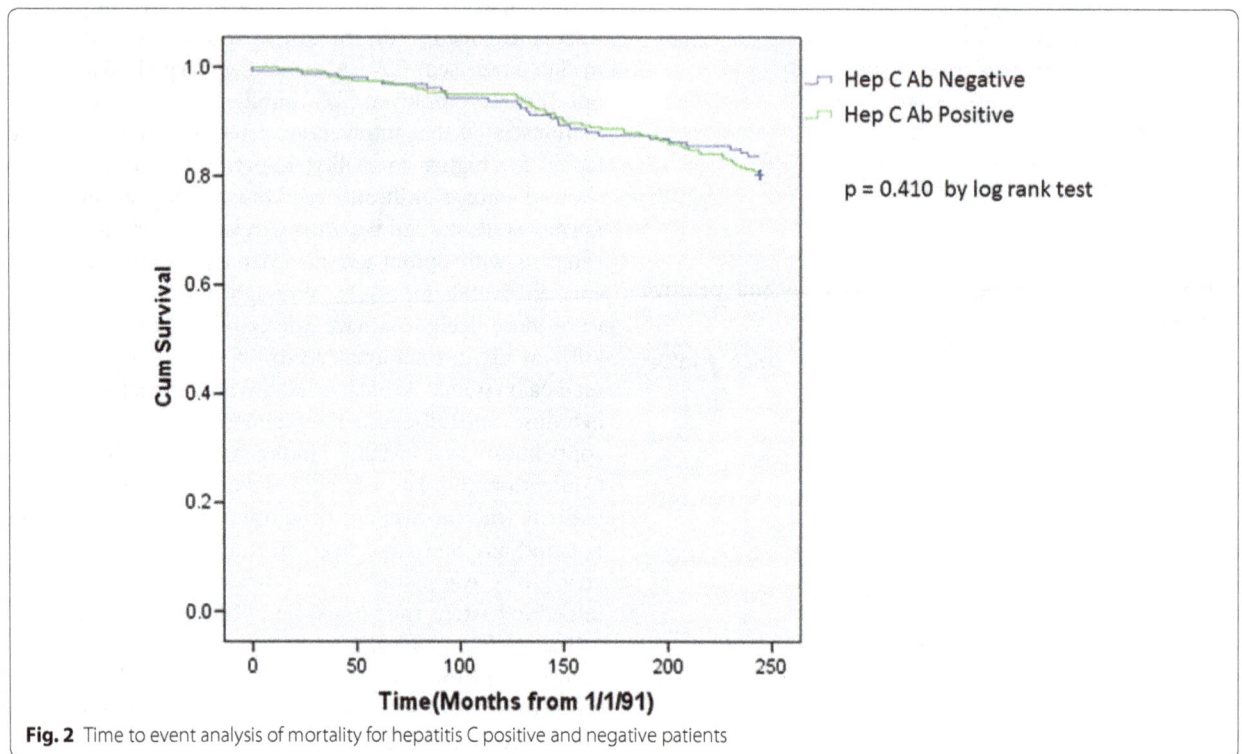

Fig. 2 Time to event analysis of mortality for hepatitis C positive and negative patients

also possible that some of the patients were deceased but not reported to the Social Security administration, but this should not bias the results.

Our study has implications for health policy-related questions. Current medical practice has begun to shift attention toward stewardship and the allocation of medical resources, with campaigns such as *Choosing Wisely* gaining increased popularity [44]. Given a system with limited financial resources, it may be reasonable to question which therapies would provide the greatest health benefit to patients with substance use disorders. The average cost per treatment episode for outpatient substance use disorder is $2000–7000 [45]. The cost of new

oral treatment for hepatitis C infection has been estimated at $84,000 per 12-week course of therapy [24]. Our study suggests that substance use disorders alone increase mortality, a finding that is consistent with prior research [46–48]. It does not, however, support the idea that hepatitis C virus was responsible for a significant fraction of that mortality. Although in a perfect system all patients would be treated for both, our study suggests that younger patients with substance use disorders may derive more mortality benefit from addiction treatment than they would derive from treatment of hepatitis C virus. This effect may shift over time as patients get older. Further research is necessary to establish which patients would be best served by treatment for one or both conditions.

Conclusions

Hepatitis C antibody positivity was not associated with a statistically significant change in 20 years mortality among a cohort of patients with substance use disorders within an urban setting. The overall mortality of the cohort was higher than that of the general population in both hepatitis C positive and hepatitis C negative patients. The relative effect of hepatitis C status on mortality, if present, is likely quite small in comparison to the effect of substance use disorder within the population studied.

Authors' contributions
AA is responsible for the majority of the writing and the creation of the tables and figures. MF was the author of the original study, the source of the patient data, and the originator of the study concept. DR gave specific feedback and oversight for data analysis in regard to the regression analysis and the adjusted odds ratios and aided greatly with revisions and edits. SG performed the initial statistical analysis. All authors read and approved the final manuscript.

Acknowledgements
All of the authors had full access to all of the data in the study. Anthony Accurso takes responsibility for the integrity of the data and the accuracy of the data analysis.

Competing interests
The authors declare that they have no competing interests.

Financial disclosures
None of the authors have any financial disclosures or conflicts of interest.

References
1. Fingerhood MI. Prevalence of hepatitis C in a chemically dependent population. Arch Intern Med. 1993;153:2025.
2. Thomas DL, Vlahov D, Solomon L, et al. Correlates of hepatitis C virus infections among injection drug users. Medicine (Baltimore). 1995;74:212–20.
3. Lorvick J, Kral AH, Seal K, Gee L, Edlin BR. Prevalence and duration of hepatitis C among injection drug users in San Francisco, Calif. Am J Public Health. 2001;91:46–7.
4. Garfein RS, Doherty MC, Monterroso ER, Thomas DL, Nelson KE, Vlahov D. Prevalence and incidence of hepatitis C virus infection among young adult injection drug users. J Acquir Immune Defic Syndr Hum Retrovirol. 1998;18(Suppl 1):S11–9.
5. Thomas DL, Astemborski J, Rai RM, et al. The natural history of hepatitis C virus infection: host, viral, and environmental factors. JAMA. 2000;284:450–6.
6. Alberti A, Chemello L, Benvegnu L. Natural history of hepatitis C. J Hepatol. 1999;31(Suppl 1):17–24.
7. Seeff LB. Natural history of chronic hepatitis C. Hepatology. 2002;36:S35–46.
8. Benhamou Y, Bochet M, Di Martino V, et al. Liver fibrosis progression in human immunodeficiency virus and hepatitis C virus coinfected patients. The multivirc group. Hepatology. 1999;30:1054–8.
9. Di Bisceglie AM, Martin P, Kassianides C, et al. Recombinant interferon alfa therapy for chronic hepatitis C. A randomized, double-blind, placebo-controlled trial. N Engl J Med. 1989;321:1506–10.
10. Davis GL, Balart LA, Schiff ER, et al. Treatment of chronic hepatitis C with recombinant interferon alfa. A multicenter randomized, controlled trial. Hepatitis interventional therapy group. N Engl J Med. 1989;321:1501–6.
11. Everson GT, Sims KD, Rodriguez-Torres M, et al. Efficacy of an interferon- and ribavirin-free regimen of daclatasvir, asunaprevir, and BMS-791325 in treatment-naive patients with HCV genotype 1 infection. Gastroenterology. 2014;146:420–9.
12. Kowdley KV, Lawitz E, Poordad F, et al. Phase 2b trial of interferon-free therapy for hepatitis C virus genotype 1. N Engl J Med. 2014;370:222–32.
13. Osinusi A, Meissner EG, Lee YJ, et al. Sofosbuvir and ribavirin for hepatitis C genotype 1 in patients with unfavorable treatment characteristics: a randomized clinical trial. JAMA. 2013;310:804–11.
14. Poordad F, Lawitz E, Kowdley KV, et al. Exploratory study of oral combination antiviral therapy for hepatitis C. N Engl J Med. 2013;368:45–53.
15. Zeuzem S, Soriano V, Asselah T, et al. Faldaprevir and deleobuvir for HCV genotype 1 infection. N Engl J Med. 2013;369:630–9.
16. Chou R, Cottrell EB, Wasson N, Rahman B, Guise JM. Screening for hepatitis C virus infection in adults: a systematic review for the U.S. preventive services task force. Ann Intern Med. 2013;158:101–8.
17. Moyer VA. U.S. Preventive Services Task Force. Screening for hepatitis C virus infection in adults: U.S. preventive services task force recommendation statement. Ann Intern Med. 2013;159:349–57.
18. Ngo-Metzger Q, Ward JW, Valdiserri RO. Expanded hepatitis C virus screening recommendations promote opportunities for care and cure. Ann Intern Med. 2013;159:364–5.
19. Smith BD, Morgan RL, Beckett GA, Falck-Ytter Y, Holtzman D, Ward JW. Hepatitis C virus testing of persons born during 1945–1965: recommendations from the centers for disease control and prevention. Ann Intern Med. 2012;157:817–22.
20. [Anonymous]. Summaries for patients: Screening for hepatitis C virus infection in adults: U.S. preventive services task force recommendation statement. Ann Intern Med. 2013; 159:I-32.
21. [Anonymous]. Summaries for patients. hepatitis C virus testing of persons born during 1945–1965: Recommendations from the centers for disease control and prevention. Ann Intern Med. 2012; 157:I-38.
22. Kowdley KV, Gordon SC, Reddy KR, et al. Ledipasvir and sofosbuvir for 8 or 12 weeks for chronic HCV without cirrhosis. N Engl J Med. 2014;370:1879–88.
23. Hezode C, Hirschfield GM, Ghesquiere W, et al. Daclatasvir plus peginterferon alfa and ribavirin for treatment-naive chronic hepatitis C genotype 1 or 4 infection: a randomised study. Gut. 2015;64:948–56.
24. Reau NS, Jensen DM. Sticker shock and the price of new therapies for hepatitis C: is it worth it? Hepatology. 2014;59:1246–9.
25. Smyth B, Hoffman V, Fan J, Hser YI. Years of potential life lost among heroin addicts 33 years after treatment. Prev Med. 2007;44:369–74.
26. CDC National Center for Health Statistics. 1993 ABRIDGED LIFE TABLE—TOTAL POPULATION. http://www.cdc.gov/nchs/data/statab/lewk1_93.pdf. Accessed 9 Dec 14.
27. Muhuri PK, Gfroerer JC. Mortality associated with illegal drug use among adults in the United States. Am J Drug Alcohol Abuse. 2011;37:155–64.
28. Fredheim OMS, et al. Clinical pharmacology of methadone for pain. Acta Anaesthesiol Scand. 2008;52:879–89.
29. Krantz MJ. QTc interval screening in methadone treatment. Ann Intern Med. 2009;150:387.
30. Bell JR, Butler B, Lawrance A, Batey R, Salmelainen P. Comparing overdose mortality associated with methadone and buprenorphine treatment. Drug Alcohol Depend. 2009;104:73–7.
31. Ray WA, Chung CP, Murray KT, Cooper WO, Hall K, Stein CM. Out-of-hospital mortality among patients receiving methadone for noncancer pain. JAMA Intern Med. 2015;175:420.
32. Grady B, van den Berg C, van der Helm J, et al. No impact of hepatitis C virus infection on mortality among drug users during the first decade after seroconversion. Clin Gastroenterol Hepatol. 2011;9(786–792):e1.
33. Gibson A, Randall D, Degenhardt L. The increasing mortality burden of liver disease among opioid-dependent people: Cohort study. Addiction. 2011;106:2186–92.
34. Grebely J, Raffa JD, Lai C, et al. Impact of hepatitis C virus infection on all-cause and liver-related mortality in a large community-based cohort of inner city residents. J Viral Hepat. 2011;18:32–41.

35. Kielland KB, Skaug K, Amundsen EJ, Dalgard O. All-cause and liver-related mortality in hepatitis C infected drug users followed for 33 years: a controlled study. J Hepatol. 2013;58:31–7.

36. Lee MH, Yang HI, Lu SN, et al. Chronic hepatitis C virus infection increases mortality from hepatic and extrahepatic diseases: a community-based long-term prospective study. J Infect Dis. 2012;206:469–77.

37. Evans JL, Tsui JI, Hahn JA, Davidson PJ, Lum PJ, Page K. Mortality among young injection drug users in San Francisco: a 10-year follow-up of the UFO study. Am J Epidemiol. 2012;175:302–8.

38. Larney S, Bohnert AS, Ganoczy D, et al. Mortality among older adults with opioid use disorders in the veteran's health administration, 2000–2011. Drug Alcohol Depend. 2015;147:32–7.

39. Aspinall EJ, Hutchinson SJ, Janjua NZ, et al. Trends in mortality after diagnosis of hepatitis C virus infection: an international comparison and implications for monitoring the population impact of treatment. J Hepatol. 2015;62:269–77.

40. Hayashi K, Milloy MJ, Wood E, Dong H, Montaner JS, Kerr T. Predictors of liver-related death among people who inject drugs in vancouver, canada: a 15-year prospective cohort study. J Int AIDS Soc. 2014;17:19296.

41. Fuster D, Cheng DM, Quinn EK, et al. Chronic hepatitis C virus infection is associated with all-cause and liver-related mortality in a cohort of HIV-infected patients with alcohol problems. Addiction. 2014;2013(109):62–70.

42. Hernando V, Perez-Cachafeiro S, Lewden C, et al. All-cause and liver-related mortality in HIV positive subjects compared to the general population: differences by HCV co-infection. J Hepatol. 2012;57:743–75.

43. Klein MB, Rollet-Kurhajec KC, Moodie EE, et al. Mortality in HIV-hepatitis C co-infected patients in canada compared to the general canadian population (2003–2013). AIDS. 2014;28:1957–65.

44. Morden NE, Colla CH, Sequist TD, Rosenthal MB. Choosing wisely—the politics and economics of labeling low-value services. N Engl J Med. 2014;370:589–92.

45. French MT, Popovici I, Tapsell L. The economic costs of substance abuse treatment: Updated estimates and cost bands for program assessment and reimbursement. J Subst Abuse Treat. 2008;35:462–9.

46. Hser YI, Hoffman V, Grella CE, Anglin MD. A 33-year follow-up of narcotics addicts. Arch Gen Psychiatry. 2001;58:503–8.

47. Joe GW, Simpson DD. Mortality rates among opioid addicts in a longitudinal study. Am J Public Health. 1987;77(3):347–8.

48. Scott CK, Dennis ML, Laudet A, Funk RR, Simeone RS. Surviving drug addiction: the effect of treatment and abstinence on mortality. Am J Public Health. 2011;101:737–44.

11

Acceptability of a mobile health intervention to enhance HIV care coordination for patients with substance use disorders

Ryan P. Westergaard[1,7]* ⓘ, Andrew Genz[2], Kristen Panico[3], Pamela J. Surkan[4], Jeanne Keruly[5], Heidi E. Hutton[6], Larry W. Chang[5] and Gregory D. Kirk[2,5]

Abstract

Background: Persons living with HIV and substance use disorders face barriers to sustained engagement in medical care, leading to suboptimal antiretroviral treatment outcomes. Innovative mobile technology tools such as customizable smartphone applications have the potential to enhance existing care coordination programs, but have not been rigorously studied.

Methods: We developed and implemented a two-component intervention consisting of peer health navigation supported by a smartphone application conducting ecologic momentary assessment (EMA) of barriers to care and medication adherence. Patients with a history of antiretroviral treatment failure and substance use were recruited to participate in the 9-month pilot intervention. Three peer health navigators were trained to provide social and logistical support while participants re-engaged in HIV care. We assessed the acceptability of the intervention components using qualitative analysis of in-depth interviews conducted with study participants and peer navigators.

Results: Of 19 patients enrolled in the study, 17 participated for at least 2 months and 15 completed the entire 9-month study protocol. The acceptability of the peer navigation intervention was rated favorably by all participants interviewed, who felt that peer support was instrumental in helping them re-engage in HIV care. Participants also responded favorably to the smartphone application, but described its usefulness mostly as providing reminders to take medications and attend appointments, rather than as a facilitator of patient navigation.

Conclusions: Peer health navigation and smartphone-based EMA are acceptable approaches to facilitating engagement in HIV care for drug using populations. Future studies to evaluate the efficacy of this approach for improving long-term retention in care and antiretroviral treatment outcomes are warranted.

ClinicalTrials.gov Identifier NCT01941108; registered on September 4, 2013

Introduction

Background

The development of combination antiretroviral therapy (ART) has had a dramatic impact on the global rate of deaths due to HIV/AIDS. By the end of 2015, an estimated 15.8 million people were receiving ART globally, the large majority of whom reside in low and middle-income countries [1]. When taken consistently as part of a comprehensive package of medical care, ART is highly effective for preventing progression to AIDS and also reduces sexual transmission of HIV, making it a powerful prevention tool.

HIV care is a complex, life-long intervention that requires sustained engagement in care and high-levels of medication adherence in order to confer optimal benefit [2, 3]. These requirements can contribute to health disparities, whereby patients with range of vulnerabilities including mental illnesses, [4] substance use disorders [5] and other challenges [6–8] are less likely to achieve

*Correspondence: rpw@medicine.wisc.edu
[7] University of Wisconsin-Madison, 1685 Highland Ave, MFCB 5223, Madison, WI 53705-2281, USA
Full list of author information is available at the end of the article

HIV viral suppression. In large cohort studies, people who inject drugs have been demonstrated to have inferior virologic outcomes and higher mortality than other patients receiving ART [9]. To ensure maximal benefit for these populations, social support and/or care coordination strategies are needed to address the specific barriers encountered by people who use drugs when they receive HIV care.

The determinants of poor engagement in HIV care among people who use drugs are heterogeneous and complex. Improving HIV care therefore requires interventions that are individually tailored and flexible. An example of such a strategy is case management, which has been adopted in many HIV care settings as a means to coordinate care for patients with psychosocial needs [10]. Case management, while demonstrated to be effective linking patients to needed services and support, [11] is typically *clinic-based*, and therefore may have limited impact for the most highly marginalized patients who have difficulty attending clinic appointments. Patient navigation, an alternative care coordination strategy developed in cancer care settings, provides comparable support using staff who are often para-professional, peer, or lay health workers. Patient navigators are frequently *community-based*, and therefore may be able to provide individualized support in the context of patients' daily lives, rather than primarily inside clinic environments [12].

While more flexible and responsive than traditional case managers, patient navigators typically support a relatively small number of clients, a limitation that may reduce the affordability and scalability of this approach in resource-limited settings. A recent randomized trial showed that patient navigation improved short-term HIV treatment outcomes for hospitalized patients with substance use disorders, but failed to show a significant benefit compared to treatment as usual after 1 year of follow-up [13]. Strategies to improve the efficiency and geographic reach of patient navigators could strengthen their impact on populations at high risk for poor treatment outcomes.

Electronic health (eHealth) and mobile health (mHealth) tools hold promise to move these efforts forward. Mobile phone ownership and use has expanded among people in all income strata [14], including those affected by substance abuse [15] and mental illness, [16] suggesting that mHealth interventions may be increasingly feasible among marginalized groups. Our team's prior work showed that individuals who report daily drug use are willing to adhere to research protocols involving frequent use of electronic diaries or smartphones for reporting symptoms and responding to surveys [17–19]. Trials of longer-term mHealth interventions have shown

benefit for reducing unhealthy alcohol use, [20] and are currently underway to evaluate effectiveness for reducing relapse among individuals with opioid use disorder [21]. Pilot feasibility studies of smartphone applications for self-monitoring of risk behaviors [22] and antiretroviral treatment adherence [23] among HIV-infected substance users have been completed, but larger studies are needed to determine their effectiveness for improving HIV treatment outcomes.

Study objectives

mPeer2Peer was a two-component intervention that used a smartphone application and patient navigation delivered by peer health workers ("peer navigators") to support HIV treatment for patients who had been marginally engaged in care. Peer navigators were trained to deliver intensive psychosocial and logistical support for patients with substance use and other barriers to HIV care. Both patients and peer navigators used a smartphone-based mHealth application, which was developed specifically for this study as a means to enhance communication and enable timely, individually tailored support interventions.

This study targeted patients with past or current illicit drug use, whom our prior research has shown to experience frequent lapses in HIV care [24]. Specifically, we aimed to recruit adult patients who were aware of their HIV status, had been linked to HIV care and were prescribed ART, but had not successfully achieved viral suppression. In this paper, we describe the development, implementation and acceptability of the mPeer2Peer intervention, and then discuss implications of the findings from this pilot study to the development of future, larger-scale clinical trials in this population.

Methods
Study setting

This study was conducted in Baltimore, Maryland, a city located in the Mid-Atlantic United States with a population of 620,000 and an HIV prevalence of 2377 per 100,000. Over 50% of people diagnosed with HIV in Baltimore report a history of injection drug use, a percentage substantially higher than the general HIV-infected US population [25]. The main clinical site for the study was the Johns Hopkins Moore Clinic, an academic HIV clinical practice serving approximately 2000 patients annually [26]. The mPeer2Peer study protocol was nested within the AIDS Linked to the IntraVenous Experience (ALIVE) study, an ongoing, NIH-funded observational cohort of current and former injection drug users [27].

Study population

Current and former patients of the Moore Clinic were eligible for mPeer2Peer if they were older than 18, had an

HIV viral load greater than 1000 copies/mL, attended no clinic visits with an HIV care provider in the preceding six months, and were willing to attend at least one HIV care visit at the Moore Clinic after enrollment. A formal diagnosis of substance use disorder was an inclusion criterion in the original study protocol, but this requirement was removed mid-study because of difficulty meeting recruitment goals. Exclusion criteria were any medical or psychiatric conditions that would interfere with the participant's ability to comply with study procedures (e.g., eyesight conditions that would make it difficult to read the smartphone screen) and concurrent participation in other studies focusing on retention in HIV care. Active drug use was not an exclusion criterion.

Intervention development

The mPeer2Peer intervention featured two components, mHealth and peer navigation, which were based on the situated Information, Motivation and Behavioral Skills (sIMB) model of care initiation and maintenance [28]. In this theoretical framework, relevant information, motivation, and behavioral skills interact to determine engagement in care and HIV-related behaviors and outcomes. In the context of this study, the IMB model is influenced by moderating patient and peer factors, as well as structural/health systems and clinical domains, as illustrated in Fig. 1.

The peer navigation intervention was adapted from procedures implemented in a large, multi-site HIV Prevention Trials Network study (HPTN 061), the methods of which have been described previously [29]. The specific duties of the peer navigator were to evaluate patients' barriers to engagement in HIV care and antiretroviral medication adherence and provide individually tailored support [30]. Three peer navigators were hired who were familiar with the communities in East Baltimore where participants lived, and had experience assisting patients access and utilize health care and social services. All patient navigators received training related to the study procedures, the mHealth application, and basic counseling strategies based on motivational interviewing. Peer navigators were expected to meet face to face with participants in the intervention group at least twice during the first month after enrollment, and interacted with participants in person or via phone calls and text messages on an as needed-basis thereafter.

The different components of the mHealth intervention are illustrated in Fig. 2. Intervention group participants and peer navigators each received a smartphone running the Android operating system. The research budget provided for service plans allowing unlimited voice, text and mobile data service throughout the study. Participant data entered at the baseline study encounter and updated regularly by the patient and peer navigator was stored on an encrypted server, which could be accessed and edited via smartphone or using an internet-based application ("dashboard") by peer navigators. The participant interface of the mHealth application consisted

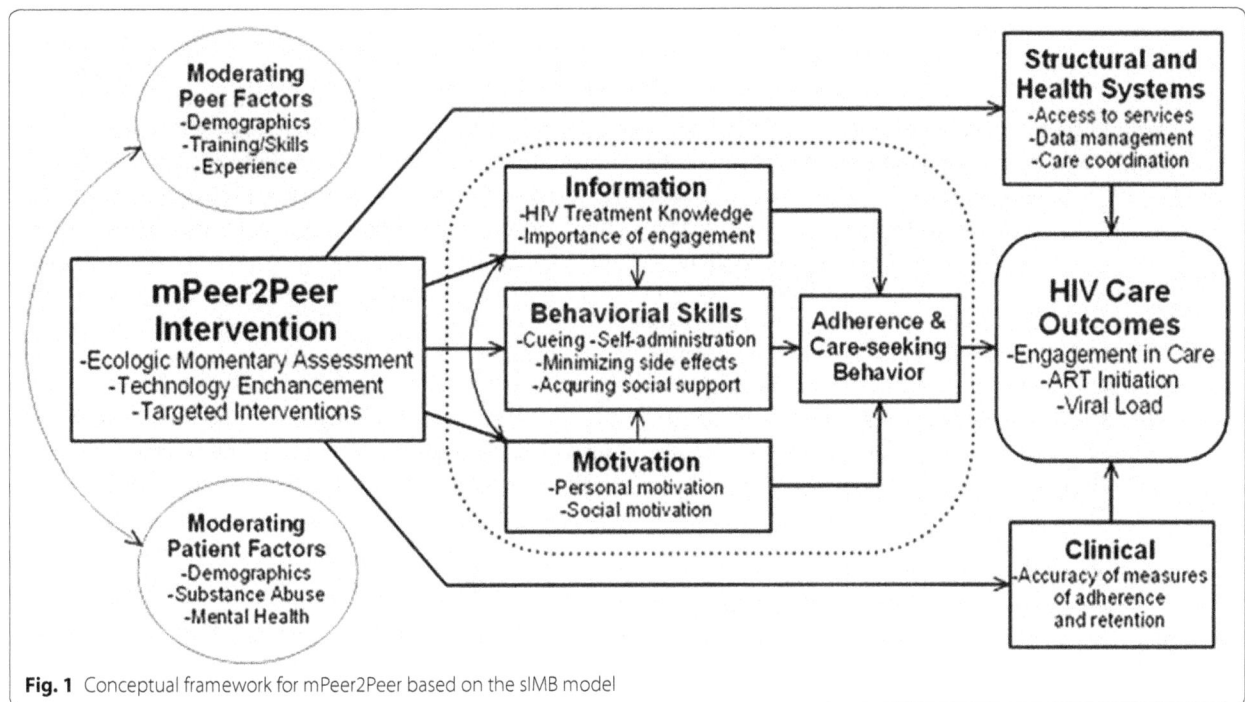

Fig. 1 Conceptual framework for mPeer2Peer based on the sIMB model

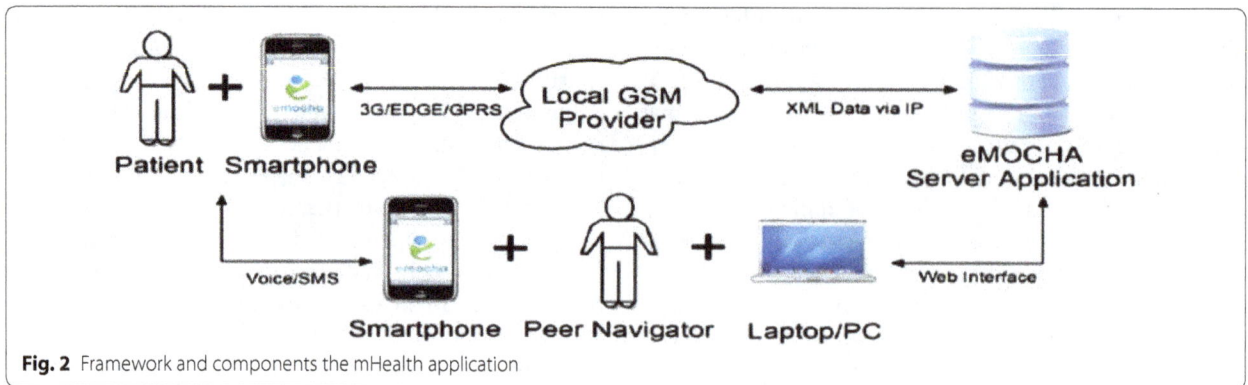
Fig. 2 Framework and components the mHealth application

of a password-protected, personalized HIV care summary screen, which displayed updated information about upcoming clinic appointments, recent laboratory results, and contact information for clinic staff on their care team. Participants also had the option of inserting text describing their personal goals or brief motivating statements to be displayed on the summary screen every time the application was launched.

Ecological momentary assessment

Ecological momentary assessment (EMA) is a method of studying target behaviors and their antecedents by collecting data from research subjects in real time, typically through the use smartphones or other types of electronic diaries. The smartphone application prompted participants to complete brief surveys via the smartphone interface twice daily. One prompt was delivered at a random time of day between 9:00 a.m. and 9:00 p.m. and the second prompt occurred at the end of the day, typically between 9:00 and 10:00 p.m. The precise schedule of prompts could be modified based on participant preferences. The dual purposes of the prompts were (1) to provide reminders about adherence to medications and HIV care visits, and (2) to briefly assess symptoms or behaviors that pose potential threats to ongoing engagement in care, thereby facilitating brief message-based interventions or peer navigator contact. Care engagement surveys were tailored to each participant's schedule of upcoming appointments using pre-defined algorithms and data fields populated by participants' responses to prior surveys, and included assessments of medication adherence specific to each participant's prescribed regimen.

Other variables assessed via daily surveys included craving for drugs or alcohol, use of drugs or alcohol, and mood states. Mood was assessed weekly using the Profile of Mood States-Short Form (POMS-SF) [31], and daily using an abbreviated version of POMS-SF that was limited to symptoms of depression, anxiety, irritability and

exhaustion. Under the supervision of the research team and a clinical psychologist, peer navigators reviewed participant-generated data using the web-based interface. Concerning patterns of survey responses related to drug use (e.g. relapsing heroin use after a period of sobriety), or sustained high levels of negative mood states would serve as a trigger for a peer navigator to initiate contact with participants and offer support and linkage to needed services, as appropriate.

Recruitment and enrollment

A pool of potentially eligible patients was generated using the electronic health records system of the Moore Clinic as part of a clinic-wide initiative to identify and re-engage patients who had lapsed in their HIV care. The mPeer2Peer study inclusion criteria served as the basis of the query, which was conducted using Epic Systems software (Epic Systems Corp., Verona, WI). Clinic staff contacted patients by phone using the contact information contained in their medical records. Patients meeting eligibility criteria who expressed willingness to re-engage in care were invited to meet with the study coordinator in a private off-site research office. After providing demographic and locator data, consenting participants were randomized in equal proportions to receive either (1) usual care or (2) the mPeer2Peer intervention. The experiences of the intervention participants are presented here; a forthcoming manuscript will describe the control group participants and the results from the pilot intervention trial. Participants assigned to the intervention were loaned a smartphone and provided with standardized training on how to use the mHealth application. Afterwards, the study coordinator facilitated a face-to-face meeting between participants and their peer navigator, which typically occurred on the same day as the baseline study visit.

Participants received remuneration in the amount of $25 for completion of the baseline study visit and for each of 3 follow-up study assessments scheduled at 3, 6, and 9 months after enrollment. Additional incentives of $2 per week was offered for responding to 60% or more of their EMA prompts and $5 per week for responding to at least 80% of their EMA prompts. If a participant lost a study smartphone, one replacement device would be dispensed. As a deterrent to device loss, intervention participants received $100 if they returned their original smartphone device at the end of the study and $50 for returning a replacement device. Participants were informed at enrollment that loss of two study devices would result in their dismissal from the study.

Qualitative evaluation

Acceptability of the intervention was evaluated with one-on-one, in-depth interviews with the first 12 study participants and the 3 peer navigators. Interviews were digitally recorded and professionally transcribed for qualitative analysis by an interdisciplinary research team. Semi-structured interview guides were designed to elicit perceptions about the usefulness of each intervention component, specific needs met by the intervention, and the ease of use of the smartphone application. Interview transcripts were imported into Atlas.ti, a software program for managing and analyzing qualitative data (ATLAS.ti:. Version 7. Statistical Software. (2012) Berlin, Germany: Scientific Software Development). Qualitative data analysis was based on thematic analysis, which aimed to discover themes, as defined as patterns of responses or meaning within the data, through a process of coding, analysis, and thematic mapping [32]. A preliminary codebook was developed based on topics addressed in the interview guides. One of the authors independently coded the transcripts and results were summarized and shared among investigators as a written report after the conclusion of the intervention period.

Results

Between September 2013 and November 2014, 19 individuals were enrolled and randomly assigned to receive the mPeer2Peer intervention. The baseline characteristics of the intervention recipients are shown in Table 1. The study sample was reflective of the population living with HIV in Baltimore, i.e., predominantly Black, male, and low-income, with a median age of 49. 3 years. Most participants reported they were taking antiretroviral therapy at the time of enrollment, yet all but one had an HIV viral load greater than 1000 copies/mL.

Study retention and losses to follow-up

Of the 19 patients randomized into the intervention group, 15 (78.9%) were followed for the entire 9-month study period. Two participants were immediately lost to

Table 1 Baseline characteristics of intervention sample (N = 19)

Characteristic	N (%)
Sociodemographic variables	
Median age, years (IQR)	49.3 (45.0–54.6)
African American (%)	17 (89%)
Male (%)	12 (63%)
High school/GED (%)	14 (74%)
Ever married (%)	5 (26%)
Income, yearly < $5000 (%)	8 (42%)
In prison, ever (%)	9 (47%)
Homeless, ever (%)	5 (26%)
Substance use variables*	
Cigarette use (%)	14 (74%)
Alcohol use (%)	8 (42%)
Marijuana use (%)	10 (53%)
Cocaine use (%)	3 (15%)
Heroin use (%)	4 (26%)
Injecting drug use, any (%)	3 (16%)
Clinical variables†	
Prescribed ART at enrollment (%)	16 (84%)
Hepatitis C virus seropositive (%)	7 (37%)
Median CD4 (IQR)	171 (95–262)
CD4 < 200 cells/mcL (%)	10 (53%)
Median HIV viral Load (copies/mL) (IQR)	18,938 (3458–103,437)

* Represents self-reported exposure during the 6 months prior to enrollment. *IQR* Intra-quartile range, *GED* graduation equivalence degree, *ART* antiretroviral therapy

† From health records at time of enrollment

follow-up and had no contact with the study team after the enrollment visit; two others were lost to follow-up after month 2 and 6, respectively. Collectively, these 19 participants contributed 143 person-months of follow-up after enrollment.

Acceptability of intervention components

Of the 15 participants who completed the study, twelve were interviewed at the end of the study. Interviews elicited uniformly positive assessments of both intervention components, and reported that they found the intervention helpful for supporting their engagement in HIV care. All 12 rated the smartphone application as easy to use or very easy to use. One sixty-two year-old woman reported the system was somewhat difficult in the beginning because she had never used a smartphone before; by the end of the study she reported it was easy to use.

When asked to describe the unmet needs that were addressed by the mHealth application, the most common benefit reported by participants was that it provided reminders to take medications and attend appointments. Participants who described their daily lives as disorganized or chaotic indicated that prompts to complete EMA surveys helped them focus on their HIV care at times when they felt distracted by other sources of stress, as described by one participant as follows:

> "It was helping me stay a grip with things that was going on in my life, which was drugs, and it was a reminder because it would ask me, 'Did you use?' And I was able to say, 'No, no,' you know, so it did help me, especially with my appointments and what my goals was it did help.... I'm gonna miss that now. I just hope and pray that everything goes still smooth. I haven't missed an appointment since then." (Participant, 58 year-old woman)

Several participants expressed disappointment that they would no longer have access to the emocha application after their participation in the study ended. Several asked for assistance to find and download a freely available smartphone application that would allow them a way to continue to receive reminders.

> "They told me about the app and it was a free download and I downloaded it on my regular phone. 'Cause I liked it so much. It just it doesn't feed into your database.... 'cause it's a whole different app itself. But I did set up a reminder for it." (Participant, 48 year-old man)

Participants expressed the belief that the intervention would be beneficial for other patients facing similar challenges, and even felt that their experience in the study would empower them to provide support for other patients.

> "By me helping myself I will help others, because I had some associates that was dealing with stuff by not being compliant, and I had this phone. It was like, 'How can I get in this program? Because I need something.' Because they go through a lot throughout the day and you forget, like I forgot things today. So having that phone, that reminder is so good. It was so good." (Participant, 37 year-old man)

The peer navigation intervention component was also very well-received by participants, who strongly believed that the social support they received facilitated their engagement in HIV care. As described by participants, the nature of the support provided by peer navigators appeared multi-faceted. Some participants valued the presence of a peer who is available to listen and provide encouragement in in a non-judgmental way, while at other times the peer navigator served as an advocate for their health care in a more direct way.

> "She's very smart, she works with you not against you, you know, and that's what I like about her...

they're the kind of people I like to have in my life." (Participant, 55 year old man)

> "[My Peer Navigator] is one of those people that you just know she's in your corner. [She] listened. She didn't judge. She didn't nag. She just listened to what you have to say." (Participant, 48 year old man)

> "I had to go in the hospital and she was right there. She walked it through everything that I needed. Thank God she was there because she helped the hospital process move along. So they wouldn't forget me in the emergency room where—I remember one time I was in there and they kept me on a bedpan for almost an hour and a half. And when [peer navigator] called and she said, "How's it going," and I told her, and before I knew it somebody was in that room. She's really helpful, and I appreciate it and I love her. That's my girl." (Participant, 58 year-old woman)

From the perspective of peer navigators, both intervention components appeared to provide important support for patients who had historically struggled to remain engaged in HIV care. The most frequently mentioned benefits perceived by peer navigators were their roles as a peer educator and as a source of support that mitigated against patients' experiences of depression and social isolation:

> "For some of them, some of their barriers were depression. So they just weren't self-motivated to do things. And just having me call them once a week to check in, just to have a conversation, and to show them other outlets of where they can go and talk to people was helpful too." (Peer-navigator, 36 year-old woman)

All 3 peer navigators interviewed agreed that EMA prompts served as medication reminders, which were important facilitators of improved antiretroviral adherence.

> "The navigation worked well. For most of them, the phone worked well. A lot of them more than anything appreciated the reminders. The appointment reminders and the take their medication [reminders] 'cause some of 'em just forget to take their meds." (Peer Navigator, 68 year-old woman)

Not clearly reflected in the interviews was the hoped-for impression that the mHealth application was *integrated* into the peer navigation intervention. Specifically, we did not observe that the data collected using EMA informed the peer navigators' activity on a regular basis. One of the peer navigators acknowledged how the content of the EMA surveys addressed more upstream determinants of medication adherence and overall engagement in HIV care, but perceived that the surveys were beneficial in their own right, rather than as a tool to improve her ability to support patients:

"The ones that suffered with mental health issues, depression mostly, they really liked the mood questions. It helped them gauge how they were feeling and it was a way of getting it out, you know what I mean, it was a way of expressing themselves, it made them feel a little bit better, even if it was temporary relief. (Peer Navigator, 36 year-old woman)

One of the three peer navigators described an instance in which data collected through an EMA survey informed her interactions with a participant in a meaningful way. The peer navigator, who periodically reviewed the EMA survey results of her clients, discovered that one had reported using drugs at a time she had previously believed he was in recovery. This provided an impetus to contact the participant by phone and discuss the issues surrounding his relapse, and to ensure the patient was continuing to take his medications and would attend his next clinic appointment. The other two peer navigators reported that they found it difficult to find time to log into the emocha server application to review participant data in real time, and did not find it to be a useful resource for their interactions with participants. Rather, they viewed the mHealth component as a distinct intervention that offered benefits that were different from peer navigation

"I know they liked the phone they did find it useful... they also appreciated more the human contact. Knowing somebody cared. Knowing that if I got an issue I can call this person up.

Discussion

In this pilot study, we implemented a novel mHealth-supported patient navigation intervention designed to improve HIV treatment utilization and outcomes among people with substance use disorders. Our findings suggest that people living with HIV in urban communities characterized by high levels of poverty and substance abuse find both intervention components acceptable and responsive to the types of barriers encountered when accessing HIV care.

Electronic health (eHealth) and mobile health (mHealth) strategies are new and potentially powerful approaches to coordinating complex, longitudinal medical care. Technology can empower patients, with direct delivery of individualized motivation, education, and support. Internet-based tools can facilitate communication among patients, providers, and supportive peers. Wireless technologies remove the barriers of time and distance between patients and providers. These advantages are especially important for substance-using patients and other populations that are hard to reach and difficult to keep engaged in care. Technology-based interventions may therefore serve as valuable adjuncts to case management and patient navigation programs, which deliver high-impact support but are expensive and challenging to disseminate on a large scale.

Our study adds to the growing literature suggesting that patient navigation and mHealth interventions are acceptable, client-centered strategies to improve engagement in health care. Patient navigation has been implemented among groups with shared experiences and challenges, such as HIV-positive women of color, [33], adults undergoing complex evaluations for cancer, [34] and persons leaving correctional facilities [35]. The high-level of acceptability of the smartphone intervention in this sample of older adults (i.e., half were older than 50) is notable. Social isolation is an important risk factor for adverse health outcomes among aging individuals living with HIV [36]. Prior research has suggested the benefits of mHealth and eHealth for improving care for chronic conditions are mediated by enhancement of social support [37, 38]. If true, this provides reason for optimism that the now ubiquitous opportunities or online social networking can be leveraged to fill unmet social support needs among people who are aging and have complex health needs.

Most participants endorsed the peer navigation intervention as a source of needed support, and believed that having a phone provided by the study facilitated their interactions with the peer navigators. Whether a standard mobile phone without the mHealth application would have served this purpose equally well is not clear. Some participants enjoyed receiving the EMA surveys, and even found the periodic monitoring of mood and drug cravings to be a source of support in and of itself. We did not find strong evidence that peer navigators reviewed and acted upon the EMA data provided by participants on a regular basis, which was one of rationales for developing this two-component intervention. This may reflect several limitations of our approach. For example, the internet-based dashboard did not display participants' EMA data in a way that was easy for peer navigators to visualize and interpret. While peer navigators had dedicated office space and internet access, the majority of their work was done outside of the clinic, and reviewing EMA data was not incorporated into their workflow on a consistent basis. Increasing the nature or intensity of peer navigator training and oversight may improve this aspect of the intervention, and should be explored in future projects of this type.

Other potential limitations of this study deserve mention. Based on the query of electronic health records, there were a number of patients who had lapsed in their HIV care who could not be contacted or were not willing to participate in the study. It is therefore possible that the participants in this study represent a subset of out-of-care patients who are more responsive to interventions such as mPeer2Peer, and that this approach may be less acceptable to patients with more intractable barriers to engagement in HIV care. Participants received modest financial incentives for responding to EMA surveys. While this was felt to be necessary to ensure the pilot study generated useful data, this approach may have biased participants' perceptions of the acceptability of the intervention. Whether adherence to the intervention protocol would be similar in routine practice settings as we observed in this research study is not known. A criticism of the mHealth field in general is that findings from small pilot studies have not been translated to larger scale projects that can make an impact on a population level [39].

Conclusions

This study demonstrates that interventions using patient navigation bundled with an mHealth application are feasible and acceptable to patients with substance use disorders who have failed to remain consistently engaged in HIV care in the past. Challenges highlighted by our research include the potential difficulty of integrating technology-based tools into the workflow of lay treatment supporters such as peer navigators. Additional research to inform implementation strategies, and ultimately to determine the efficacy of these interventions for improving engagement in HIV care and viral suppression, is warranted.

Abbreviations
HIV: human immunodeficiency virus; EMA: ecologic momentary assessment; ART: antiretroviral therapy; AIDS: acquired immunodeficiency syndrome; ALIVE: AIDS Linked to the IntraVenous Experience study; NIH: National Institutes of Health; sIMB: situated information, motivation, and behavioral skills model; GPS: global positioning systems; HPTN:: HIV Prevention Trials Network; POMS-SF: profile of mood states-short form; eHealth: electronic health; mHealth: mobile health.

Authors' contributions
RPW, LWC and GDK conceived of and designed the study. AG, JK, HEH oversaw conduct of the study intervention and were responsible for data collection. KP and PJS conducted interviews and conducted qualitative data analysis. RPW wrote the first draft of the manuscript and incorporated reviewers' comments into the final manuscript version. All authors read and approved the final manuscript.

Author details
[1] Department of Medicine, University of Wisconsin School of Medicine and Public Health, Madison, WI, USA. [2] Department of Epidemiology, Johns Hopkins Bloomberg School of Public Health, Baltimore, MD, USA. [3] Department of Population, Family and Reproductive Health, Johns Hopkins Bloomberg School of Public Health, Baltimore, MD, USA. [4] Department of International Health, Johns Hopkins Bloomberg School of Public Health, Baltimore, MD, USA. [5] Department of Medicine, Johns Hopkins School of Medicine, Baltimore, MD, USA. [6] Department of Psychiatry and Behavioral Sciences, Johns Hopkins School of Medicine, Baltimore, MD, USA. [7] University of Wisconsin-Madison, 1685 Highland Ave, MFCB 5223, Madison, WI 53705-2281, USA.

Acknowledgements
The authors are grateful to the patients, staff and providers at the Johns Hopkins Moore Clinic and the staff of the ALIVE Study, without whose support this study would not have been possible.

Competing interests
Larry Chang has a financial interest in emocha Mobile Health Inc., a company licensing an invention (emocha) from Johns Hopkins University which LC helped invent and is described in this publication. All other authors have no competing interests to declare.

Consent for publication
Written informed consent for publication of direct quotations was obtained from individual study participants at the time of enrollment.

Ethics approval and consent to participate
The study protocol was approved by the Institutional Review Board at the Johns Hopkins Bloomberg School of Public Health. A Certificate of Confidentiality was obtained through the National Institute on Drug Abuse.

Funding
This study was funded by the National Institutes of Health/National Institute on Drug Abuse Grants R34DA033181, U01DA036297 and K23DA032306. The funders had no role in the study design, data collection and analysis, decision to publish, or preparation of this manuscript. The article processing charge for this article was funded by the National Institute on Drug Abuse (NIDA), the National Drug Abuse Treatment Clinical Trials Network and the NIDA/SAMHSA Blending Initiative.

References
1. UNAIDS: UNAIDS fact sheet 2015. In Geneva: Joint United Nations Programme on HIV/AIDS (UNAIDS); http://www.unaids.org/sites/default/files/media_asset/20150901_FactSheet_2015_en.pdf. Archived at http://www.webcitation.org/6ehnTuiGs on 01/21/16; 2015.
2. Bangsberg DR, Hecht FM, Charlebois ED, Zolopa AR, Holodniy M, Sheiner L, Bamberger JD, Chesney MA, Moss A. Adherence to protease inhibitors, HIV-1 viral load, and development of drug resistance in an indigent population. AIDS. 2000;14(4):357–66.
3. Paterson DL, Swindells S, Mohr J, Brester M, Vergis EN, Squier C, Wagener MM, Singh N. Adherence to protease inhibitor therapy and outcomes in patients with HIV infection. Ann Intern Med. 2000;133(1):21–30.
4. Huang YF, Kuo HS, Lew-Ting CY, Tian F, Yang CH, Tsai TI, Gange SJ, Nelson KE. Mortality among a cohort of drug users after their release from prison: an evaluation of the effectiveness of a harm reduction program in Taiwan. Addiction. 2011;106(8):1437–45.
5. Nakimuli-Mpungu E, Bass JK, Alexandre P, Mills EJ, Musisi S, Ram M, Katabira E, Nachega JB. Depression, alcohol use and adherence to antiretroviral therapy in sub-Saharan Africa: a systematic review. AIDS Behav. 2012;16(8):2101–18.

6. Rachlis BS, Mills EJ, Cole DC. Livelihood security and adherence to antiretroviral therapy in low and middle income settings: a systematic review. PLoS One. 2011;6(5):e18948.

7. Leaver CA, Bargh G, Dunn JR, Hwang SW. The effects of housing status on health-related outcomes in people living with HIV: a systematic review of the literature. AIDS Behav. 2007;11(6 Suppl):85–100.

8. Singer AW, Weiser SD, McCoy SI. Does food insecurity undermine adherence to antiretroviral therapy? A systematic review. AIDS Behav. 2015;19(8):1510–26.

9. Samji H, Cescon A, Hogg RS, Modur SP, Althoff KN, Buchacz K, Burchell AN, Cohen M, Gebo KA, Gill MJ, et al. Closing the gap: increases in life expectancy among treated HIV-positive individuals in the United States and Canada. PLoS One. 2013;8(12):e81355.

10. Gardner LI, Metsch LR, Anderson-Mahoney P, Loughlin AM, del Rio C, Strathdee S, Sansom SL, Siegal HA, Greenberg AE, Holmberg SD. Efficacy of a brief case management intervention to link recently diagnosed HIV-infected persons to care. Aids. 2005;19(4):423–31.

11. Kushel MB, Colfax G, Ragland K, Heineman A, Palacio H, Bangsberg DR. Case management is associated with improved antiretroviral adherence and CD4 + cell counts in homeless and marginally housed individuals with HIV infection. Clin Infect Dis. 2006;43(2):234–42.

12. Bradford JB, Coleman S, Cunningham W. HIV system navigation: an emerging model to improve HIV care access. Aids Patient Care STDS. 2007;21(Suppl 1):S49–58.

13. Metsch LR, Feaster DJ, Gooden L, Matheson T, Stitzer M, Das M, Jain MK, Rodriguez AE, Armstrong WS, Lucas GM, et al. Effect of patient navigation with or without financial incentives on viral suppression among hospitalized patients with HIV infection and substance use: a randomized clinical trial. JAMA. 2016;316(2):156–70.

14. Pew Research Center: The smartphone difference. http://www.pewinternet.org/2015/04/01/us-smartphone-use-in-2015/. 2015.

15. Kirk GD, Himelhoch SS, Westergaard RP, Beckwith CG. Using mobile health technology to improve HIV care for persons living with HIV and substance abuse. AIDS Res Treat. 2013;2013:194613.

16. Naslund JA, Marsch LA, McHugo GJ, Bartels SJ. Emerging mHealth and eHealth interventions for serious mental illness: a review of the literature. J Ment Health. 2015;24(5):321–32.

17. Kirk GD, Linas BS, Westergaard RP, Piggott D, Bollinger RC, Chang LW, Genz A. The exposure assessment in current time study: implementation, feasibility, and acceptability of real-time data collection in a community cohort of illicit drug users. AIDS Res Treat. 2013;2013:594671. doi:10.1155/2013/594671.

18. Linas BS, Latkin C, Genz A, Westergaard RP, Chang LW, Bollinger RC, Kirk GD. Utilizing mHealth methods to identify patterns of high risk illicit drug use. Drug Alcohol Depend. 2015;151:250–7. doi:10.1016/j.drugalcdep.2015.03.031.

19. Linas BS, Latkin C, Westergaard RP, Chang LW, Bollinger RC, Genz A, Kirk GD. Capturing illicit drug use where and when it happens: an ecological momentary assessment of the social, physical and activity environment of using versus craving illicit drugs. Addiction. 2015;110(2):315–25.

20. Gustafson DH, McTavish FM, Chih MY, Atwood AK, Johnson RA, Boyle MG, Levy MS, Driscoll H, Chisholm SM, Dillenburg L, et al. A smartphone application to support recovery from alcoholism: a randomized clinical trial. JAMA Psychiatry. 2014;71(5):566–72.

21. Gustafson DH Sr, Landucci G, McTavish F, Kornfield R, Johnson RA, Mares ML, Westergaard RP, Quanbeck A, Alagoz E, Pe-Romashko K, et al. The effect of bundling medication-assisted treatment for opioid addiction with mHealth: study protocol for a randomized clinical trial. Trials. 2016;17(1):592.

22. Swendeman D, Ramanathan N, Baetscher L, Medich M, Scheffler A, Comulada WS, Estrin D. Smartphone self-monitoring to support self-management among people living with HIV: perceived benefits and theory of change from a mixed-methods randomized pilot study. J Acquir Immune Defic Syndr. 2015;69(Suppl 1):S80–91.

23. Himelhoch S, Kreyenbuhl J, Palmer-Bacon J, Chu M, Brown C, Potts W. Pilot feasibility study of Heart2HAART: a smartphone application to assist with adherence among substance users living with HIV. AIDS Care. 2017;1–7. doi:10.1080/09540121.2016.1259454.

24. Westergaard RP, Hess T, Astemborski J, Mehta SH, Kirk GD. Longitudinal changes in engagement in care and viral suppression for HIV-infected injection drug users. AIDS. 2013;27(16):2559–66.

25. Maryland Dept. of Health and Mental Hygiene. Baltimore City HIV/AIDS Epidemiological Profile. http://phpa.dhmh.maryland.gov/OIDEOR/CHSE/Shared%20Documents/Baltimore-City.pdf. Archived at http://www.webcitation.org/6ehosBQUE on 01/21/16. 2013.

26. Moore RD, Bartlett JG. Dramatic decline in the HIV-1 RNA level over calendar time in a large urban HIV practice. Clin Infect Dis. 2011;53(6):600–4.

27. Vlahov D, Anthony JC, Munoz A, Margolick J, Nelson KE, Celentano DD, Solomon L, Polk BF. The ALIVE study, a longitudinal study of HIV-1 infection in intravenous drug users: description of methods and characteristics of participants. NIDA Res Monogr. 1991;109:75–100.

28. Amico KR. A situated-information motivation behavioral skills model of care initiation and maintenance (sIMB-CIM): an IMB model based approach to understanding and intervening in engagement in care for chronic medical conditions. J Health Psychol. 2011;16(7):1071–81.

29. Magnus M, Franks J, Griffith S, Arnold MP, Goodman K, Wheeler DP. Engaging, recruiting, and retaining black men who have sex with men in research studies: don't underestimate the importance of staffing—lessons learned from HPTN 061, the BROTHERS study. J Public Health Manag Pract: JPHMP. 2014;20(6):E1–9.

30. HPTN 061 Study Group: HPTN 061 Peer Health Navigation Operations Manual. http://www.hptn.org/web%20documents/HPTN061/App_E_PHNOpsCombov2.0.pdf; Archived at http://www.webcitation.org/6eXGtWWGI on 01/14/16. 2009.

31. Curran SL, Andrykowski MA, Studts JL. Short form of the profile of mood states (POMS-SF): psychometric information. Psychol Assess. 1995;7(1):80–3.

32. Braun V, Clarke V. Using thematic analysis in psychology. Qual Res Psychol. 2006;3(2):77–101.

33. Sullivan KA, Schultz K, Ramaiya M, Berger M, Parnell H, Quinlivan EB. Experiences of women of color with a nurse patient navigation program for linkage and engagement in HIV care. AIDS Patient Care STDs. 2015;29(Suppl 1):S49–54.

34. Paskett ED, Katz ML, Post DM, Pennell ML, Young GS, Seiber EE, Harrop JP, DeGraffinreid CR, Tatum CM, Dean JA, et al. The Ohio patient navigation research program: does the american cancer society patient navigation model improve time to resolution in patients with abnormal screening tests? Cancer Epidemiol Biomarkers Prev. 2012;21(10):1620–8.

35. Koester KA, Morewitz M, Pearson C, Weeks J, Packard R, Estes M, Tulsky J, Kang-Dufour MS, Myers JJ. Patient navigation facilitates medical and social services engagement among HIV-infected individuals leaving jail and returning to the community. AIDS Patient Care STDS. 2014;28(2):82–90.

36. Greysen SR, Horwitz LI, Covinsky KE, Gordon K, Ohl ME, Justice AC. Does social isolation predict hospitalization and mortality among HIV + and uninfected older veterans? J Am Geriatr Soc. 2013;61(9):1456–63.

37. Gustafson D, Wise M, Bhattacharya A, Pulvermacher A, Shanovich K, Phillips B, Lehman E, Chinchilli V, Hawkins R, Kim JS. The effects of combining web-based eHealth with telephone nurse case management for pediatric asthma control: a randomized controlled trial. J Med Internet Res. 2012;14(4):e101.

38. Hull SJ, Abril EP, Shah DV, Choi M, Chih MY, Kim SC, Namkoong K, McTavish F, Gustafson DH. Self-determination theory and computer-mediated support: modeling effects on breast cancer patient's quality-of-life. Health Commun. 2016;31(10):1205–14.

39. Tomlinson M, Rotheram-Borus MJ, Swartz L, Tsai AC. Scaling up mHealth: where is the evidence? PLoS Med. 2013;10(2):e1001382.

12

Eligibility for heroin-assisted treatment (HAT) among people who inject opioids and are living with HIV in a Canadian setting

Jan Klimas[1,2,3] (iD), Huiru Dong[1], Nadia Fairbairn[1,3], Eugenia Socías[1,3], Rolando Barrios[1], Evan Wood[1,2], Thomas Kerr[1,2], Julio Montaner[1,2] and M.-J. Milloy[1,2]*

Abstract

Objectives: A growing body of evidence supports the effectiveness of injectable diacetylmorphine (i.e., heroin) for individuals with treatment-refractory opioid use disorder. Despite this evidence, and the increasing toll of opioid-associated morbidity and mortality, it remains controversial in some settings. To investigate the possible contribution of heroin-assisted treatment (HAT) to HIV treatment-related outcomes, we sought to estimate the proportion and characteristics of HIV-positive people who inject opioids that might be eligible for HAT in Vancouver, Canada.

Methods: We used data from a prospective cohort of people living with HIV who use illicit drugs in Vancouver, Canada. Using generalized estimating equations (GEE), we assessed the longitudinal relationships between eligibility for HAT, using criteria from previous clinical trials and guidelines, with behavioural, social, and clinical characteristics.

Results: Between 2005 and 2014, 478 participants were included in these analyses, contributing 1927 person-years of observation. Of those, 94 (19.7%) met eligibility for HAT at least once during the study period. In a multivariable GEE model, after adjusting for clinical characteristics, being eligible for HAT was positively associated with homelessness, female gender, high-intensity illicit drug use, drug dealing and higher CD4 count.

Conclusions: In our study of HIV-positive people with a history of injection drug use, approximately 20% of participants were eligible for HAT at ≥ 1 follow-up period. Eligibility was linked to risk factors for sub-optimal HIV/AIDS treatment outcomes, such as homelessness and involvement in the local illicit drug trade, suggesting that scaling-up access to HAT might contribute to achieving optimal HIV treatment in this setting.

Keywords: Substance-related disorders, Heroin, HIV/AIDS, Illicit drug use, Opioid agonist treatment

Background

A growing body of evidence, including findings from randomised controlled trials (RCT) in Europe and North America, and systematic reviews by the Cochrane Collaboration and others, supports the effectiveness of injectable diacetylmorphine (i.e., prescribed heroin) for treatment-refractory opioid use disorder [1–3]. Despite this support, heroin-assisted treatment (HAT) remains controversial and unavailable in most settings [4]. However, given the growing amount of evidence and the increasing toll of opioid-associated morbidity and mortality, efforts to develop guidance on injectable opioid agonist treatments for opioid use disorder, including medications that do not face the same regulatory barriers as diacetylmorphine (e.g., hydromorphone), are under way in some settings [5].

Medical management of people living with HIV (PLHIV), with co-occurring substance use disorder (SUD), poses many challenges. There remains low coverage of medically-proven treatment for SUD in many settings [6, 7]; furthermore, HIV-positive people who use illicit drugs (PWID) have not fully benefitted from scale-up of HIV testing and antiretroviral treatment (ART), a

*Correspondence: bccsu-mjsm@cfenet.ubc.ca
[1] British Columbia Centres on Substance Use and Excellence in HIV/AIDS, St. Paul's Hospital, 608-1081 Burrard Street, Vancouver, BC V6Z 1Y6, Canada
Full list of author information is available at the end of the article

strategy commonly referred to treatment-as-prevention (TasP), has resulted in reduced rates of HIV-associated morbidity, mortality and viral transmission [8]. As a result of sub-optimal HIV treatment outcomes and barriers to accessing harm reduction supplies, such as sterile syringes, HIV outbreaks among PWID are common and ongoing in many settings [9, 10].

Despite the demonstrated benefits of oral opioid agonist therapy (OAT, i.e. methadone, buprenorphine/naloxone) on reducing illicit opioid use and HIV risk behaviours and promoting optimal HIV treatment outcomes [11, 12], gaps in SUD treatment persist, especially for PWID living with HIV [6, 13]. The limitations of oral OAT are many and significant, specifically the attrition that has been shown to increase the mortality risk during the induction phase onto methadone treatment, during the first year and during the time immediately after leaving treatment.[ENTER REF SORDO] In this respect, several RCTs (e.g., NAOMI, SALOME) have demonstrated the potential benefits of HAT for people with treatment-refractory opioid use disorder, including decreased levels of used syringe sharing, reduced illicit drug use, criminal activity and increased engagement with healthcare [1–3, 14]. However, we are unaware of any study to explore the potential uptake of HAT in the HIV-positive population. Thus, we sought to estimate the prevalence and characteristics of HIV-positive individuals that might be eligible for HAT in Vancouver, Canada.

Methods

Data for these analyses were derived from a prospective cohort of people who use illicit drugs and live with HIV in Vancouver, Canada, the AIDS Care Cohort to evaluate Exposure to Survival Services (ACCESS), which has been described elsewhere [15–17]. In brief, ACCESS is a cohort of HIV-seropositive adults who have used at least one illicit drug (other than or in addition to cannabis) in the month prior to recruitment. Individuals are recruited from community settings via snowball sampling and outreach techniques. At baseline and each biannual follow-up interview, participants complete interviewer-administered questionnaires that assess sociodemographic, drug use and other related behaviours, characteristics, or exposures. This includes a nursing examination and phlebotomy for HIV clinical monitoring. In addition to the interview data, we also accessed linked (using a government-issued identifier, i.e., Personal Health Number—PHN) data from a comprehensive retrospective and prospective HIV clinical monitoring profile, including all plasma HIV-1 RNA viral loads, CD4 cell counts and records of all antiretroviral therapy (ART) dispensations, available from the Drug Treatment Program at the BC Centre for Excellence in HIV/AIDS

(BC-CfE), as described previously [18]. The BC-CfE is responsible for dispensing ART, provided at no charge, to all people living with HIV in the province. The records include all clinical measures conducted through the study or by a participant's physician or healthcare provider.

Participants are compensated at each study interview with a $30 CDN stipend. The University of British Columbia/Providence Healthcare Research Ethics Board approved the study and all participants provided written informed consent at baseline.

We included all participants who completed at least one study visit between December 1, 2005 and May 31, 2014 and who were older than 18 years old and reported ever injecting drugs at least once at the baseline interview. Our primary outcome of interest was being eligible for HAT as per the historical criteria from previous published RCTs [1–3], that defined HAT eligibility variably as: (a) currently residing in the study area (i.e., the city of Vancouver); (b) current regular injection of illicit opioids (i.e., $\geq$ one time in the previous 6 months); (c) at least two self-reported prior SUD treatment attempts, including one episode of OAT (i.e., methadone or buprenorphine/naloxone); (d) at least 5 years of illicit opioid use; and (e) poor health, or psychosocial functioning, defined as a self-reported mental health diagnosis. At each interview period of the present study, we determined if an individual was eligible for HAT during that period by evaluating each criterion using responses given to relevant interview questions, specifically: (a) current residence in the City of Vancouver; (b) $\geq$ weekly injection of an opioid (e.g., heroin, methadone, prescription opioids, etc.) in the last 6 months (yes vs. no); (c) number of times during the study period reporting being engaged in any SUD treatment and any OAT included if (1) positive response to at least two of the options, or at least two positive responses for "number of times in treatment" at baseline, including one MMT programme, or included if (2) participants reported at least two prior "attempts at treatment" over follow-up, defined as not being currently in treatment but treatment in the last 6 months ($\geq$ 2 vs. < 2); (d) number of years since initiation of illicit opioid use ($\geq$ 5 vs. < 5 years); and (e) reporting a mental health diagnosis (Have you been diagnosed with a mental health issue in the last 6 months? Yes vs. no), or baseline depression, as measured by the Center for Epidemiologic Studies Depression scale (CES-D) (score of $\geq$ 16 vs. score of < 16). Participants had to fulfill all the above criteria to be deemed eligible for HAT.

We also defined a number of explanatory variables, including: age (per year older); gender (male vs. non-male); Caucasian ethnicity/ancestry (yes vs. no); hepatitis C virus antibody status (positive vs. negative); number of years of using injection heroin at baseline; homelessness (yes vs. no); relationship status (legally married/common law/regular partner vs. other); highest level of education completed (≥ high school diploma vs. < high school diploma); formal employment (yes vs. no, i.e., regular job, temporary job, or self-employed); money spent on drugs per day (≥ \$50 per day vs. < \$50 per day); drug dealing (yes vs. no); ≥ daily non-injection cocaine use (yes vs. no); ≥ daily non-injection heroin use (yes vs. no); ≥ daily crack use (yes vs. no); ≥ daily methamphetamine use (yes vs. no); non-fatal overdose (yes vs. no); lent used syringe (yes vs. no); recent incarceration (yes vs. no); engagement in any form of unprotected sex (yes vs. no); exchange of sex for gifts, food, shelter, clothes, etc. (yes vs. no); being a victim of violence, defined as having been attacked or assaulted (yes vs. no) [19–21]. All time-updated variables refer to behaviours or exposures in the 6-month period prior to the study interview.

We also included the following data based on the confidential linkage (using PHN identifier) to the local HIV clinical monitoring registry and ART dispensary: HIV-1 RNA plasma viral load (VL), using the median of all observations in the previous 6 months or, if none, the most recent observation, dichotomised at > 50 versus ≤ 50 copies/mL; ART engagement, using the number of days of ART dispensed in the previous 6 months (dichotomized at ≥ 1 vs. 0 day); and CD4 cell count, using the median of all observations in the previous 6 months or, if none, the most recent observation (expressed per 100 cells/mL) [22].

As a first step, we described the study sample at baseline stratified by eligibility for HAT. We used Chi square test and Fisher's exact test to compare categorical variables and Wilcoxon's rank-sum test to compare continuous variables.

To evaluate the association between eligibility for HAT and each of the explanatory variables of interest, we built a statistical model, using generalised estimating equation (GEE), assuming a binomial distribution, a logit-link function and an exchangeable working correlation structure. We first build bivariable GEE to examine the association between being eligible for HAT and each of the explanatory variables. To fit the final multivariable model, we applied an a priori-defined backward model selection approach based on examination of quasilikelihood under the independence model criterion statistic (QIC). We first included all explanatory variables that were associated with the outcome at the level of $p < 0.10$ in bivariable analyses in a full model. From the QIC of the model, we excluded the variable with the largest p value and constructed a reduced model. We proceeded this iterative method and chose the multivariable model with the lowest QIC value [23]. All p values were two-sided.

All statistical analyses were performed using the SAS software version 9.4 (SAS, Cary, NC, USA).

Results

Between December 2005 and May 2014, 852 individuals were recruited into the cohort, of whom 478 (56.1%) participants satisfied all criteria, including age and injection drug use, and were included in the analysis. They contributed 3495 observations, or a median of 7 interviews [inter-quartile range (IQR): 3–11] during follow-up. Of those, 94 (19.7%) were deemed to be eligible for HAT at least once through study period: 32 reported eligible for once, 19 twice, 11 thrice, and 32 more than thrice. Baseline characteristics are reported in Table 1. As shown, most participants included in this analysis were Caucasian (273, 57.1%), males (321, 67.2%), with median age of 43.1 (IQR 36.7–47.9) years.

As shown in Table 2, the following variables were positively associated with being eligible for HAT: homelessness [adjusted odds ratio (AOR) 1.47; 95% confidence interval (CI) 1.07–2.01]; drug dealing in the last 6 months (AOR 1.76; 95% CI 1.33–2.31); ≥ daily non-injection heroin use (AOR 8.18; 95% CI 1.25–53.56); ≥ daily crack use (AOR1.35; 95% CI 1.01–1.82); and CD4 cell count (per 100 cells/mL increase, AOR 1.08; 95% CI 1.00–1.17). Male gender was negatively associated with the outcome (AOR 0.50; 95% CI 0.31–0.82).

Discussion

In this study to estimate the prevalence and characteristics of PLHIV who inject drugs that might be eligible for HAT, we observed that approximately one-fifth of all participants were eligible at least once during study follow-up. Periods of HAT eligibility were associated with important factors that have been linked with sub-optimal HIV treatment outcomes in previous studies, including markers of severe SUD, such as high-intensity illicit drug use, homelessness and drug dealing [3, 4, 17]. These associations signal that expanding HAT to this population might influence the factors linked with sub-optimal HIV treatment and improve HIV treatment outcomes, thus contributing to TasP goals [15]. Moreover, they provide further support for the potential role of HAT in decreasing opioid-associated morbidity and mortality.

The links between HAT eligibility and various drug-related (e.g., high-intensity illicit drug use and survival dealing as markers of severe SUD), and socio-structural determinants of health (e.g., homelessness), indicate that HAT-eligible individuals face numerous barriers to optimal HIV treatment outcomes, even in a setting where HIV treatment and care is delivered at no cost [16, 24]. Admittedly, HAT eligibility can impact markers of severe

Table 1 Baseline characteristics of participants who inject opioids and live with HIV in Vancouver, BC, stratified by the baseline HAT eligibility status

Characteristic	Total (%) (n = 478)	HAT eligibility		p value
		Yes (%) 45 (9.4)	No (%) 433 (90.6)	
Age (median, inter-quartile range-IQR)[b]	43.1 (36.7–47.9)	36.7 (34.2–43.7)	43.5 (37.9–48.1)	< 0.001
Gender				
Male	321 (67.2)	23 (51.1)	298 (68.8)	0.016
Non-male	157 (32.8)	22 (48.9)	135 (31.2)	
Ethnicity				
Caucasian	273 (57.1)	29 (64.4)	244 (56.4)	0.296
Non-Caucasian	205 (42.9)	16 (35.6)	189 (43.6)	
Homelessness[a]				
Yes	169 (35.4)	22 (48.9)	147 (33.9)	0.026
No	305 (63.8)	21 (46.7)	284 (65.6)	
Relationship status[a]				
Legally married/common law/regular partner	126 (26.4)	15 (33.3)	111 (25.6)	0.228
Other	339 (70.9)	28 (62.2)	311 (71.8)	
Highest level of education completed				
≥ high school diploma	229 (47.9)	23 (51.1)	206 (47.6)	0.512
< high school diploma	241 (50.4)	20 (44.4)	221 (51.0)	
Employment[a,c]				
Yes	101 (21.1)	4 (8.9)	97 (22.4)	0.035
No	377 (78.9)	41 (91.1)	336 (77.6)	
Money spent on drugs p/day[c]				
≥ $50 p/day	315 (65.9)	39 (86.7)	276 (63.7)	< 0.001
< $50 p/day	158 (33.1)	5 (11.1)	153 (35.3)	
Drug dealing[a]				
Yes	148 (31.0)	25 (55.6)	123 (28.4)	< 0.001
No	330 (69.0)	20 (44.4)	310 (71.6)	
Years of using heroin injection heroin at baseline (median, IQR)[b]				
Number of years	14.8 (7.3–22.6)	15.7 (8.7–20.4)	14.4 (7.3–22.7)	0.640
Daily non-injection cocaine use[a,c]				
Yes	2 (0.4)	0 (0.0)	2 (0.5)	1.000
No	476 (99.6)	45 (100.0)	431 (99.5)	
Daily non-injection heroin use[a,c]				
Yes	4 (0.8)	1 (2.2)	3 (0.7)	0.328
No	474 (99.2)	44 (97.8)	430 (99.3)	
Daily crack use[a]				
Yes	181 (37.9)	25 (55.6)	156 (36.0)	0.010
No	297 (62.1)	20 (44.4)	277 (64.0)	
Daily crystal meth use[a]				
Yes	19 (4.0)	5 (11.1)	14 (3.2)	0.025
No	459 (96.0)	40 (88.9)	419 (96.8)	
Overdose[a]				
Yes	32 (6.7)	7 (15.6)	25 (5.8)	0.012
No	446 (93.3)	38 (84.4)	408 (94.2)	
Lent syringe[a,c]				
Yes	17 (3.6)	3 (6.7)	14 (3.2)	0.210
No	460 (96.2)	42 (93.3)	418 (96.5)	

Table 1 continued

Characteristic	Total (%) (n = 478)	HAT eligibility		p value
		Yes (%) 45 (9.4)	No (%) 433 (90.6)	
Recent incarceration[a]				
Yes	75 (15.7)	12 (26.7)	63 (14.5)	0.034
No	402 (84.1)	33 (73.3)	369 (85.2)	
Engaged in any form of unprotected sex[a,c]				
Yes	46 (9.6)	5 (11.1)	41 (9.5)	0.790
No	429 (89.7)	40 (88.9)	389 (89.8)	
Exchanged sex for gifts, food, shelter, clothes, etc.[a]				
Yes	72 (15.1)	15 (33.3)	57 (13.2)	< 0.001
No	403 (84.3)	30 (66.7)	373 (86.1)	
Attacked, assaulted, or suffered violence[a]				
Yes	98 (20.5)	12 (26.7)	86 (19.9)	0.293
No	377 (78.9)	33 (73.3)	344 (79.4)	
HCV[c]				
Yes	429 (89.7)	40 (88.9)	389 (89.8)	0.797
No	49 (10.3)	5 (11.1)	44 (10.2)	
Plasma HIV-1 RNA viral load > 50 c/mL				
Yes	313 (65.5)	31 (68.9)	282 (65.1)	0.656
No	162 (33.9)	14 (31.1)	148 (34.2)	
On ART (≥ 1 day)[a]				
Yes	283 (59.2)	28 (62.2)	255 (58.9)	0.665
No	195 (40.8)	17 (37.8)	178 (41.1)	
CD4+ cell count per 100 cells[a,b]				
Median, IQR	3.2 (2.0–4.8)	3.2 (1.6–5.0)	3.2 (2.0–4.8)	0.696

[a] All behavioural variables refer to the 6 months prior to the follow-up questionnaire

[b] Continuous variable, p value is generated from Wilcoxon rank-sum test

[c] p value is generated from Fisher's exact test because of small cell count

SUD (and indirectly HIV treatment outcomes) but no direct associations with indicators of HIV status were observed. Nevertheless, because a noteworthy proportion of PLHIV met the HAT eligibility criteria in the current study, investment into HAT, and other intensive treatments of this targeted group, might also improve their general medical care outcomes as their commonly comorbid diseases (e.g., HCV) can require intense care and frequent follow-up [1]. Similar impact has been demonstrated through protective effect of methadone maintenance therapy on hepatitis C and HIV incidence among PWIDs in this setting [25, 26]. Another justification for expanding access to HAT among this population lies in the growing body of evidence that confirms that many people who do not respond to typical treatment of opioid use disorder (OUD) improve in HAT in areas such as treatment retention, reduced use of illicit drugs, and social functioning [3]. In response, some settings have started developing guidelines for injectable OAT as a treatment for OUD [27].

We have identified a cohort of PWID with indicators of severe SUD suggesting treatment-refractory opioid use disorders, who could benefit from combined treatment of SUD and concurrent chronic diseases, such as HIV. The association with homelessness, as another potential marker of severe SUD, could suggest that HAT eligible PWIDs cannot afford to stay in housing or access services to facilitate housing [28, 29]. Males in our HIV-positive sample were less likely to be deemed HAT eligible, which is a novel finding, given that men are disproportionately being represented in the opioid epidemic in terms of overdose deaths and in the SUD treatment [30]. In this respect, longitudinal research has identified an adherence gap whereby women living with HIV had lower ART adherence than men which suggest that targeted research into a potential role of HAT in facilitating HAT adherence among women is needed [31]. Studies have shown HIV risk reduction with oral opioid agonist treatment (OAT) [32, 33]. Aligned with the scientific literature, these findings suggest that treatment of

Table 2 Bivariable and multivariable GEE analysis of factors associated with HAT eligibility among people who live with HIV

Characteristic	Bivariable		Multivariable	
	Odds ratio (95% CI)	p value	Odds ratio (95% CI)	p value
Age				
(Per 10 years older)	0.97 (0.94–1.01)	0.101		
Gender				
(Male vs. female/non-male)	0.49 (0.31–0.80)	0.004	0.50 (0.31–0.82)	0.006
Ethnicity				
(Caucasian vs. other)	1.39 (0.84–2.28)	0.198		
Homelessness[a]				
(Yes vs. no)	1.61 (1.21–2.16)	0.001	1.47 (1.07–2.01)	0.016
Relationship status[a]				
(Legally married/common law/regular partner vs. other)	0.82 (0.60–1.12)	0.213		
Highest level of education completed				
(≥ high school diploma vs. < high school diploma)	1.01 (0.62–1.65)	0.957		
Employment[a]				
(Yes vs. no)	0.73 (0.56–0.95)	0.018		
Money spent on drugs p/day				
(= $50 per day vs. < $50 per day)	1.53 (1.15–2.02)	0.003		
Drug dealing[a]				
(Yes vs. no)	1.93 (1.50–2.49)	< 0.001	1.76 (1.33–2.31)	< 0.001
Years of using injection heroin at baseline				
(Per year increase)	1.00 (0.98–1.02)	0.781		
Daily non-injection cocaine use[a]				
(Yes vs. no)	1.76 (0.54–5.68)	0.347		
Daily non-injection heroin use[a]				
(Yes vs. no)	7.45 (1.50–37.05)	0.014	8.18 (1.25–53.56)	0.028
Daily crack use[a]				
(Yes vs. no)	1.56 (1.17–2.09)	0.003	1.35 (1.01–1.82)	0.045
Daily meth use[a]				
(Yes vs. no)	1.79 (0.97–3.30)	0.061		
Overdose[a]				
(Yes vs. no)	1.29 (0.77–2.15)	0.328		
Lent syringe[a]				
(Yes vs. no)	0.93 (0.24–3.59)	0.915		
Recent incarceration[a]				
(Yes vs. no)	1.34 (0.83–2.18)	0.233		
Engaged in any form of unprotected sex[a]				
(Yes vs. no)	1.07 (0.64–1.81)	0.787		
Exchanged sex for gifts, food, shelter, clothes, etc.[a]				
(Yes vs. no)	1.30 (0.73–2.32)	0.378		
Attacked, assaulted, or suffered violence[a]				
(Yes vs. no)	1.10 (0.76–1.58)	0.613		
HCV[a]				
(Yes vs. no)	1.05 (0.53–2.05)	0.898		
Plasma HIV-1 RNA viral load > 50 c/mL[a]				
(Yes vs. no)	0.98 (0.76–1.25)	0.853		
On ART (≥ 1 day)[a]				
(Yes vs. no)	0.79 (0.56–1.10)	0.162		
CD4+ cell count[a]				
(Per 100 cells/mL increase)	1.07 (0.99–1.15)	0.096	1.08 (1.00–1.17)	0.042

[a] All behavioural variables refer to the 6 months prior to the follow-up questionnaire

SUD should be tailored to the needs of the individuals, including providing supervised injectable HAT to people with treatment-refractory OUD that does not respond to first and second-line oral OAT alternatives [4]. Oral OAT has been shown effective, but not for everyone [34]. For example, between 46 and 65% of patients who initiate methadone OAT discontinue treatment in the first year and relapse to opioid use—a period of high risk for fatal overdose [35]. Furthermore, adherence to therapeutic dose guidelines, which is independently associated with retention, remains problematic in many settings [36]. The benefits of providing concomitant HAT and ART to people with treatment-refractory opioid use disorder, and the potential synergetic effects on treatment outcomes of both diseases, have yet to be established.

This study is limited by several factors. Our sample was not recruited at random and cannot be assumed to represent the larger population of PWID in Vancouver. We did not confirm the diagnoses of mental health and opioid use disorder and did not retrieve provider-level data for treatment episodes. However, the results from previous HAT research did not suggest that a group of PLHIV might not benefit from HAT, because they were not excluded from those studies [2]. Potential risk factors for opioid overdose, such as current co-use of benzodiazepines, alcohol or non-injection heroin, should be explored in future as well. The omission of these factors may have inflated the potentially eligible group. Finally, it is possible that we underestimated the rates of risky behaviours and drug use, such as syringe sharing, due to the effects of social desirability.

To conclude, in our 10-year longitudinal study of PLHIV, approximately 20% of participants would have been eligible for HAT at least once during the study period. Being eligible for HAT was linked to a number of important risk factors for sub-optimal HIV treatment outcomes, and onward viral transmission, suggesting that more evidence is needed for scaling-up access to HAT and how it might contribute to treatment-as-prevention goals.

Authors' contributions
JK and MJM conceived the study and hypothesis. HD analysed the data. TK, EW conceived the cohorts that provided the data for this analysis. NF, ES, RB, EW, TK, JM, MJM participated in the study design and drafting the manuscript. All authors read and approved the final manuscript.

Author details
[1] British Columbia Centres on Substance Use and Excellence in HIV/AIDS, St. Paul's Hospital, 608-1081 Burrard Street, Vancouver, BC V6Z 1Y6, Canada. [2] Department of Medicine, University of British Columbia, St. Paul's Hospital, 608-1081 Burrard Street, Vancouver, BC V6Z 1Y6, Canada. [3] School of Medicine, University College Dublin, Health Sciences Centre, Belfield, Dublin 4, Ireland.

Acknowledgements
The authors thank the study participants for their contribution to the research, as well as current and past researchers and staff. The study was supported by the US National Institutes of Health (R25DA037756, U01DA021525, U01DA038886). This research was undertaken, in part, thanks to funding from the Canada Research Chairs program through a Tier 1 Canada Research Chair in Inner City Medicine that supports Dr. Evan Wood. Dr. Milloy is supported by the United States National Institutes of Health (U01-DA021525), a New Investigator award from the Canadian Institutes of Health Research and a Scholar award from the Michael Smith Foundation for Health Research. His institution has received unstructured funds from National Green Biomed, Ltd., to support him. ELEVATE: Irish Research Council International Career Development Fellowship—co-funded by Marie Cure Actions (ELEVATEPD/2014/6); and European Commission (701698)—supported Dr. Jan Klimas. Dr. Eugenia Socías is supported by Michael Smith Foundation for Health Research and Canadian Institute for Health Research fellowship awards and a Canada Addiction Medicine Research Fellowship (US National Institute on Drug Abuse, R25-DA037756). Dr. Nadia Fairbairn is supported by a Scholar award from the Michael Smith Foundation for Health Research and the Research in Addiction Medicine Scholars Program from the United States National Institutes of Health (R25DA033211).

Competing interests
The authors declare that they have no competing interests.

References
1. Nosyk B, Guh DP, Bansback NJ, Oviedo-Joekes E, Brissette S, Marsh DC, Meikleham E, Schechter MT, Anis AH. Cost-effectiveness of diacetylmorphine versus methadone for chronic opioid dependence refractory to treatment. Can Med Assoc J. 2012;184:E317–28.
2. Oviedo-Joekes E, Marchand K, Lock K, MacDonald S, Guh D, Schechter MT. The SALOME study: recruitment experiences in a clinical trial offering injectable diacetylmorphine and hydromorphone for opioid dependency. Subst Abuse Treat Prev Policy. 2015;10:3.
3. Ferri M, Davoli M, Perucci CA. Heroin maintenance for chronic heroin-dependent individuals. Cochrane Database Syst Rev. 2011;8:CD003410.
4. Strang J, Groshkova T, Uchtenhagen A, van den Brink W, Haasen C, Schechter MT, Lintzeris N, Bell J, Pirona A, Oviedo-Joekes E, et al. Heroin on trial: systematic review and meta-analysis of randomised trials of diamorphine-prescribing as treatment for refractory heroin addiction. Br J Psychiatry. 2015;207:5–14.
5. Dunlap B, Cifu AS. Clinical management of opioid use disorder. JAMA. 2016;316:338–9.
6. Milloy M-J, Montaner J, Wood E. Barriers to HIV treatment among people who use injection drugs: implications for 'treatment as prevention'. Curr Opin HIV AIDS. 2012;7:332–8.
7. Meyer JP, Althoff AL, Altice FL. Optimizing care for HIV-infected people who use drugs: evidence-based approaches to overcoming healthcare disparities. Clin Infect Dis. 2013;57(9):1309–17.
8. Montaner JS, Hogg R, Wood E, Kerr T, Tyndall M, Levy AR, Harrigan PR. The case for expanding access to highly active antiretroviral therapy to curb the growth of the HIV epidemic. Lancet. 2006;368:531–6.
9. Mesquita F, Jacka D, Ricard D, Shaw G, Tieru H, Yifei H, Poundstone K, Salva M, Fujita M, Singh N. Accelerating harm reduction interventions to confront the HIV epidemic in the Western Pacific and Asia: the role of WHO (WPRO). Harm Reduct J. 2008;5:1.
10. Ratliff EA, McCurdy SA, Mbwambo JK, Lambdin BH, Voets A, Pont S, Maruyama H, Kilonzo GP. An overview of HIV prevention interventions for people who inject drugs in Tanzania. Adv Prev Med. 2013;2013:183187.
11. Mattick RP, Breen C, Kimber J, Davoli M. Buprenorphine maintenance versus placebo or methadone maintenance for opioid dependence. Cochrane Database Syst Rev. 2014;2:CD002207.
12. Amato L, Davoli M, Perucci CA, Ferri M, Faggiano F, Mattick RP. An overview of systematic reviews of the effectiveness of opiate maintenance therapies: available evidence to inform clinical practice and research. J Subst Abuse Treat. 2005;28:321–9.
13. Altice FL, Kamarulzaman A, Soriano VV, Schechter M, Friedland GH. Treatment of medical, psychiatric, and substance-use comorbidities in people infected with HIV who use drugs. Lancet. 2010;376:367–87.
14. Oviedo-Joekes E, Nosyk B, Brissette S, Chettiar J, Schneeberger P, Marsh DC, Krausz M, Anis A, Schechter MT. The North American Opiate Medication Initiative (NAOMI): profile of participants in North America's first trial of heroin-assisted treatment. J Urban Health. 2008;85:812–25.

15. Strathdee SA, Palepu A, Cornelisse PG, Yip B, O'Shaughnessy MV, Montaner JS, Schechter MT, Hogg RS. Barriers to use of free antiretroviral therapy in injection drug users. JAMA. 1998;280:547–9.

16. Wood E, Hogg RS, Bonner S, Kerr T, Li K, Palepu A, Guillemi S, Schechter MT, Montaner JS. Staging for antiretroviral therapy among HIV-infected drug users. JAMA. 2004;292:1175–7.

17. Kerr T, Small W, Johnston C, Li K, Montaner JS, Wood E. Characteristics of injection drug users who participate in drug dealing: implications for drug policy. J Psychoact Drugs. 2008;40:147–52.

18. Hogg RS, Heath KV, Yip B, Craib KJ, O'Shaughnessy MV, Schechter MT, Montaner JS. Improved survival among HIV-infected individuals following initiation of antiretroviral therapy. JAMA. 1998;279:450–4.

19. Lucas GM. Substance abuse, adherence with antiretroviral therapy, and clinical outcomes among HIV-infected individuals. Life Sci. 2011;88:948–52.

20. Spire B, Lucas GM, Carrieri MP. Adherence to HIV treatment among IDUs and the role of opioid substitution treatment (OST). Int J Drug Policy. 2007;18:262–70.

21. Erickson A, Becker M, Shaw S, Kasper K, Keynan Y. Substance use and its impact on care outcomes among HIV-infected individuals in Manitoba. AIDS Care. 2015;27:1168–73.

22. Lee WK, Milloy MJ, Walsh J, Nguyen P, Wood E, Kerr T. Psychosocial factors in adherence to antiretroviral therapy among HIV-positive people who use drugs. Health Psychol. 2016;35:290–7.

23. Pan W. Akaike's information criterion in generalized estimating equations. Biometrics. 2001;57:120–5.

24. Wood E, Hogg RS, Lima VD, Kerr T, Yip B, Marshall BD, Montaner JS. Highly active antiretroviral therapy and survival in HIV-infected injection drug users. JAMA. 2008;300:550–4.

25. Nolan S, Dias Lima V, Fairbairn N, Kerr T, Montaner J, Grebely J, Wood E. The impact of methadone maintenance therapy on hepatitis C incidence among illicit drug users. Addiction. 2014;109:2053–9.

26. Ahamad K, Hayashi K, Nguyen P, Dobrer S, Kerr T, Schutz CG, Montaner JS, Wood E. Effect of low-threshold methadone maintenance therapy for people who inject drugs on HIV incidence in Vancouver, BC, Canada: an observational cohort study. Lancet HIV. 2015;2:e445–50.

27. Woo A. B.C. mulls framework for expanded heroin-assisted treatment. In: The Globe and Mail. Vancouver; 2017.

28. Cheng T, Wood E, Nguyen P, Kerr T, DeBeck K. Increases and decreases in drug use attributed to housing status among street-involved youth in a Canadian setting. Harm Reduct J. 2014;11:12.

29. Zivanovic R, Milloy MJ, Hayashi K, Dong H, Sutherland C, Kerr T, Wood E. Impact of unstable housing on all-cause mortality among persons who inject drugs. BMC Public Health. 2015;15:106.

30. Iversen J, Page K, Madden A, Maher L. HIV, HCV, and health-related harms among women who inject drugs: implications for prevention and treatment. J Acquir Immune Defic Syndr. 2015;69(Suppl 2):S176–81.

31. Puskas CM, Kaida A, Miller CL, Zhang W, Yip B, Pick N, Montaner JS, Hogg RS. The adherence gap: a longitudinal examination of men's and women's antiretroviral therapy adherence in British Columbia, 2000–2014. AIDS. 2017;31:827–33.

32. Metsch LR, Feaster DJ, Gooden L, Matheson T, Mandler RN, Haynes L, Tross S, Kyle T, Gallup D, Kosinski AS, et al. Implementing rapid HIV testing with or without risk-reduction counseling in drug treatment centers: results of a randomized trial. Am J Public Health. 2012;102:1160–7.

33. Woody GE, Bruce D, Korthuis PT, Chhatre S, Poole S, Hillhouse M, Jacobs P, Sorensen J, Saxon AJ, Metzger D, Ling W. HIV risk reduction with buprenorphine-naloxone or methadone: findings from a randomized trial. J Acquir Immune Defic Syndr. 2014;66:288–93.

34. Caputo F, Addolorato G, Domenicali M, Mosti A, Viaggi M, Trevisani F, Gasbarrini G, Bernardi M, Stefanini GF, Treatment TSFA. Short-term methadone administration reduces alcohol consumption in non-alcoholic heroin addicts. Alcohol Alcohol. 2002;37:164–8.

35. Sordo L, Barrio G, Bravo MJ, Indave BI, Degenhardt L, Wiessing L, Ferri M, Pastor-Barriuso R. Mortality risk during and after opioid substitution treatment: systematic review and meta-analysis of cohort studies. BMJ. 2017;357:j1550.

36. Nosyk B, Marsh DC, Sun H, Schechter MT, Anis AH. Trends in methadone maintenance treatment participation, retention, and compliance to dosing guidelines in British Columbia, Canada: 1996–2006. J Subst Abuse Treat. 2010;39:22–31.

13

Integrated HIV care is associated with improved engagement in treatment in an urban methadone clinic

Claire Simeone[1*], Brad Shapiro[2] and Paula J. Lum[3]

Abstract

Background: Persons living with HIV and unhealthy substance use are often less engaged in HIV care, have higher morbidity and mortality and are at increased risk of transmitting HIV to uninfected partners. We developed a quality-improvement tracking system at an urban methadone clinic to monitor patients along the HIV care continuum and identify patients needing intervention.

Objective: To evaluate patient outcomes along the HIV Care Continuum at an urban methadone clinic and explore the relationship of HIV primary care site and patient demographic characteristics with retention in HIV treatment and viral suppression.

Methods: We reviewed electronic medical record data from 2015 for all methadone clinic patients with known HIV disease, including age, gender, race, HIV care sites, HIV care visit dates and HIV viral load. Patients received either HIV primary care at the methadone clinic, an HIV specialty clinic located in the adjacent building, or a community clinic. Retention was defined as an HIV primary care visit in both halves of the year. Viral suppression was defined as an HIV viral load <40 copies/ml at the last lab draw.

Results: The population (n = 65) was 63% male, 82% age 45 or older and 60% non-Caucasian. Of these 65 patients 77% (n = 50) were retained in care and 80% (n = 52) were virologically suppressed. Viral suppression was significantly higher for women ($p = .022$) and patients 45 years or older ($p = .034$). There was a trend towards greater retention in care and viral suppression among patients receiving HIV care at the methadone clinic (93, 93%) compared to the HIV clinic (74, 79%) or community clinics (62, 62%).

Conclusions: Retention in HIV care and viral suppression are high in an urban methadone clinic providing integrated HIV services. This quality improvement analysis supports integrating HIV primary care with methadone treatment services for this at-risk population.

Keywords: Methadone treatment, Retention, Viral suppression, HIV, Engagement, Care continuum

Background

Persons living with HIV and unhealthy substance use are often less engaged in HIV care, have higher morbidity and mortality and are at increased risk of transmitting

*Correspondence: csimeone@att.net; claire.simeone@ucsf.edu
[1] Opiate Treatment Outpatient Program, Division of Substance Abuse and Addiction Medicine, Zuckerberg San Francisco General Hospital and Trauma Center, University of California San Francisco School of Nursing, 995 Potrero Ave, Building 90, Ward 93, San Francisco, CA 94110, USA
Full list of author information is available at the end of the article

HIV to uninfected partners [1–4]. The HIV Care Continuum describes key steps to achieve HIV treatment success, from diagnosis to linkage to care, retention in care and finally viral suppression [5]. HIV treatment is considered successful when patients are retained in medical care and achieve viral suppression [6]. According to the most recent published data for the United States, an estimated 86% of people living with HIV had been diagnosed, 40% were engaged in care (defined as having had an HIV medical care visit during the four month sampling period), and 30% achieved viral suppression of HIV (defined as HIV RNA < 200 copies/ml) [7]. UNAIDS set the "90-90-90" goal to end the global AIDS epidemic by 2030, whereby 90% of people living with HIV are diagnosed, 90% of those diagnosed access treatment and 90% on treatment have achieved viral suppression [8]. Current global estimates indicate that 53% of people living with HIV are diagnosed, 41% are in care and 32% are virally suppressed [9–11] with persons who inject drugs identified as a key population for screening and treatment intervention.

Samet et al. [12] described the benefits of linking primary medical care with substance use treatment services which included improved patient access to and satisfaction with both types of health services and better patient outcomes through coordination of care. The authors described models for successful centralized care that integrate medical and psychiatric services into substance use treatment settings.

Subsequent studies have described the impact of methadone and buprenorphine treatment of comorbid opioid use disorder on HIV treatment outcomes. Analyses of a cohort of people who inject drugs (PWID) in Vancouver, British Colombia found an association between methadone maintenance treatment and higher rates of antiretroviral initiation, medication adherence, and viral suppression [13, 14]. In France, better antiretroviral adherence was demonstrated among patients who had ceased injecting drugs while prescribed opioid agonist therapy (methadone or buprenorphine) compared with people who continued to inject drugs. In addition, duration of opioid agonist therapy (OAT) was significantly associated with viral suppression [15]. This research suggests the importance of linking HIV primary care with OAT in order to achieve treatment success in this population.

The Opiate Treatment Outpatient Program (OTOP) is a publicly funded methadone treatment program for patients with opioid use disorder at a large safety net hospital in San Francisco. OTOP serves a patient population with high rates of homelessness, poly-substance use and psychiatric co-morbidities. In addition to methadone treatment, OTOP provides onsite opt-out HIV screening, integrated HIV primary care and psychiatric services, directly observed antiretroviral therapy (DAART), and medical and social HIV case management. Throughout 2015, OTOP provided methadone treatment services to 704 individual patients, 11% of whom had HIV infection based on OTOP's universal opt-out HIV testing procedures. An HIV prevalence of 11% is similar to that among PWID nationally (11%) [4] and in San Francisco (12%) [16].

OTOP patients infected with HIV have the option to receive their HIV primary care at the methadone clinic from an HIV primary care provider, at a large multidisciplinary HIV specialty clinic located in a building adjacent to the OTOP clinic, or at any number of clinics in the San Francisco community. OTOP patients who receive their HIV primary care onsite at OTOP or at the HIV specialty clinic also have the option of receiving their antiretroviral treatments as DAART along with their methadone dose, an adherence support strategy that was associated with improved viral suppression in a 2007 pilot study at OTOP [17].

At our urban methadone clinic, we developed a quality-improvement tracking system to monitor patients along the HIV care continuum in order to evaluate retention in care and viral suppression for our HIV-infected patients. A second goal of our tracking system was to identify patients who did not meet retention and viral suppression criteria and target those patients for interventions in order to improve treatment success. The purpose of this study was to evaluate patient outcomes associated with OTOP's HIV Care Continuum and explore the relationship of HIV primary care site and patient demographic characteristics with retention in treatment and viral suppression.

Methods

We reviewed electronic medical record (EMR) data from 2015 for all OTOP patients with known HIV disease (n = 73) including age, gender, race, HIV care sites, HIV care visit dates and HIV viral load. Patients who left OTOP treatment before the final month of the study year (n = 5) or whose medical records were in a different healthcare system and unavailable (n = 3) were excluded, leaving 65 patients in the final analysis.

Retention was defined as having an HIV primary care visit in both halves of the study year. Viral Suppression (VS) was defined as having an HIV viral load <40 copies/ml at the last determination within the study year (2015). Patients who had their most recent viral load prior to 2015 were classified as not meeting viral suppression criteria. Primary care visit dates and viral load values were transformed into dichotomous variables (yes/no) for meeting the indicator criteria. Age was categorized as <45 and ≥45 years old. Race was extracted from the patient profile in the medical record and was collapsed into three categorical variables (African American, Caucasian and other) to allow for statistical analysis with the small sample size. Site of care was also collapsed into three categorical variables (methadone clinic, HIV clinic and community clinics). Using IBM SPSS [18], data were analyzed with Fisher's exact test. Expedited IRB approval for this study was granted by the University of California San Francisco Committee on Human Research as a retrospective records review without subject contact or consent.

Results

The study population was mostly male, over the age of 45 and non-Caucasian (Table 1). Among all patients diagnosed with HIV in treatment at OTOP at the end of the study year who were eligible for analysis (n = 65), 50 (77%) met retention criteria and 52 (80%) were virologically suppressed. Viral suppression was significantly higher for women ($p = .022$) and patients 45 years or older ($p = .034$). A larger proportion of patients receiving care at the methadone clinic compared to the HIV specialty clinic or community clinics were retained in care (93 vs. 74 vs. 63%, $p = .150$) and achieved viral suppression (93 vs. 79 vs. 62%, $p = .164$), although these comparisons did not reach statistical significance.

Discussion

In a quality improvement clinical investigation, we found that HIV-infected patients enrolled in a publicly-funded methadone treatment program in San Francisco had high rates of retention in HIV care and viral suppression, both markers of HIV treatment success along the HIV care continuum. HIV engagement outcomes assessed in 2015 for OTOP patients diagnosed with HIV far exceeded the most recently reported national HIV care continuum data for retention in care (77 vs. 40%) and viral suppression (80 vs. 30%) [7]. This is an encouraging result given

Table 1 Outcomes by demographic characteristics

Characteristic	Variable (N)	Retention in care[a] N (%)		Viral suppression[b] N (%)	
		Yes	No	Yes	No
Gender	Female (24)	19 (79%)	5 (21%)	23 (96%)*	1 (4%)
	Male (41)	31 (76%)	10 (24%)	29 (71%)	12 (29%)
Age	<45 years (12)	8 (64%)	4 (33%)	6 (50%)*	6 (50%)
	≥45 years (53)	43 (81%)	10 (19%)	43 (81%)	10 (19%)
Race	African American (27)	20 (74%)	7 (26%)	21 (78%)	6 (22%)
	Caucasian (26)	20 (77%)	6 (23%)	17 (65%)	9 (35%)
	Other (12)	11 (92%)	1 (8%)	11 (92%)	1 (8%)
Site of care	Methadone clinic (15)	14 (93%)	1 (7%)	14 (93%)	1 (7%)
	HIV clinic (42)	31 (74%)	11 (26%)	33 (79%)	9 (21%)
	Community clinics (8)	5 (62%)	3 (38%)	5 (62%)	3 (38%)

[a] Retention in care = meets criteria of having a primary care visit in 1st and 2nd halves of the study year

[b] Viral suppression = meets criteria of HIV viral load <40 copies/ml at most recent laboratory draw

* Significant relationships for (a) viral suppression and gender (Fisher's exact test (2-sided), $p = .022$), and (b) viral suppression and age (Fisher's exact test (2-sided), $p = .034$)

the high frequency of homelessness, poly-substance use and psychiatric co-morbidities among OTOP patients and the known negative impact of these psychosocial circumstances on successful HIV treatment [19, 20].

The extent to which integrated HIV and addiction care may play a role in achieving better outcomes along the care cascade and achieving the U.N. targets of 90-90-90 by 2030, is of considerable interest to this study. We measured a 19 and 31% difference, respectively, in retention in care for patients who received their HIV primary care onsite at OTOP (93%) compared to patients who received their HIV care from the large HIV specialty clinic next door (74%) and compared to patients receiving HIV care from other community clinics (62%). Viral suppression in OTOP primary care patients (93%) also was 14 and 31% higher compared to HIV clinic (79%) and community clinic patients (62%), respectively. These notable differences may reflect the "one-stop shopping" convenience of integrated HIV and methadone treatment or patients' perceptions of OTOP as a less stigmatizing medical home. Most patients visit an opioid treatment program daily for directly observed methadone dosing, which is very likely to improve retention in co-located HIV care. Furthermore, the opportunity for our HIV-infected patients at highest risk for poor medication adherence to receive their treatment through DAART may contribute to OTOP's high viral suppression rate. In this regard, Rothman et al. [21] found that co-locating HIV treatment in a variety of New York's substance use treatment programs was acceptable, effective and efficient in delivering HIV care to this high-risk population. Our research similarly suggests that HIV treatment in methadone clinics may have high levels of acceptance and effectiveness for persons living with HIV and opioid use disorders. While the small size of our patient sample required observing very large differences in order to reach statistical significance, our findings suggest that those differences may be much larger than clinically significant differences. A multi-site study with a larger sample size could be conducted to further explore this relationship. Qualitative research that explores factors that influence patients' choice of where locate their HIV care could also contribute to the understanding and design of care systems to serve people in treatment with OAT.

The 2016 *Surgeon General's Report on Alcohol, Drugs and Health* [22] calls for an evidence-based approach to increase integration of substance use disorder treatment and general health care services, as have the Centers for Disease Control and Prevention [23, 24] and the Substance Abuse and Mental Health Services Administration [25]. The primary focus for integrated services nationally has been the addition of behavioral health into general health care services, in particular substance use screening and treatment in primary care settings. While this direction is critically important to expand both awareness of and access to substance use treatment and prevention services, our findings suggest that a "reverse integration" strategy, the incorporation of medical services into substance use treatment programs, offers another useful approach to integrated care for a patient population with historically low levels of engagement with preventive and routine health care [1, 4, 20].

Other examples of reverse integration models include screening as well as treatment services. Integration of HIV testing within substance use treatment programs, including methadone programs, has been shown to be feasible, acceptable to patients, and effective [26–28]. Participants attending community-based drug treatment programs were significantly more likely to receive their HIV results if testing was conducted on-site compared with a referral for off-site testing ($p < .001$, aRR = 4.52, 97.5% confidence interval = 3.57, 5.72) [28]. In a pilot study of HIV-infected PWID attending a syringe access program and not engaged in drug or HIV treatment at baseline (n = 13), on-site HIV treatment resulted in 85 and 54% of participants achieving viral suppression at 6 and 12 months, respectively [29]. Sylla et al. [30] proposed a model for integrated substance use, tuberculosis and HIV services that included screening and testing for each condition, co-location of services, provision of effective substance use treatment, enhanced monitoring for adverse events and cross-training of generalists and specialists in the target conditions in order to address the disparities in health care access and clinical outcomes for PWID. Smith-Rohrberg et al. [31] demonstrated that improved HIV virologic success (HIV viral load ≤ 400 copies/ml or a decrease from baseline viral load $\geq 1.0 \log_{10}$ copies/ml) among PWID who received DAART at a mobile community health van providing syringe access services was associated with higher use of on-site medical and case management services compared with lower use of on-site services (89 vs. 64%, OR = 4.4, $p = .03$ for medical and 79 vs. 50%, OR = 4.0, $p = .06$ for case management services). They proposed that the proximity of services as well as strong interpersonal relationships between patients and staff may have contributed to successful treatment outcomes. Umbricht-Schneiter et al. [32] found that patients attending a methadone treatment program presenting with one of four key acute or chronic medical conditions (hypertension, purified protein derivative conversion, asymptomatic HIV infection and sexually transmitted infections) were more likely to receive medical care if treatment was onsite compared with referral for treatment (92 vs. 32%, $p < .001$).

In this study, we also found that a significantly higher proportion of HIV-infected women (96%) were virologically suppressed compared to men (71%), but that there was no sex difference in retention in HIV care. Historically, women have been less engaged in HIV care than men, which has been attributed to prioritization of family responsibilities, stigma, intimate partner violence, mental health and substance use disorders, and poverty [33]. However, 2011 United States data for all persons living with HIV from the National HIV Surveillance System and the Medical Monitoring Project showed no significant sex differences in viral suppression (32% for women, 29% for men) [7]. At OTOP, HIV-infected women demonstrated a significantly higher rate of treatment success (viral suppression) than men. Further research with OAT patients into the relationships of sex and housing stability and abstinence from alcohol and illicit substances, both associated with HIV treatment success [19, 34], may provide insight into the significantly higher viral suppression among women.

Our data also showed decreased viral suppression among OTOP patients <45 years old. Younger age is a known risk factor for poor engagement in care and worse treatment outcomes [7, 35]. In the SMILE collaborative, just 7% of HIV-infected youth between 12 and 24 years old obtained viral suppression [35]. Our data confirmed decreased viral suppression for our patients <45 years old. Young adults face particular challenges with engagement in care and medication adherence due to factors that include their stage of psychosocial and cognitive development, distrust of medical institutions and risk behavior [36]. At OTOP, our young adult patients are impacted by severe substance use disorders, social instability including homelessness, trauma and violence, and a lack of support during key developmental milestones. Our finding of worse treatment outcomes for our younger patients, though a small group, highlights the need to design integrated services that support engagement, adherence and ultimately viral suppression for this at-risk group.

The overall high levels of retention in care and viral suppression among OTOP patients living with HIV should also be viewed within the larger context of the wide availability of HIV primary care services across the city of San Francisco. Healthy San Francisco, a program of the San Francisco Department of Public Health and its community partners was started in 2007 to address the health care needs of uninsured residents [37, 38] and provides San Franciscans access to comprehensive preventive and primary care services, regardless of income and legal status. Health care access was further expanded in 2012 with Medicaid (MediCal) expansion and Covered California, the state's health insurance marketplace.

Policies supporting expanded access to care have facilitated linkage to HIV treatment for new patients entering OTOP who are not engaged in HIV care. OTOP is also the recipient of Ryan White Care Act funding that supports our efforts to improve engagement in care for our HIV-infected patients. However challenges to linkage and engagement in care remain, including patients with out-of-county MediCal, a history of distrust of medical systems, the stigmatization of substance use disorders, and recent federal threats to Medicaid expansion. Additional analyses that examine OTOP's linkage data and explore the engagement status for HIV-infected patients at other methadone treatment programs in San Francisco would further our understanding of and guide interventions for these challenges.

Finally, HIV prevalence among OTOP patients (11%) may be higher than expected when compared with city and national prevalence among PWID alone (San Francisco 12%, USA 11%). The fact that OTOP enrolls persons with opioid use disorder who do not inject drugs in addition to people who do, as well as the anticipated HIV prevention impact of our city's longstanding commitment to syringe service programs and a policy of substance use treatment on demand (factors associated with decreased risk for HIV transmission), suggests we might find a lower prevalence among OTOP patients. Possible explanations for OTOP's HIV prevalence could be a high level of sexual risk behavior among our patient population or a greater tendency for people living with HIV and opioid use disorder to enter methadone treatment programs compared with their HIV uninfected counterparts. Further research is needed to explore these hypotheses.

This report has a number of limitations. Conducted as part of a quality improvement project, this descriptive study relied on retrospective chart reviews as data sources. Not only is our study design unable to establish causal relationships, but also the analysis is constrained by the types of variables available in the medical record. In addition, our analysis was limited by the group size of OTOP's HIV-infected population in the study year. A challenge with a sample size of n = 68 is that fairly large differences need to be observed in order to reach statistical significance, which may be much larger than what we might think of as a clinically significant difference. This is evident in the differences we found in our analyses. An analysis with larger numbers of patients could be conducted by a consortium of methadone treatment programs offering integrated models of care to further examine our findings. Despite these limitations, our analysis provides valuable information about engagement in care for HIV-infected patients with opioid use disorder and a foundation from which to build individualized, targeted interventions.

Conclusions
Retention in HIV care and viral suppression are high in this urban, publicly-funded, non-profit methadone clinic with integrated HIV primary care services. In addition to finding that female and older patients had significantly higher rates of viral suppression, this research supports the benefit of integrating HIV primary care and support services with methadone treatment services for this at-risk population.

Abbreviations
EMR: electronic medical record; HIV: human immunodeficiency virus; OST: opioid substitution therapy; OTOP: Opiate Treatment Outpatient Program; SPSS: statistical package for the social sciences; VS: viral suppression.

Authors' contributions
CS conceived and designed the study, collected, analyzed and interpreted the data, and drafted the manuscript. BS contributed to the study design and conception, interpretation of data and drafting and revising the manuscript. PL contributed to the study design and conception, interpretation of data and drafting and revising the manuscript. All authors read and approved the final manuscript.

Author details
[1] Opiate Treatment Outpatient Program, Division of Substance Abuse and Addiction Medicine, Zuckerberg San Francisco General Hospital and Trauma Center, University of California San Francisco School of Nursing, 995 Potrero Ave, Building 90, Ward 93, San Francisco, CA 94110, USA. [2] Opiate Treatment Outpatient Program, Division of Substance Abuse and Addiction Medicine, Departments of Psychiatry and Family and Community Medicine, Zuckerberg San Francisco General Hospital and Trauma Center, University of California San Francisco, San Francisco, CA, USA. [3] Division of HIV, Infectious Diseases, and Global Medicine, Department of Medicine, Zuckerberg San Francisco General Hospital and Trauma Center, University of California San Francisco, San Francisco, CA, USA.

Acknowledgements
The authors would like to thank the following individuals and organizations for their support of this project: OTOP patients and staff, Dr. Jacqueline Tulsky, Dr. Laura Samuel, Johns Hopkins School of Nursing, Ryan White Care Act, SBIRT Interdisciplinary Training Program (1U79TI025386-01, PI: Dawson-Rose) from SAMHSA, the Association for Medical Education and Research in Substance Abuse, the Marguerite Aue Rankin Graduate Education Scholarship and the Jonas Center for Nursing and Veterans Healthcare for scholarship support.

Competing interests
The authors declare that they have no competing interests.

Funding
The study was unfunded.

References
1. Altice FL, Kamarulzaman A, Soriano VV, Schechter M, Freidland GH. Treatment of medical, psychiatric and substance-use comorbidities in people infected with HIV who use drugs. Lancet. 2010;376(9738):50–79.
2. Campbell AC, Tross S, Calysn DA. Substance use disorders and HIV/AIDS prevention and treatment intervention: research and practice considerations. Soc Work Pub Health. 2012;28:333–48.
3. Skarbinski J, Rosenberg E, Paz-Bailey G, et al. Human immunodeficiency virus transmission at each step of the care continuum in the United States. JAMA Int Med. 2015;175(4):588–96. doi:10.1001/jamainternmed.2014.8180.
4. Spiller MW, Broz D, Wenjert C, Nerlander L, Paz-Bailey G. HIV infection and HIV-associated behaviors among persons who inject drugs- 20 cities, United States, 2012. MMWR. 2015;64(10):270–5.

5. Gardner EM, McLees MP, Steiner JF, del Rio C, Burman WJ. The spectrum of engagement in HIV care and its relevance to test-and-treat strategies for HIV prevention. Clin Infect Dis. 2011;52:793–800.

6. Office of National AIDS Policy. National HIV/AIDS strategy for the United States: Updated to 2020. http://www.whitehouse.gov/onap. Accessed 2 Nov 2016.

7. Bradley H, Hall IH, Wolitski RJ, et al. Vital signs: HIV diagnosis, care and treatment among persons living with HIV-United States, 2011. MMWR. 2014;63(47):1113–7.

8. UNAIDS. Global AIDS update 2016. [http://www.unaids.org/sites/default/files/media_asset/global-AIDS-update-2016_en.pdf. Accessed 25 Apr 2016.

9. Levi J, Raymond A, Pozniak A, et al. Can the UNAIDS 90-90-90 target be reached? Analysis of national treatment cascades. In: 8th International AIDS Society Conference on HIV Pathogenesis, Treatment, and Prevention (IAS 2015), Vancouver, BC. Presented 20 July 2015.

10. McMahon JH, Elliott JH, Bertagnolio S, et al. Viral suppression after 12 months of antiretroviral therapy in low- and middle-income countries: a systematic review. Bull World Health Org. 2013;91:377–85.

11. UNAIDS. The gap report. Joint United Nations Programme on HIV/AIDS. 2014. Geneva, Switzerland.

12. Samet JH, Freidmann P, Saitz R. Benefits of linking primary medical care and substance abuse services. Arch Int Med. 2001;161:85–91.

13. Palepu A, Tyndall MW, Joy R, et al. Antiretroviral adherence and HIV treatment outcomes among HIV/HCV co-infected injection drug users: the role of methadone maintenance therapy. Drug Alc Dep. 2006;84:188–94.

14. Uhlmann S, Milloy MJ, Kerr T, et al. Methadone maintenance therapy promotes initiation of antiretroviral therapy among injection drug users. Addiction. 2010;105(5):907–13.

15. Roux P, Carrieri MP, Villes V, et al. The impact of methadone or buprenorphine treatment and ongoing injection on highly active antiretroviral therapy (HAART) adherence: evidence from the MANIF2000 cohort study. Addiction. 2008;103:1828–36.

16. San Francisco Department of Public Health. HIV/AIDS epidemiology annual report 2012. https://www.sfdph.org/dph/comupg/oprograms/hivepisec/HIVepiSecReports.asp. Accessed 22 May 2017.

17. Sorenson JL, Haug NA, Larios S, et al. Directly administered antiretroviral therapy: a pilot study of a structural intervention in methadone maintenance. J Subst Abuse Treat. 2012;43(4):418–23. doi:10.1016/j.jsat.2012.08.014.

18. IBM Corp. IBM SPSS Statistics, Version 23.0.0.2. Armonk, NY: IBM Corp; 2015.

19. Milloy MJ, Marshall BD, Montaner J, Wood E. Housing status and the health of people living with HIV/AIDS. Curr HIV/AIDS Rep. 2012;9(4):364–74. doi:10.1007/s11904-012-0137-5.

20. Chandler G, Himelhoch S, Moore RD. Substance abuse and psychiatric disorders in HIV-positive patients: epidemiology and impact on antiretroviral therapy. Drugs. 2006;66(6):769–89.

21. Rothman J, Rudnick D, Slifer M, Agins B, Heiner K, Birkhead G. Co-located substance use treatment and HIV prevention and primary care services, New York State, 1990-2002: a model for effective service delivery to high risk population. J Urb Health. 2012;84(2):226–42.

22. U.S. Department of Health and Human Services (HHS), Office of the Surgeon General. Facing addiction in America: The Surgeon General's Report on Alcohol, Drugs and Health. Washington, DC: HHS, November 2016.

23. Belani H, Chorba T, Fletcher F, et al. Integrated prevention services for HIV infection, viral hepatitis, sexually transmitted diseases, and tuberculosis for persons who use drugs illicitly: summary guidance from the CDC and the U.S. Department of Health and Human Services. MMWR. 2012;61(RR05):1–40.

24. Centers for Disease Control and Prevention. Program collaboration and service integration: enhancing the prevention and control of HIV/AIDS, viral hepatitis, sexually transmitted diseases, and tuberculosis in the United States. Atlanta: U.S. Department of Health and Human Services; 2009.

25. Substance Abuse and Mental Health Services Administration. Innovations in addictions treatment: addiction treatment providers working with primary care services. Washington: Center for Integrated Health Solutions; 2013.

26. Haynes LF, Kortbe JE, Holmes BE, et al. HIV rapid testing in substance abuse treatment: implementation following a clinical trial. Eval Prog Plan. 2011;34(4):399–406.

27. Hood KB, Robertson AA, Baird-Thomas C. Implementing solutions to barriers to on-site HIV testing in substance abuse treatment: a tale of three facilities. Eval Program Plan. 2015;49:1–9.

28. Metsch LR, Feaster DJ, Gooden L, et al. Implementing rapid HIV testing with or without risk-reduction counseling in drug treatment centers: results of a randomized trial. Am J Pub Health. 2012;102(6):1160–7.

29. Altice FL, Springer S, Buitrago M, Hunt DP, Friedland GH. Pilot study to enhance HIV care using needle exchange-based health services for out-of-treatment injecting drug users. J Urban Health. 2003;80(3):416–27.

30. Sylla L, Bruce RD, Kamarulzaman A, Altice FL. Integration and co-location of HIV/AIDS, tuberculosis and drug treatment services. Int J Drug Policy. 2007;18:306–12.

31. Smith-Rohrberg D, Mezger J, Walton M, Bruce D, Altice F. Impact of enhanced services on virologic outcomes in a directly administered antiretroviral therapy trail for HIV = infected drug users. J Acquir Immune Defic Syndr. 2006;43(S1):S48–53.

32. Umbricht-Schneiter A, Ginn DH, Pabst KM, Bigelow GE. Providing medical care to methadone clinic patients: referral vs on-site care. Am J Pub Health. 1994;84(2):207–10.

33. Aziz M, Smith KY. Challenges and successes in linking HIV-infected women to care in the United States. Clin Inf Dis. 2011;52(Suppl 2):S231–7.

34. Palepu A, Milloy MJ, Kerr T, Zhang R, Wood E. Homelessness and adherence to antiretroviral therapy among a cohort of HIV-infected injection drug users. J Urban Health. 2011;88(3):545–55. doi:10.1007/s11524-011-9562-9.

35. Kapogiannis BG, Xu J, Mayer KH. The HIV continuum of care for adolescents and young adults (12–24 years) attending 13 urban US centers of the NICHD-ATN-CDC-HRSA SMILE collaborative. In 8th international AIDS society conference on HIV pathogenesis, treatment, and prevention (IAS 2015), Vancouver, BC. Abstract WELBPE16, 2015. http://www.natap.org/2015/IAS/IAS_42.htm. Accessed 10 March 2016.

36. Centers for Disease Control and Prevention. Guidelines for the use of antiretroviral agents in HIV-1-infected adults and adolescents. Considerations for antiretroviral use in special patient populations—HIV-infected adolescents and young adults. https://aidsinfo.nih.gov/guidelines/html/1/adult-and-adolescent-arv-guidelines/21/hiv-infected-adolescents-and-young-adults. Accessed 20 Jan 2017.

37. Grimaldi S. 2016. Health San Francisco application assistor eligibility reference manual. Ed. 6.2016. http://healthysanfrancisco.org/. Accessed 10 May 2017.

38. Ngyuen QC, Miller M. Health San Francisco: a case study of city-level health reform. Boston MA: Community Catalyst; 2008.

14

Factors influencing the long-term sustainment of quality improvements made in addiction treatment facilities

Scott P. Stumbo[1*], James H. Ford II[2] and Carla A. Green[1]

Abstract

Background: A greater understanding of the factors that influence long-term sustainment of quality improvement (QI) initiatives is needed to promote organizational ability to sustain QI practices over time, help improve future interventions, and increase the value of QI investments.

Methods: We approached 83 of 201 executive sponsors or change leaders at addiction treatment organizations that participated in the 2007–2009 NIATx200 QI intervention. We completed semi-structured interviews with 33 individuals between November 2015 and April 2016. NIATx200 goals were to decrease wait time, increase admissions and improve retention in treatment. Interviews sought to understand factors that either facilitated or impeded long-term sustainment of organizational QI practices made during the intervention. We used thematic analysis to organize the data and group patterns of responses. We assessed available quantitative outcome data and intervention engagement data to corroborate qualitative results.

Results: We used narrative analysis to group four important themes related to long-term sustainment of QI practices: (1) finding alignment between business- and client-centered practices; (2) staff engagement early in QI process added legitimacy which facilitated sustainment; (3) commitment to integrating data into monitoring practices and the identification of a data champion; and (4) adequate organizational human resources devoted to sustainment. We found four corollary factors among agencies which did not sustain practices: (1) lack of evidence of impact on business practices led to discontinuation; (2) disengaged staff and lack of organizational capacity during implementation period led to lack of sustainment; (3) no data integration into overall business practices and no identified data champion; and (4) high staff turnover. In addition, we found that many agencies' current use of NIATx methods and tools suggested a legacy effect that might improve quality elsewhere, even absent overall sustainment of original study outcome goals. Available quantitative data on wait-time reduction demonstrated general concordance between agency perceptions of, and evidence for, sustainment 2 years following the end of the intervention. Additional quantitative data suggested that greater engagement during the intervention period showed some association with sustainment.

Conclusions: Factors identified in QI frameworks as important for short-term sustainment—organizational capacity (e.g. staffing and leadership) and intervention characteristics (e.g. flexibility and fit)—are also important to long-term sustainment.

*Correspondence: scott.p.stumbo@kpchr.org
[1] Kaiser Permanente Northwest, Center for Health Research, 3800 N. Interstate Avenue, Portland, OR 97227-1110, USA
Full list of author information is available at the end of the article

Keywords: Quality improvement, Long-term sustainment, Addiction treatment, Organizational behavior, NIATx200, Qualitative methods

Background

Funders and stakeholders are increasingly asking for evidence that public health investments have meaningful effects that are sustained over time. Recent research has provided some evidence of the impact and sustainment of health interventions [1–3], and leaders in the field have proposed an agenda for additional public health sustainability research [4]. To date, interventions to improve organizational performance and increase capacity to deliver medical and behavioral health interventions often show no results or mixed results, or show short- but not long-term improvements [2, 5, 6].

Broadly defined, sustainment is the maintenance of program components or outcomes once an initial intervention is completed, or funding is withdrawn [1]. In recent years, researchers have improved methods for assessing sustainability and in the process have described factors that increase the likelihood of sustainability or the capacity to sustain improvements [7, 8]. Three factors important to sustainment have been described across numerous studies: agency characteristics, intervention characteristics, and the external environment. Agency characteristics include staff stability [9], leadership [10], the presence of intervention champions [11], and the capacity to routinize innovations and processes [12]. Important intervention characteristics include the value of innovations to the agency [13], and the flexibility to adapt intervention components to fit within an agency [14]. Finally, external factors include funding availability [13] and institutional climate [12]. How these factors coalesce into sustainment, and in which circumstances each component is a necessary precondition for sustainment, is a matter of debate [4, 7, 14, 15]. Further, many studies of sustainment have focused on a relatively short period of time directly following intervention completion. However, some studies have utilized interviews or administrative data to examine sustainability one to 3 years post-intervention [16–18] or even over a longer-term [19–21].

NIATx200 (formerly the Network for the Improvement of Addiction Treatment) was designed to increase the organizational capacity of addiction treatment centers to reduce waitlists for services, increase enrollment, and improve retention of clients engaged in services. The intervention included four separate intervention arms: (1) "coaching" which included a process improvement expert working directly with each agency; (2) "learning sessions" which brought participants together in twice yearly conferences involving process change experts; (3) "interest circle calls" which used monthly conference calls to discuss process improvement activities; and (4) a "combination" arm which included access to all three intervention activities. 201 agencies that admitted > 60 clients in the prior year and received public funding were randomized [22]; 82% of agencies were privately owned and 83% were located in urban areas [23]. All participating agencies had access to the same web-based toolkit, which contained specific instructions on how to conduct a walk-through of the agency to identify improvement opportunities [24], how to use Plan-Do-Study-Act (PDSA) cycles to identify and enact changes, and a list of promising practices specific to each outcome. Agencies in all intervention arms were free to try whichever promising practices were both practical for their agency or they believed would have the most impact. The intervention arms varied on the type and amount of support provided to each agency to adapt and implement promising practices and other intervention tools. Final intervention results showed variability in associations between intervention type and the three main outcomes: (a) coaching, learning session and combination arms were associated with reduced wait time; (b) coaching and combination arms were associated with improvement in admissions; (c) interest circle calls had no association with any outcome; and (d) no intervention type improved patient retention [25]. An exploratory analysis (unpublished) did not identify any significant relationships between the level of agency participation in their assigned NIATx200 intervention arm and improvements in outcomes.

The goal of the current study was to assess from participating agencies which, if any, organizational practices or outcomes were sustained 6–7 years following the completion of the NIATx200 intervention. We wanted to learn what internal organizational factors were important to sustaining practices implemented during the intervention, and what internal factors served as barriers to sustainment. The interviews were also meant to provide context for, and enhance interpretation of, quantitative sustainment outcome and methods data being assessed as part of the larger follow-up project [26]. The study team was interested in external barriers to sustainment encountered by agencies in the post-intervention period, but the variability across state and within-state (e.g. county) policies and payment methods coupled with our relatively small sample size made it difficult to generalize those barriers. In this paper we describe agency and intervention characteristics associated with long-term sustainment of QI practices.

Methods

Recruitment

We recruited individuals whose agency participated in the NIATx200 intervention. In most cases this was the executive sponsor of the intervention within the agency or the "change leader" (who was the champion during the intervention). Interviews were conducted between November 2015 and April 2016, approximately 6–7 years after the intervention program ended in 2009.

We identified 83 potential interviewees using a convenience sample with a focus on ensuring representation from each of the four original intervention arms. Our initial goal was to recruit individuals from only 3 states (those with the most complete administrative data available for quantitative verification) but we were unable to meet our recruitment goals and opened up interviews to agencies from the two additional states that participated in the NIATx intervention. We completed interviews with 33 individuals (approximately a 40% response rate); we stopped recruiting when we felt we had reached sufficient saturation and no new codes or themes emerged. See Additional File 1 for a recruitment diagram. Reasons for refusing to participate included: (a) lack of interest or time, (b) not remembering enough about the intervention, or (c) no staff member left at organization who participated in NIATx. Though these last two reasons were not specifically disqualifying, we were unable to convince some potential participants that their insights would still be valuable. Interviews were conducted by phone and typically lasted 45 min. Participants received a $10 gift card to a national coffee chain as a token of appreciation. The University of Wisconsin Institutional Review Board approved and monitored the study.

Interview guide

We developed the semi-structured interview guide to first ground interviewees in the original intervention by having them describe their role during the intervention and elaborate on their recollections of what transpired during the intervention. Second, we reviewed a list of promising practices with participants who could describe their current use of those practices and also their use during the intervention period. The list of promising practices was organized by outcome (wait time, retention, admissions) and was developed as part of the NIATx200 study [22]. The promising practices were originally provided to participating agencies during the intervention period. It included practices which agencies could adopt during the participation period to improve each outcome, but were meant merely as suggestions. Agencies were free to use other practices to achieve outcome goals. During the interviews, the list of promising practices were a helpful trigger for placing the individual back in the intervention context. Further questions assessed (1) what changes the organization had maintained at the time of the interview that they implemented as part of NIATx200 participation; (2) what changes were made as part of intervention participation that had not been maintained; (3) attributes of practices that made some more sustainable than others; (4) infrastructure changes made to enhance sustainability; and (5) other barriers or facilitators of sustainment. The interview guide is available from the authors upon request.

Qualitative analytic approach

All interviews were conducted by phone, recorded using encrypted audio-recorders, and transcribed verbatim. Following a pilot test of the interview guide, and completion of the first five interviews, we began reading transcripts to develop the codebook. Other than the general concept of "sustainment" we had no a priori codes in mind when reviewing transcripts, and did not use conceptual domains from extant literature to develop codes to fit participant narratives into predetermined concepts. This modified grounded theory approach [27, 28] encouraged us to use open coding techniques to establish codes and definitions [29]. Open coding began with reading text and noting the broad concepts expressed. In the process we wrote short memos outlining how we believed those concepts were conveyed in the text [29]. From this we created a list of descriptive codes to be applied to the narratives using Atlas.ti [30]. Descriptive codes were applied to portions of text that offered examples, or contra-examples, of concepts that were relevant to themes of sustainability [31]. We developed definitions for all codes once the final list of descriptive codes was complete. We wrote brief case summaries for all 33 completed interviews. The lead author developed initial codes and was responsible for coding all interviews. We used a consensus process (SS and CG) to further refine codes and to assure that coded text aligned with established code definitions.

The results presented in this paper come from the case summaries and focused queries of coded text on topics that participants reported as important to sustainment. Using thematic analysis [32, 33], and elements of grounded theory [27, 29, 31] and constant comparative methods [27], we re-read all queries, searching for patterns in the narratives. This allowed us to develop sub-themes to help explain elements or processes that participants believed were related to intervention sustainment (or lack of sustainment). The themes presented here were developed by sticking closely to the narrative data we collected. No single threshold was used to determine the themes; salience to interviewees and their belief in themes' relationship to sustainment was critical. The lead author developed initial themes; CG and JF provided refinement of themes and helped situate findings in the sustainment literature.

Quantitative data

We used available quantitative data to provide a face validity check on our narrative findings, and to contextualize our interviewees as a subset of all intervention participants. First, as a check on narrative sustainment categorization we used observed wait-time outcome data. "Sustainers" were defined as those with a shorter wait time post-intervention compared to baseline values with a p value < .05. We calculated the level of long-term engagement with NIATx by assessing the mean level of survey responses (a post-intervention activity) up to 27 months following the intervention. Higher responses indicated greater continued engagement with NIATx. We also calculated participation level in the original intervention using number of sessions attended (arm-specific), and used those results to compare interviewees with individuals we did not interview, and also to compare sustainers versus non-sustainers in our data. All t-tests were calculated using SPSS v.22 (IBM).

Results

We completed interviews with 25 women and 8 men representing agencies in five states, including nine individuals whose organizations had received the "coaching" intervention during the main trial, seven from the "learning session" arm, ten from the "interest circle" arm, and seven who were in the "combination" arm.

Written case summaries allowed us to group the 33 interviews into two overall categories: agencies which reported sustaining improvements ($n = 13$) and those which reported low/no sustainment ($n = 20$). Agencies were coded as sustainers by using their stated beliefs that they had sustained practices initiated during the intervention period, and that those sustained practices were associated with sustained (or improved) outcomes over time. Sustainment of practices and/or outcomes could have come in any of the three outcome goals (wait-time, retention, admissions) but did not have to be uniform across all three. We corroborated these findings by using data measuring reduction in wait-time for 20 agencies (those with sufficient data approximately 3 years following completion of the wait-time reduction portion of the intervention) to assess congruence with the narrative data. We found that 16 of 20 agencies reported narrative data which matched the measured wait-time data: there was agreement in six cases where both the narrative and observed data pointed to overall wait-time reduction sustainment and agreement in 10 cases where both the narrative and observed data suggested a lack of sustainment. We found four cases where the narrative data suggested sustainment that was not corroborated by the numerical data. Our final results, therefore, include nine agencies which reported sustainment (6 agencies where the reported and observed data were in agreement, and 3 agencies with reported sustainment). See Table 1 for additional information.

Our analyses of the narrative data were grouped to describe four overarching factors that influenced the long-term sustainability of programmatic investments made during NIATx: impact on business practices; staff engagement; data integration into monitoring activities; and organizational human resources devoted to sustainment. In order to highlight how each of these themes operates within sustaining and non-sustaining agencies, we present the results by sustainment status to describe

Table 1 Agreement between narrative description of sustainment and data measuring post-intervention wait-list reduction by intervention arm

| | Observed wait list data (n = 20) | | Observed wait list data not available (n = 13) |
	Sustained	Not sustained	
Narrative			
Report sustained	3 combination 1 coaching 1 interest circle 1 learning session	2 interest circle 1 combination 1 coaching	2 coaching 1 learning session
Report not sustained		4 interest circle 2 combination 2 coaching 2 learning session	3 coaching 3 learning session 3 interest circle 1 combination

The post-intervention measurement period was more than 2 years following the cessation of all intervention activities, and more than 3 years after the completion of the intervention segment where wait-time reduction was the primary focus. For the observed data, "sustainers" were defined as those with a shorter wait time post-intervention compared to baseline values with a p value < .05. Thirteen agencies we interviewed did not have sufficient data available from that time period to categorize. Later time periods had even greater amounts of missing data

how each of the four factors influenced or hindered sustainment.

Agencies that sustained improvements

In this section we describe the role played by the four factors we identified in agencies which sustained improvement after the intervention had ended (n = 9).

Impact on business practices: finding alignment between business-centered and client-centered practices

Agencies that reported sustainment described finding an affinity between NIATx's client-centered principles and the organization's business practices, and most agencies reporting sustainment had adopted client-centeredness as a core value. As described by one sustaining agency, NIATx encouraged the agency to think about business practices and client-centeredness together, rather than as mutually exclusive goals:

> "I would say that it was jointly client-focused and organization-focused. It sort of allowed us to say it's okay, as an organization, for us to think about our business, and for us to be focusing on the business case for doing these things as opposed to just doing good in the community...We're allowed to be a business. And we want to be a successful business...And providing good customer service and meeting clients' needs and being a good business can be the same" (Agency#1, sustainer).

Staff engagement: early staff buy-in added legitimacy; legitimacy helped with sustainment

Successfully engaging staff in intervention and QI processes is often critical for their immediate success. Several sustaining agencies reported that getting staff buy-in, early in the process, was critical to legitimizing the roll-out of the intervention in what could have been seen as simply a leadership or top-down business decision. Without such staff engagement some were doubtful that the intervention principles would have taken hold in the first place or been sustained in the long run. As one participant explained, knowing when to broaden the QI team to add legitimacy was critical:

> "I was running up against a lot of resistance from staff and other people. [So] I brought onboard our clinical supervisor...who was a very influential leader...[and] had that ability to bring people onboard with these changes and reduce some of this discomfort...I was banging my head up against a wall for a long time before I finally realized I need other support to kind of bring the buy-in from the staff...I just think that they're more comfort-

able working together in that way as opposed to me coming to them and saying, hey, I want to try this because I think it will really help improve services" (Agency #6, sustainer).

Bringing existing, respected staff onto the change team gave the agency a long-term work group in which to discuss "shifting workload around and establishing priorities of services...then once we know [something is] a good practice, we just do it."

Embedding data integration: making the connection with quality improvement

Agencies made use of a "change project form" to implement promising practices by identifying areas for improvement, proposing changes, assigning responsible parties, engaging in PDSA steps, and documenting results of the rapid test cycle. Collecting and monitoring change project data were key components of the NIATx intervention; agencies were encouraged to develop simple tools (pencil/paper, spreadsheets) to monitor the impact of their change projects. Study researchers did not provide feedback to the agencies about their outcome performance during the active intervention period.

In our interviews, agencies that reported sustaining intervention improvements described how deeply embedded the philosophy of this data collection and monitoring became during, and following, the intervention period. Some agencies described an individual who was their data champion, and that this role facilitated sustainment. Several agencies reported that monitoring data closely and consistently allowed them to get ahead of any problems (e.g. an increase in waitlist time), rather than falling behind the problem.

> "So in the past, we would see a drop in revenue and say, oh, what's going on...We really learned, as a result of NIATx, that we need to do this on a very consistent basis. And this has become a lot of my job—I'm looking all the time; I'm pulling data. And when I see that there's an issue, we will say, okay, where do we think it is? What is the date it's showing [as] of? And then we take a look at that and say, okay, what do we need to tweak? Or what do we need to improve?...[This is] primarily now what I do...it's something that we definitely prioritized...probably three quarters of [my] job is now doing something related to [data]" (Agency #18, sustainer).

Committing organizational human resources: building on the initial investment

Organizational leadership and commitment of human resources also played a role in sustaining changes.

Though the NIATx intervention encouraged agencies to develop a "sustainability plan," no one we interviewed reported that their agency actually developed such a plan. Absent such a plan, one interviewee described the agency's initial investment in NIATx and the leadership's subsequent expectation to see something develop from that investment. This participant describes how the agency established and maintained new procedures related to expanding walk-in hours:

"I think...it was the accountability. I really do...I think it was an investment in [organization] that they [leadership] wanted...You know, they'd kind of given up these resources [to accommodate NIATx]. And they were focusing on it...everybody was invested in it. We spent a long time...making sure that we wanted it to work...And, you know, we prioritized it. I think that was the big piece..." (Agency #8, sustainer).

Agencies that did not sustain improvements

We found four important factors—many the inverse of positive factors associated with sustainment noted above—common among agencies (n = 24) reporting lack of sustainment.

Impact on business practices: lack of evidence of impact on bottom line led to discontinuation

For some agencies the lack of ability to sustain improvements was related to lack of evidence that it continued to have an impact on the bottom line. One agency reported that doing reminder calls worked during the intervention, but that it was too labor-intensive to continue given that it is not a reimbursable activity.

"And we're operating in the black...just barely...And we do that by being very sparse on our admin and management staff...[And] we were tracking our no-show rate, which was generally under 20%...sometimes down around 12%...even without doing the [reminder calls] anymore. So we weren't feeling like that's the most urgent thing we had to deal with" (Agency #14, non-sustainer).

Lack of agency capacity or lack of buy-in during implementation period led to lack of sustainment

In the course of implementing the NIATx intervention, managers often asked staff—from frontline administrators to counselors—to take on new tasks in order to improve efficiency. Without a general buy-in on intervention goals, however, these requests were sometimes met with resistance. From our interviewees' perspectives (all of whom were managers), some felt that staff were resistant to shifting work onto their plates, such as requiring them to make the reminder calls. For example, after saying that doing reminder calls "proved onerous," one interviewee went on to say: "Well, the front desk didn't like doing it. They usually didn't have the time to do it. And counselors resisted doing it" (Agency #13, non-sustainer).

In another agency, the lack of tone-setting to get organizational buy-in came directly from the top. Following randomization to the "interest circle calls," one agency CEO became uninterested in the intervention: "We were told that we would get the face-to-face [coaching] intervention." Following that, her agency did not participate much in the program. She described the interest circle calls as "worthless" and of the PDSA cycle she said "We all got that [training], but we didn't do it." This lack of leadership commitment to NIATx ensured that the agency subsequently devoted no time or resources to engaging in the intervention (Agency # 25, non-sustainer).

Finally, some agencies simply lacked capacity to expand practices, especially practices that staff assumed would increase their workload. For example, when asked why providing walk-in hours did not work, one interviewee said:

"Generally, it was fear on the part of clinicians that they would become overwhelmed...To increase access, doesn't that mean that my case load will triple?...Clinicians, by and large, are [saying] I can't make the time...My caseload is full. I can't see anybody else" (Agency #13, non-sustainer).

Running into data roadblocks

Several agencies that were unable to sustain improvements struggled with continued access to data that would allow them to monitor ongoing activities. For some it was that the data was never quite how they needed it; it required too much "massaging" to make it useful. Some agencies mentioned competing reporting requirements from different funders, which took up a lot of time but still did not leave them with the data they really wanted. When describing what she thought her agency needed to sustain or regain improvements made during the intervention period, one interviewee reported:

"More data. More data on the access center, more data on the call volumes, more data...there's some things that we could track that we're not tracking because of priority and limitations to resources. So in a perfect world, I would be able to quadruple the IT Department and have a couple of guys in there who really knew how to write these reports in our electronic health record...And maybe someday we'll

get there...I know that this organization really wants to be data driven and to use that to make decisions..." (Agency#11, non-sustainer).

Organizational human resources: high levels of staff turnover
If committing organizational human resources is important to sustainment, then high staff turnover is problematic for sustainment. Turnover at community-based agencies is a problem for many organizations. Staff turnover at all levels can be problematic, but agencies reported that it was particularly difficult to sustain improvements when their data analyst left:

"At the time, we had someone who was our data person who was really good with the files and medical records. And she's no longer with us...[That's why] there's not actual data as much...It's more monthly, quarterly or annually, which is not rapid change..." (Agency #16, non-sustainer).

Further evidence of the relationship between staff turnover and low reports of sustainment in our data can also be seen in the interviews we conducted with individuals (n = 6) who were not there during NIATx intervention period. These individuals agreed to be interviewed because no one currently employed at their agency participated in NIATx. All six agencies were in the non-sustainment group, suggesting anecdotally that lack of organizational staff continuity is inconsistent with sustainment.

Sustaining the principles if not the outcomes: the legacy of the NIATx intervention
In addition to coding sustainment of specific practices and outcomes, we coded any mention that an agency might still be adhering to any of the guiding principles of NIATx (e.g. using the PDSA cycle, doing regular walk-throughs to identify areas for improvement, using the change project form to assess new activities). We found that 50% (n = 12) of agencies which we classified as non-sustainers still mentioned one or more philosophical tenets of the NIATx intervention as being used within the agency. One individual, who was not at the agency during the intervention period, said:

"We have quarterly meetings to discuss business strengths and weaknesses and...address areas of concern or risk...[O]ne approach that we frequently used these quarterly meetings to explore was Plan, Do, Study, Act, which is a NIATx thing...So that was sort of a nice framework for us to...identify areas that were not as effective or that we felt needed our attention, and then do brief... periods of determining whether any long-term changes would benefit us" (Agency #17, non-sustainer).

Another interviewee reported:

"What I really liked about NIATx is...that we got that worksheet [change form]...We've always had some quality improvement we use [here]. But we didn't document [it]...it wasn't so formal...The form itself really helped put structure to it. Otherwise, it was kind of chaotic [for] us. So we use that form even today" (Agency #16, non-sustainer).

Finally, it should be noted that agencies (both sustainers and non-sustainers) did report on external barriers to sustainment. However, due to the relatively limited sample and the within- and between-state variability of policy and payment systems, it would be difficult to characterize coherent themes. For example, there were roughly equal numbers of agencies reporting that the implementation of the Affordable Care Act was either a positive change in environment (in that it expanded the eligible population and thus could increase admissions) or a negative change (in that many states capped Medicaid payments at low rates). Some agencies reported that it was both helpful in increasing admissions and unhelpful in reducing overall revenue.

Quantitative analyses
We conducted additional analyses using available data to assess the generalizability of our narrative data. First, as a measure of overall engagement in the intervention and whether that differed among individuals we enrolled for interviews, we tested the survey completion rate at each of four survey time periods. Participating individuals within all agencies were surveyed at four time points (baseline and three additional times at 9-month intervals) to assess their use of promising practices within their agency. Individuals who agreed to participate in our interviews were more likely to be from agencies with high survey participation rates at both 18 months (mean survey completion = 7.1 vs. 5.6, $p = .042$) and 27 months (mean survey completion = 6.5 vs. 4.7, $p = .021$) following baseline, suggesting an association between higher levels of continued intervention engagement and willingness to participate in an interview (Table 2).

Next we tested whether individuals who participated in our interviews were more or less likely to be from agencies which were more engaged in their respective intervention arms. NIATx measured the amount of engagement as the total participation activity, by arm, relative to the amount of intervention activities offered. Table 3 column A shows a secular trend toward higher levels of engagement in the intervention comparing current interviewees to non-interviewees, but they did not differ statistically.

Table 2 Association between agency survey completion and interview participation, n = 194

	Agencies interviewed (n = 33)	Agencies not interviewed (n = 161)	p
	Mean (SD)	Mean (SD)	
Baseline	8.2 (3.8)	7.2 (3.5)	.134
+ 9 months	6.3 (3.6)	5.4 (4.1)	.257
+ 18 months	7.1 (3.9)	5.6 (4.0)	.042
+ 27 months	6.5 (4.5)	4.7 (4.0)	.021

Surveys asked agency staff about the use of promising practices and other measures of intervention engagement. Multiple respondents at each agency were encouraged. Means represent the number of agency staff completing surveys at each time period

Finally, we tested the association between intervention engagement and sustainment status among agencies we interviewed. For three intervention arms we saw higher arm-level engagement among sustainers compared with non-sustainers, though the results were not significant. Among participants in the combination arm, we found higher levels of intervention engagement among those who were able to sustain improvements (27.33 vs. 18.75, $p = .045$). See Table 3 column B for additional results. This suggests that a high level of engagement in intervention activities among those assigned to the combination arm may be associated with sustainment.

Discussion

We found variability in sustainment at addiction treatment facilities 7 years after the completion of a quality improvement intervention. Four factors were found to influence long-term sustainment: impact on business practices, staff buy-in and engagement, an organizational commitment to sustainment, and the ability to embed new data processes into an overall organizational QI strategy. These findings on the long-term sustainment of intervention improvements share several common factors with previously published studies on short-term sustainment, and sustainment in other organizational contexts. For example, our findings on the importance of intervention characteristics to sustainment are similar to those described elsewhere [2, 7, 9]. Specifically, our work documents that the intervention's positive impact on business efficiency, and concomitant improvements to the bottom line, was more common among agencies which sustained practices.

Also similar to findings from short-term sustainment studies, we found that agency capacity played a critical role in long-term sustainment of intervention effects [2, 9–11]. In our study this included the capacity to elicit staff buy-in and engagement early in the intervention [13, 34], and the capacity to sustain staffing to maintain practice changes. Conversely, staff turnover, previously identified as a barrier to implementing an intervention [35] and also as a barrier to sustainment [2, 13], was a factor related to non-sustainment in our findings. We found that no agencies reported documenting all intervention efforts for future staff thus underscoring the importance of staff continuity.

Our finding on the importance of the use of data to monitor and improve activities demonstrates the dynamic interplay between intervention characteristics and agency capacity, and their relationship to sustainment. Data collection to monitor and review intervention-related improvements was a key characteristic of the intervention for all participating agencies. An agency's capacity to develop and maintain the person who could serve as a data champion was also critical. However, the ability to sustain data monitoring efforts was related not just to the person but to a process. Agencies which embedded data review into their QI teams, or used intervention participation to spur the creation of such a team, were more likely

Table 3 Associations between intervention engagement and interview status, and between intervention engagement and sustainment among interviewees

Intervention arm (maximum number of engagement activities in arm)	A			B		
	Among all agencies, n = 201			Among interviewees, n = 33		
	Agencies interviewed (n = 33)	Agencies not interviewed (n = 168)		Sustained improvements (n = 9)	Did not sustain improvements (n = 24)	
	Mean	Mean	p	Mean	Mean	p
Learning sessions (max = 3)	2.57	1.96	.163	3.00	2.44	.119
Interest circle (max = 18)	6.20	5.05	.408	9.25	5.85	.136
Coaching (max = 18)	12.50	10.26	.201	14.29	11,20	.101
Combo (max = 39)	22.43	17.15	.084	27.33	18.75	.045

to report sustaining improvements over time. Some agencies found they had an individual with this capacity while other agencies nurtured the development of a person to play this role; agencies who lacked such a person, or who lost their data person, showed a lack of sustainment. The importance of a champion, in this case a data champion, is something that others have noted as critical to the routinization of sustainment [7, 9, 11].

Our quantitative results she light on additional areas of interest to the sustainment field. Intervention arm assignment did not show a strong association with sustainment status in our data; agencies enrolled in all four arms were distributed across the sustainer and non-sustainer groups. NIATx practices were available to all agencies regardless of intervention arm, and some agencies sustained practices (e.g. use of PDSA cycle) despite lack of overall sustainment and independent of the facilitative support offered as part of the intervention arm. These findings suggest that the relationship between intervention strength, intervention engagement, and sustainment is complex. Sustainment may best be seen as a dynamic process on a continuum rather than as all or nothing at a fixed point in time, something others have noted [2]. Agencies which sustained practices, regardless of intervention arm, may share another trait in common: agency capacity. Certainly our results demonstrate the overall importance of agency capacity in getting staff buy-in and maintaining staff, including a data champion. Future research could explore, quantitatively, the relationship between intervention engagement, agency capacity, and long-term sustainment.

Finally, we found that the total "impact" of an intervention is difficult to measure. For example, how should one define and measure an agency's perception that tools and methods learned during the intervention (e.g. using PDSA or walk-throughs to improve services), are still important to the agency and, in fact, still being used, even absent measureable improvement in the outcomes studied? Agencies, and researchers, wishing to extend intervention investments need to understand the value of continuing any portion of an intervention, and how to measure those latent effects [12]. Such improvements to measuring the full impact of an intervention could focus not just on the diffusion and replication of activities in other settings [4], but on other QI activities within the same organization. Future work could explore identifying unmeasured effects of sustained intervention practices, or measuring sustainment of QI practices and activities within agencies that were unrelated to the original intervention outcomes.

A few limitations in our study should be noted. First, our narrative themes are based on self-reported sustainment; retrospective assessment years after the fact may be subject to recall bias. We tried to mitigate this limitation by including observed post-intervention wait-time

data; however, data from some agencies was lacking. Second, our results may be subject to self-selection bias: some agencies we approached opted out of participating because no current employee remembered the intervention. This could potentially under-report barriers to sustainment; however, we did interview six individuals who revealed they were not at the agency and, thus, captured sustainment from agencies that experienced staff turnover. Interviewing additional agencies who reported no sustainment, or additional agencies who had no staff remaining from the NIATx period, would undoubtedly have revealed additional barriers to sustainment. Our results, therefore, should be interpreted with caution and additional studies should focus on the impact of high staff turnover on QI sustainment. We also attempted to mitigate selection bias by assessing intervention engagement levels between interviewees and non-interviewees and found mixed results. We found no differences between interviewees and non-interviewees based on level of engagement (i.e. session attendance) during the intervention, but did find some differences in post-intervention study engagement (i.e. completing surveys on agency practices) and willingness to participate in an interview. Finally, we were unable to assess the impact of the external environment, including the implementation of the Affordable Care Act, on agency sustainment. Including such information may have produced somewhat different conclusions.

Conclusions

Some agencies that participated in a quality improvement intervention were able to sustain improvements over a long period of time. Agency capacity—including staff engagement during the intervention, stable staffing afterward, and an investment of human resources to maintain QI practices—were critical to extending intervention effects. Intervention characteristics that aligned with business practices in the agency were also associated with long-term sustainment. Finally, agencies which had the capacity, e.g. a data champion, to embed important intervention characteristics into their organizational QI strategy also showed signs of long-term sustainment.

Authors' contributions
SS was primarily responsible for analyzing the qualitative data and preparing the manuscript. JF was responsible for designing the study, analyzing the quantitative data, and preparing the final manuscript. CG was responsible for the qualitative study design, analyzing the qualitative data, and preparing the final manuscript. All authors read and approved the final manuscript.

Author details
[1] Kaiser Permanente Northwest, Center for Health Research, 3800 N. Interstate Avenue, Portland, OR 97227-1110, USA. [2] Center for Health Systems Research

and Analysis, University of Wisconsin – Madison, 610 Walnut Street, Madison, WI 53726, USA.

Acknowledgements
We acknowledge the important contributions made to this manuscript by Mary Ann Scheirer who passed away during its preparation. We would also like to express appreciation to the substance abuse clinics in these states who participated in the NIATx200 study.

Competing interests
The authors declare that they have no competing interests

Consent for publication
Individuals were provided with a consent information sheet. In that document they were informed that publications would result from this work and that "any quotes used for publication will not identify you, your organization or location."

Funding
The development and publishing of this manuscript was supported by a grant from the US Department of Health and Human Services, National Institutes of Health, National Institute of Drug Abuse (Grant number: R21 DA36700-01A1, PI: Ford II, JH).

References
1. Scheirer MA. Is sustainability possible? A review and commentary on empirical studies of program sustainability. Am J Eval. 2005;26(3):320–47.
2. Stirman SW, Kimberly J, Cook N, Calloway A, Castro F, Charns M. The sustainability of new programs and innovations: a review of the empirical literature and recommendations for future research. Implement Sci IS. 2012;7:17.
3. Scoville R, Little K, Rakover J, Luther K, Mate K. Sustaining improvement. IHI white paper. Cambridge: Institute for Healthcare Improvement; 2016.
4. Scheirer MA, Dearing JW. An agenda for research on the sustainability of public health programs. Am J Public Health. 2011;101(11):2059–67.
5. Lager KE, Mistri AK, Khunti K, Haunton VJ, Sett AK, Wilson AD. Interventions for improving modifiable risk factor control in the secondary prevention of stroke. Cochrane Database Syst Rev. 2014;2014(5):Cd009103.
6. Naghieh A, Montgomery P, Bonell CP, Thompson M, Aber JL. Organisational interventions for improving wellbeing and reducing work-related stress in teachers. Cochrane Database Syst Rev. 2015;4:Cd010306.
7. Fleiszer AR, Semenic SE, Ritchie JA, Richer MC, Denis JL. The sustainability of healthcare innovations: a concept analysis. J Adv Nurs. 2015;71(7):1484–98.
8. Ford JH II, Alagoz E, Dinauer S, Johnson KA, Pe-Romashko K, Gustafson DH. Successful organizational strategies to sustain use of A-CHESS: a mobile intervention for individuals with alcohol use disorders. J Med Internet Res. 2015;17(8):e201.
9. perspective on the long-term sustainability of a nursing best practice Fleiszer AR, Semenic SE, Ritchie JA, Richer MC, Denis JL. A unit-level guidelines program: an embedded multiple case study. Int J Nurs Stud. 2016;53:204–18.
10. Aarons GA, Green AE, Trott E, Willging CE, Torres EM, Ehrhart MG, Roesch SC. The roles of system and organizational leadership in system-wide evidence-based intervention sustainment: a mixed-method study. Adm Policy Ment Health. 2016;43(6):991–1008.
11. Brewster AL, Curry LA, Cherlin EJ, Talbert-Slagle K, Horwitz LI, Bradley EH. Integrating new practices: a qualitative study of how hospital innovations become routine. Implement Sci IS. 2015;10:168.
12. Pluye P, Potvin L, Denis JL. Making public health programs last: conceptualizing sustainability. Eval Program Plann. 2004;27:121–33.
13. Mancini JA, Marek LI. Sustaining community-based programs for families: conceptualization and measurement. Fam Relat. 2004;53(4):339–47.
14. Chambers DA, Glasgow RE, Stange KC. The dynamic sustainability framework: addressing the paradox of sustainment amid ongoing change. Implement Sci IS. 2013;8:117.
15. Nilsen P. Making sense of implementation theories, models and frameworks. Implement Sci IS. 2015;10:53.
16. Bond GR, Drake RE. Making the case for IPS supported employment. Adm Policy Ment Health. 2014;41(1):69–73.
17. Harris AH, Bowe T, Hagedorn H, Nevedal A, Finlay AK, Gidwani R, Rosen C, Kay C, Christopher M. Multifaceted academic detailing program to increase pharmacotherapy for alcohol use disorder: interrupted time series evaluation of effectiveness. Addict Sci Clin Pract. 2016;11(1):15.
18. Lopatto J, Keith SW, Del Canale S, Templin M, Maio V. Evaluating sustained quality improvements: long-term effectiveness of a physician-focused intervention to reduce potentially inappropriate medication prescribing in an older population. J Clin Pharm Ther. 2014;39(3):266–71.
19. Fleiszer AR, Semenic SE, Ritchie JA, Richer MC, Denis JL. Nursing unit leaders' influence on the long-term sustainability of evidence-based practice improvements. J Nurs Manag. 2016;24(3):309–18.
20. Peterson AE, Bond GR, Drake RE, McHugo GJ, Jones AM, Williams JR. Predicting the long-term sustainability of evidence-based practices in mentalhealth care: an 8-year longitudinal analysis. J Behv Health Serv Res. 2014;41(3):337–46.
21. Pronovost PJ, Watson SR, Goeschel CA, Hyzy RC, Berenholtz SM. Sustaining reductions in central line-associated bloodstream infections in Michigan intensive care units: a 10-year analysis. Am J Med Qual. 2016;31(3):197–202.
22. Quanbeck AR, Gustafson DH, Ford JH 2nd, Pulvermacher A, French MT, McConnell KJ, McCarty D. Disseminating quality improvement: study protocol for a large cluster-randomized trial. Implement Sci IS. 2011;6:44.
23. Grazier KL, Quanbeck AR, Oruongo J, Robinson J, Ford JH, 2nd, McCarty D, Pulvermacher A, Johnson RA, Gustafson DH. What influences participation in QI? A randomized trial of addiction treatment organizations. J Healthc Qual. 2015;37(6):342–53.
24. Ford JH, Green CA, Hoffman KA, Wisdom JP, Riley KJ, Bergmann L, Molfenter T. Process improvement needs in substance abuse treatment: admissions walk-through results. J Subst Abuse Treat. 2007;33(4):379–89.
25. Gustafson DH, Quanbeck AR, Robinson JM, Ford JH 2nd, Pulvermacher A, French MT, McConnell KJ, Batalden PB, Hoffman KA, McCarty D. Which elements of improvement collaborative are most effective? A cluster-randomized trial. Addiction. 2013;108(6):1145–57.
26. Ford II JH, Stumbo SP, Robinson JM: A methodological approach for assessing long-term sustainment of NIATx200 participation. Implement Sci IS Under Rev (Under review).
27. Glaser BG, Strauss AL. The discovery of grounded theory: strategies for qualitative research. Chicago: Aldine Publishing Company; 1967.
28. Strauss A, Corbin J. Grounded theory methodology: an overview. In: Denzin NK, Lincoln YS, editors. Strategies of qualitative inquiry. Thousand Oaks: Sage; 1998. p. 158–83.
29. Strauss AL, Corbin J. Open coding. In: Corbin J, Strauss A, editors. Basics of qualitative research: techniques and procedures for developing grounded theory. Thousand Oaks: SAGE Publications, Inc.; 1998, p. 101–21.
30. Friese S. User's manual for ATLAS.ti 6.0. Berlin: ATLAS.ti Scientific Software Development GmbH; 2011.
31. Saldaña J. The coding manual for qualitative researchers. London: Sage; 2009.
32. Braun V, Clarke V. Using thematic analysis in psychology. Qual Res Psychol. 2006;3(2):77–101.
33. Braun V, Clarke V. Thematic analysis. In: Cooper H, Camic PM, Long DL, Panter AT, Rindskopf D, Sher KJ, Sher KJ, editors. APA handbook of research methods in psychology, vol 2: research designs: quantitative, qualitative, neuropsychological, and biological. Washington, DC: American Psychological Association; 2012. p. 57–71.
34. Willis CD, Saul J, Bevan H, Scheirer MA, Best A, Greenhalgh T, Mannion R, Cornelissen E, Howland D, Jenkins E, et al. Sustaining organizational culture change in health systems. J Health Organ Manag. 2016;30(1):2–30.
35. Yarborough BJ, Janoff SL, Stevens VJ, Kohler D, Green CA. Delivering a lifestyle and weight loss intervention to individuals in real-world mental health settings: lessons and opportunities. Transl Behav Med. 2011;1(3):406–15.

15

Changes in Specific Substance Involvement Scores among SBIRT recipients in an HIV primary care setting

Carol Dawson-Rose[1*], Jessica E. Draughon[1,3], Yvette Cuca[1], Roland Zepf[1], Emily Huang[1], Bruce A. Cooper[1] and Paula J. Lum[2]

Abstract

Background: Substance use is common among people living with HIV (PLHIV) and is associated with worse outcomes along the HIV care continuum. One potentially effective clinic-based approach to addressing unhealthy substance use is screening, brief intervention, and referral to treatment (SBIRT).

Methods: We conducted a two-arm randomized trial to examine the effects of a self-administered, computerized SBIRT intervention compared to a clinician-administered SBIRT intervention in an HIV primary clinic. Patients were surveyed before receiving the intervention and again at 1, 3, and 6 months. We administered the WHO Alcohol, Smoking and Substance Involvement Screening Test to determine Specific Substance Involvement Scores (SSIS) and to assign participants to categories of lower, moderate, or high risk to health and other problems for each substance. We collapsed moderate or severe risk responses into a single moderate–high risk category. Based on low rates of participation in the computerized arm, we conducted an "as treated" analysis to examine 6-month changes in mean SSIS among SBIRT intervention participants.

Results: For the overall sample (n = 208), baseline mean SSIS were in the moderate risk category for alcohol, tobacco, cannabis, cocaine, amphetamine, sedatives and opioids. Of those enrolled, 134 (64.4%) received the intervention, and 109 (52.4%) completed the 6-month follow up. There was a statistically significant decline in mean SSIS for all substances except tobacco and cannabis among participants who were at moderate–high risk at baseline. We also observed a statistically significant increase in mean SSIS for all substances except amphetamines and sedatives among participants who were at lower risk at baseline.

Conclusions: Substance use among patients in this urban, safety-net, HIV primary care clinic was near universal, and moderate risk substance use was common. Among participants who received the SBIRT intervention, mean SSISs decreased among those at moderate–high risk at baseline, but increased among those at lower risk at baseline over the 6-month study period. Additional research should examine the clinical significance of SSIS changes for PLHIV, which SBIRT components drive changes in substance use scores, and what other interventions might support those patients at lower risk to maintain health and engagement along the HIV care continuum.

Trial registration ClinicalTrials.gov study NCT01300806

Keywords: SBIRT, Substance use, People living with HIV, Interventions

*Correspondence: carol.dawson-rose@ucsf.edu
[1] UCSF School of Nursing, 2 Koret Way, Box 0608, San Francisco, CA 94143-0608, USA
Full list of author information is available at the end of the article

Background

In the United States, over one million people are currently living with HIV [1]. Substance use, including both alcohol and drug use, is a significant health challenge for people living with HIV (PLHIV) as well as for those most at risk for acquiring HIV. Unhealthy alcohol and drug use is one of the major drivers of HIV acquisition [2–4] and, among people already living with HIV, it contributes to low levels of engagement in HIV care [5–7], and is linked to poor medication adherence [8]. A recent review found that only 60–79% of newly diagnosed people who inject drugs in the U.S. are linked to HIV care, with 24–59% retained in care, 20–49% on treatment, and 16–42% virally suppressed [9], rates that are well below the UNAIDS 90-90-90 goal. Other studies have found that substance-using PLHIV presented later for HIV testing and care [10]; delayed linkage to HIV care and had poorer continuous engagement in HIV care [11]; and reported lower levels of being prescribed with antiretroviral therapy [12, 13]. Additional research has shown that PLHIV who use substances have lower rates of viral suppression than those who do not use substances [14], and PLHIV who inject drugs are more than twice as likely to discontinue antiretroviral therapy compared to those who do not [13]. Despite this, many PLHIV continue to use alcohol and drugs. In a national survey of adult PLHIV, 27.9% reported binge drinking and 32.5% reported illicit substance use in the prior 30 days [15].

The relationship between unhealthy substance use and poor health outcomes along the HIV care continuum underscores the critical importance of identifying PLHIV engaged in harmful use and providing evidence-based addiction treatment. The recent U.S. Surgeon General's report on addiction calls for "integration across health care settings including primary care" [16]. A recent study showed, however, that among VA patients with alcohol use disorders, significantly fewer PLHIV received follow-up alcohol-related care compared to HIV-negative patients [17]. HIV primary care clinics may be more effective sites for screening, assessment, and intervention among those who are engaged in care [18]. In primary care, patients may present anywhere along the spectrum of substance involvement, from low risk behavior to an alcohol or substance use disorder, in recovery or during a relapse. As with other chronic illnesses, detection is an important first step, and screening can serve a dual purpose: as preventative care for those who may be at risk for problems associated with substance use, and as an opportunity for intervention for those already experiencing problems related to their substance use. Interventions may be brief counseling for those at low risk or, for those diagnosed with a substance use disorder, office-based medication-assisted treatment in the primary care setting or referral to specialty treatment by an addiction specialist. Prior studies also suggest that information technologies may be useful for improving access to behavioral interventions for substance use [19]. One strategy that has been used in various health care settings to identify harmful substance use is screening, brief intervention, and referral to treatment (SBIRT) [20].

While SBIRT has been tested in a variety of settings and populations, evidence of its efficacy as a treatment methodology for alcohol and other substance use disorders is mixed [21]. In one study conducted in four countries, SBIRT participants had lower levels of illicit substance use compared to non-SBIRT participants at follow-up, except in the United States [22]. Another meta-analysis found little evidence that SBIRT increased patients' receipt of care to reduce alcohol consumption [23]. A more recent study found no association between a brief intervention and resolution of alcohol use disorder at follow-up in PLHIV patients of the VA [24]. A qualitative study sought to identify facilitators and barriers to implementing SBIRT in primary care, and found general patient support for SBIRT, but also identified inconsistent implementation and provider lack of time as barriers [25]. SBIRT is a potentially promising method for addressing substance use in primary care settings, and could be particularly effective in HIV primary care settings where rates of substance use are high.

Therefore, in an effort to examine SBIRT specifically in an HIV primary care setting, we developed and tested a two-arm approach to delivering SBIRT (Computer vs. Clinician). We then measured changes in self-reported substance use over 6 months, using the Alcohol, Smoking and Substance Involvement Screening Test [26].

Methods
Design

We conducted a two-arm randomized trial to examine the effects of a self-administered, computerized SBIRT intervention compared to a clinician-administered SBIRT intervention in an HIV clinic. The research protocol was approved by the Institutional Review Board of the University of California, San Francisco. The study methods and rationale have been described in detail elsewhere [26, 27]. Based on low rates of participation in the computer-administered arm, we conducted an "as-treated" analysis to examine the observed changes in self-reported substance use over time in participants who received either SBIRT intervention (Computer- or Clinician-administered).

Participants

We recruited a convenience sample of patients between July 2010 and July 2011 from the waiting room of a single public hospital-based HIV clinic in San Francisco, which provides primary medical care to more than 2500 urban poor persons living with HIV/AIDS annually. Study eligibility included: (1) 18 years of age or older; (2) confirmed HIV-positive serostatus; (3) receiving HIV care at the clinic; (4) ability to provide informed consent to be a research participant and be followed over a 6-month period; and (5) ability to speak English or Spanish. All study materials were provided in both English and Spanish.

Randomization

After baseline data collection, participants were randomized in a 1:1 ratio to receive either computer-administered or clinician-administered SBIRT. The research assistants who assessed intervention outcomes and participants' primary care providers were blinded to study assignments.

Intervention

The SBIRT intervention protocol consisted of three components: Screening and Assessment; Brief Intervention; and Referral to Treatment.

Screening and assessment

All participants underwent screening and assessment for tobacco, alcohol and other drug use with the Alcohol, Smoking and Substance Involvement Screening Test (ASSIST), which was developed by the WHO for use in primary care settings [26]. Based on a participant's ASSIST responses, Specific Substance Involvement Scores (SSIS) were generated for each of the drug classes assessed; tobacco, alcohol, cannabis, cocaine, amphetamines, inhalants, sedatives, hallucinogens, opioids and other substances. These scores were used as the basis for the Brief Intervention portion of the SBIRT. Whether self-administered on a computer or administered by a clinician, the ASSIST could be completed in about 10 min [27].

Brief intervention

After screening and assessment, participants received same-day feedback in the form of a WHO ASSIST guided feedback card that detailed their substance use risk severity and received a Brief Intervention tailored to the severity of their SSIS scores and based on the principles of motivational interviewing (MI). Participants scoring at lower risk for health or other problems from their substance use received affirming, positive feedback, and safe behavior maintenance support [28]. Participants with moderate- or high-risk SSIS scores engaged in a patient-centered conversation that explored the pros and cons of continued drug use and readiness for change, and they

reviewed information about specific substance use and its health complications. Action planning was offered to those participants, who were ready to make a change.

Referral to treatment

Participants with high-risk SSIS scores also were offered appointments to meet with the clinic social worker, who had 4 h of protected time per week to meet with participants enrolled in the study. This social worker was a skilled behaviorist with expertise as a motivational interviewing trainer and extensive knowledge and experience providing referrals for different levels of substance use treatment. Treatment options ranged from office-based addiction pharmacotherapy and counseling at the HIV clinic to medically supervised withdrawal programs, intensive outpatient treatment, and inpatient residential treatment programs in the community.

Participants randomized to the Clinician Group were to receive the screening and brief intervention procedures by a trained clinic staff member either the same day or within 1 week of study enrollment. These SBI clinicians included one Nurse and one Medical Assistant, who had more than 10 years combined experience in the HIV clinic, and who participated in two 4-h SBIRT training sessions that included how to administer and score the ASSIST, delivery of the Brief Intervention utilizing WHO ASSIST materials [29], and motivational interviewing principles and practice. Fidelity of the Clinician-administered intervention was monitored through documentation of each step in SBIRT delivery and through bi-weekly supervision meetings with senior study personnel.

Participants randomized to the Computer Group were to receive a self-administered SBIRT procedure embedded in the HIV clinic's web-based personal health record [30]. Study staff assisted participants in setting up their electronic patient portal accounts, if they had not done so already. Participants were instructed to complete the self-administered SBIRT from a computer in the clinic or from a remote computer either the same day or within one week of study enrollment. Developed by the HIV clinic's lead social worker and senior study staff with SBIRT and motivational interviewing expertise, the web-based SBIRT experience was designed to replicate the flow and components of SBIRT conducted by HIV clinic staff. This included interactive web-based screening and assessment using the ASSIST, motivational phrasing for delivery of the Brief Intervention (e.g. allowing the patient to select the substance to prioritize for the Brief Intervention component), and links to substance use websites and patient resources, including referrals to in-person appointments with the HIV clinic social worker—all preprogrammed into the electronic patient portal. We did not track visits to electronic resources.

Assessment measures

Study assessments were conducted by trained research assistants. The baseline interview assessed patient demographics, including gender, sex, race/ethnicity, socioeconomic status, education, and year of HIV diagnosis, as well as frequency and severity of substance use (ASSIST). A urine specimen was collected for a urine drug screen, the results of which were not recorded in the patient's medical record nor shared with clinic staff or providers. All measures except patient demographics were repeated at 1, 3 and 6 months.

The WHO Alcohol, Smoking and Substance Involvement Screening Test (ASSIST) is a self-report measure that consists of eight items to assess lifetime and recent non-medical substance use, including injection drug use, substance use related problems, dependency levels, and risk of current or future harm. From the ASSIST, Specific Substance Involvement Scores (SSIS) were calculated for each of the drug classes assessed; tobacco, alcohol, cannabis, cocaine, amphetamines, inhalants, sedatives, hallucinogens, opioids and other substances. The SSIS is a continuous score ranging from 0 to 31 for tobacco and 0–39 for all other substances. It is the sum of responses to items 2–7: (a) frequency of use in the past 3 months, (b) strong desire or urge to use in the past 3 months, (c) health, social, legal or financial problems due to use of a substance in the past 3 months, (d) failing to do what was normally expected of you due to use of a substance in the past 3 months, (e) anyone ever expressing concern over substance use, and (f) ever trying and failing to control, cut down or stop using. Validated cut-off points stratify scores into lower risk to health and other problems (0–10 for alcohol, 0–3 for all other substances), moderate risk to health and other problems (11–26 for alcohol, 4–26 for all other substances), or high risk (health, social, financial, legal, or relationship) consistent with a diagnosis of substance dependence (27 + for all substances).

Primary outcome

Our primary outcome was change in mean SSIS between baseline and 6-month follow up. Substance use risk level was defined by the mean Specific Substance Involvement Scores assessed at baseline, 1-, 3-, and 6-month study assessments. We dichotomized risk level by previously validated cut-off points [22]: lower risk (SSIS 10 or lower for alcohol, and 3 or lower for each other substance), and collapsed moderate and high risk into a moderate–high risk category (SSIS 10 or above for alcohol, and 4 or above for each other substance). Participants' responses to the ASSIST during the SBIRT intervention procedure were not used to determine this outcome.

Analysis

Baseline demographic characteristics and SSIS were summarized with descriptive statistics. Multilevel regression models (also called hierarchical linear models, linear mixed models, random coefficient models, and random regression models) were used to examine change over time for SSIS. Major advantages of multilevel regression over traditional repeated measures analysis include the fact that cases are not dropped due to missing observations on the dependent variable at any assessment, numeric as well as categorical predictors can be used, and methods for non-normal outcomes are available. Estimation was carried out in Stata/SE Release 14.1 [31] using maximum likelihood and the Expectation–Maximization (EM) algorithm [32–34]. Models were estimated to examine unconditional change over time (linear slope) for unit-increases over the assessment months; differences in the change trajectories as a function of baseline (initial) risk of use for each substance, and differences in the change trajectories due to the intervention by initial risk interaction. Due to strong right-skewness in many of the substance use scores (many participants' reports of substance use were zero), estimation for the multilevel regression models was carried out with a nonparametric bootstrap with 5000 repetitions to obtain bias-corrected confidence intervals, unaffected by either extreme values or skewness [35–39].

The study sample size for the overall study was calculated based on the results of a prior clinic waiting room survey that measured current substance use in 33% of clinic patients (unpublished data). The sample size estimates were large enough to detect a 15% difference in alcohol use between the Computer and Clinician groups, with 80% power and 95% confidence.

Results

A total of 225 people living with HIV were assessed for eligibility to participate in the study (Fig. 1). Of these, seven were excluded because they did not meet eligibility criteria, and 10 were excluded because they did not complete the baseline survey. The remaining 208 individuals were enrolled in the study and randomized. These 208 participants were primarily male (66.4%) and largely African American (39.9%), with a mean age of 45.4 years (Table 1). The majority had a high school education or less (63.4%), were unemployed (85.3%), and reported substance use (tobacco, alcohol, marijuana, stimulants, opiates, etc.) in the past 3 months (92%). The mean time since HIV diagnosis was 12.4 years. Mean Specific Substance Involvement Scores were in the moderate risk range for all substances except inhalants, hallucinogens, and other substances. SSIS were

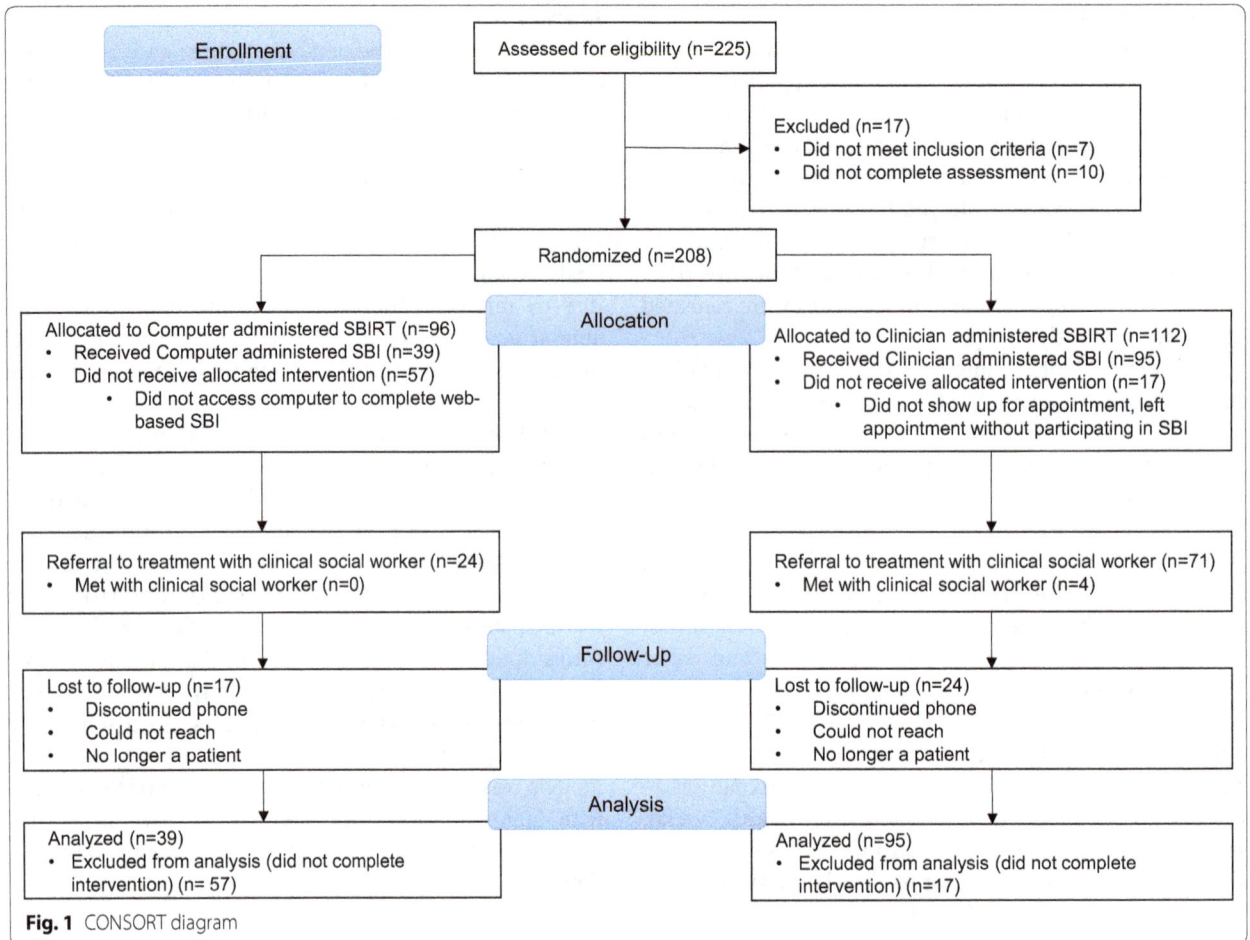

Fig. 1 CONSORT diagram

highest for tobacco, alcohol, cannabis, cocaine, and amphetamine.

Of the 208 individuals enrolled in the study, 134 (64%) individuals completed the baseline assessment visit and also received an SBIRT intervention. Of the 134, follow-up assessment rates were: 123 (92%) at 1-month, 106 (79%) at 3-month and 109 (81%) at 6-month; 92 (68.7%) completed all four study assessments and the intervention. Ninety-five participants with high SSIS accepted referrals to the clinic social worker, but only four met with the social worker. There were no significant baseline differences in sociodemographic characteristics or mean SSIS between those who received the intervention and those who did not (Table 1). Similarly, we found no differences between SBIRT treatment modality (Computer or Clinician) in our outcome measures of interest (SSIS) over time (data not shown).

For all substances, mean SSIS increased over time among those initially in the lower risk groups. The increase was statistically significant for all substances except amphetamines and sedatives (Tables 2, 3).

However, among those individuals with moderate–high risk at baseline, mean SSIS for all substances decreased at 6 months. The decrease was statistically significant for all substances except tobacco and cannabis. For all substances, the decrease in mean SSIS for the moderate–high risk group differed significantly from the increase in mean SSIS for the lower risk group.

Discussion

We conducted a screening, brief intervention, and referral to treatment (SBIRT) intervention in an urban safety-net HIV primary care clinic and detected a high prevalence of self-reported alcohol, tobacco, cannabis, cocaine, amphetamine, sedatives, and opioid use at enrollment. For all substances, the mean SSIS score for participants whose baseline substance use risk was moderate–high and who received the SBIRT intervention declined over the 6 months following the intervention, and this decrease was significant when compared to those at baseline lower risk.

While active substance use was not one of the inclusion criteria, 92% of study participants reported any substance

Table 1 Characteristics of participants enrolled in an SBIRT Study (Computer and Clinician Administered) in an HIV primary care clinic (N = 208)

Variable	Total (n = 208)	Received intervention (n = 134)	No intervention (n = 74)	P
Age (mean, SD)	45.4 ± 8.5	45.0 ± 8.5	46.1 ± 8.5	0.40
Race				
African American	83 (39.9)	54 (40.3)	29 (39.2)	0.92
Caucasian	64 (30.8)	40 (29.9)	24 (32.4)	
Hispanic	35 (16.8)	24 (17.9)	11 (14.9)	
Other	26 (12.5)	16 (11.9)	10 (13.5)	
Gender				
Female	49 (23.6)	32 (23.9)	17 (23.0)	0.51*
Male	138 (66.4)	86 (64.2)	52 (70.3)	
Other	21 (10.1)	16 (11.9)	5 (6.8)	
Education (n = 202)				
High school or GED	128 (63.4)	82 (63.6)	46 (63.0)	0.94
More than high school	74 (36.6)	47 (36.4)	27 (37.0)	
Currently employed (n = 204)				
No	174 (85.3)	112 (84.9)	62 (86.1)	0.80
Yes	30 (14.7)	20 (15.2)	10 (13.9)	
Adequate income (n = 204)				
Totally inadequate	45 (22.1)	26 (20.0)	19 (25.7)	0.34*
Barely adequate	128 (62.8)	81 (62.3)	47 (63.5)	
Enough	31 (15.2)	23 (17.7)	8 (10.8)	
Health insurance (n = 205)				
No	36 (17.6)	23 (17.6)	13 (17.6)	1.00
Yes	169 (82.4)	108 (82.4)	61 (82.4)	
Clinical				
Years positive (mean, SD)	12.4 ± 7.4	12.7 ± 7.5	11.9 ± 7.1	0.44
Undetectable viral load	128 (61.5)	85 (63.4)	43 (58.1)	0.45
CD4 count (mean, SD)	512.5 ± 333.5	503.8 ± 356.6	527.8 ± 290.5	0.68
SSIS (mean, SD)[a]				
Tobacco	14.6 ± 10.8	15.1 ± 10.7	13.8 ± 11.1	0.43
Alcohol	11.2 ± 10.8	11.4 ± 11.0	10.6 ± 10.4	0.60
Cannabis	9.9 ± 10.4	10.1 ± 10.5	9.4 ± 10.4	0.65
Cocaine	9.0 ± 11.0	9.7 ± 11.4	7.6 ± 10.1	0.20
Amphetamine	8.3 ± 11.0	9.1 ± 11.5	6.9 ± 10.2	0.19
Inhalants	1.7 ± 4.9	2.0 ± 5.6	1.2 ± 2.9	0.30
Sedatives	4.3 ± 7.6	4.5 ± 8.0	3.7 ± 6.5	0.52
Hallucinogens	1.8 ± 5.3	2.1 ± 6.1	1.1 ± 3.2	0.22
Opioids	4.3 ± 8.2	4.6 ± 8.4	3.7 ± 7.8	0.50
Other	1.2 ± 4.5	1.2 ± 4.5	1.3 ± 4.5	0.88

SSIS Specific Substance Involvement Score, from the ASSIST measure

* Fisher's exact

[a] Validated cut points: lower risk to health and other problems (0–10 for alcohol, 0–3 for all other substances), moderate risk to health and other problems (11–26 for alcohol, 4–26 for all other substances), high risk of severe problems (health, social, financial, legal, or relationship) consistent with a diagnosis of substance dependence (27 + for all substances)

use (tobacco, alcohol, marijuana, stimulants, opiates, etc.) in the prior 3 months. This finding is consistent with the known higher prevalence of substance use for PLHIV compared to the general U.S. national population [40]. Our results also show that, in an HIV primary care population, while mean SSISs were in the moderate range for most substances, a number of individuals were in the high risk range, as indicated by the large standard

Table 2 Change in mean Single Substance Involvement Scores from baseline to 6 months among 134 patient participants who received Clinician-Administered or Computer-Administered screening, brief intervention, and referral to treatment in an HIV primary care clinic

	Change in SSIS from baseline to 6-months among those at lower risk at baseline	Change in SSIS from baseline to 6-months among those at moderate–high risk at baseline
Tobacco	+ 2.25	− 0.99
Alcohol	+ 1.79	− 7.73
Cannabis	+ 3.13	− 2.38
Cocaine	+ 1.81	− 3.10
Amphetamines	+ 0.52	− 3.65
Inhalants	+ 1.02	− 4.34
Sedatives	+ 0.52	− 8.98
Hallucinogens	+ 0.98	− 10.08
Opioids	+ 1.42	− 6.76

deviations for each substance. These indicators of the severity of self-reported substance use, underscore the opportunity for detection and intervention in HIV primary care settings.

We measured a significant reduction over time in the mean SSIS for alcohol − 1.59 (95% CI − 2.19, − 1.00) among participants who scored in the medium high risk categories. Several other studies that measured self-report of substance use before and following SBIRT implementation in clinical settings have been conducted and allow for a comparison with the findings of our analysis. One of the first studies to determine the effect of SBIRT in diverse clinic populations found SBI to be associated with a decrease in self-reported alcohol use at follow-up [20]. Other studies evaluating measures of alcohol use severity before and after participating in SBIRT show similar results [41]. A more recent study among PLHIV, however, found that although alcohol use declined over time, the decline was not associated with receipt of a brief intervention [24].

We also measured moderate but statistically significant decreases in mean SSISs for illicit drugs, including reductions in cocaine − 0.82 (95% CI − 1.39, − 0.25), amphetamines − 0.69 (95% CI − 1.32, − 0.10), sedatives − 1.58 (95% CI − 2.21, − 0.92) and opioids − 1.31 (95% CI − 2.13, − 0.36). Other studies have shown mixed results of the impact of SBIRT on illicit drug use following participation in SBIRT. The ASPIRE study (Assessing Screening Plus Brief Interventions Resulting Efficacy to Stop Drug Use), a 3-group randomized controlled trial for unhealthy drug use among adults from an urban primary care setting, did not demonstrate a decrease in

unhealthy drug use following receipt of a primary care based SBIRT intervention [42]. Other studies have shown similar negative results of the effects of SBIRT on illicit substance use [43]. In contrast, Humeniuk and colleagues found significantly reduced SSISs among participants receiving a brief intervention compared to control participants, for all substances except opioids [22]. And Bernstein and colleagues found reductions in cocaine and heroin use among individuals receiving SBIRT [44].

In our study, we saw a reduction in mean SSIS for tobacco use among participants at moderate–high risk at baseline. Cropsey and colleagues also found that PLHIV who smoked at least five cigarettes per day significantly reduced their smoking over time following an SBIRT intervention that included a counseling session, nicotine replacement therapy, and follow-up visits, compared to those in usual care [45]. In a pilot study of 30 women living with HIV, those who received a motivational interviewing session reported significant reductions in the mean number of cigarettes smoked, compared to those who did not receive the MI intervention [46].

Surprisingly, we found that mean SSIS scores for participants who scored in the lower risk range at baseline increased over the 6 months for all substances at the same time that use dropped for those in the moderate–high risk group (this is the cross-level interaction between time and group, and it is equivalent to the difference between the simple slopes for each group). It is possible that the Brief Intervention that was given to those in the moderate–high risk groups had an important effect on reducing SSIS scores, but that the minimal intervention given to those in the lower risk group was not fully effective at keeping risk levels low. This was particularly the case for tobacco and cannabis; for both of these substances, mean SSISs in the lower risk group increased more than the scores decreased in the moderate–high risk group (the simple slope was greater in absolute value for the lower risk group only for tobacco and cannabis).

In some studies [22, 26, 42], ASSIST scores were reported as lower, moderate or high risk. Reporting and analyzing SSIS by risk categories is important because individuals who fall into the lower and moderate risk group may derive different benefits, and because brief interventions have previously been shown to be more effective among people with less severe substance use problems [20, 47]. In contrast to other studies, our outcome observation is based on a mean change score and on dichotomized risk groups, which may or may not be clinically useful distinctions. This area needs further study and exploring more effective interventions for people at lower risk for substance use related problems is an important area for future research.

Table 3 Estimated change in Specific Substance Involvement Scores over 6 months for PLHIV SBIRT intervention participants at lower compared to moderate–high risk at baseline

Substance	Effect[a]	Coefficient[b]	95% BC CI[b, c] Lower, upper limit
Tobacco	Months—lower	0.38	0.15, 0.65
	Months—M–H	− 0.16	− 0.44, 0.13
	Risk category	18.31	16.71, 19.90
	Month by risk	− 0.54	− 0.93, − 0.17
	Intercept[d]	1.57	
Alcohol	Months—lower	0.30	0.09, 0.51
	Months—M–H	− 1.29	− 1.84, − 0.75
	Risk category	17.44	15.44, 19.37
	Month by risk	− 1.59	− 2.19, − 1.00
	Intercept	4.06	
Cannabis	Months—lower	0.52	0.17, 1.02
	Months—M–H	− 0.40	− 0.84, 0.03
	Risk category	13.68	11.81, 15.69
	Month by risk	− 0.92	− 1.60, − 0.36
	Intercept	1.36	
Cocaine	Months—lower	0.30	0.06, 0.63
	Months—M–H	− 0.52	− 1.01, − 0.01
	Risk category	16.48	14.06, 19.03
	Month by risk	− 0.82	− 1.39, − 0.25
	Intercept	1.28	
Amphetamine	Months—lower	0.09	− 0.03, 0.21
	Months—M–H	− 0.61	− 1.22, − 0.02
	Risk category	15.95	13.56, 18.43
	Month by risk	− 0.69	− 1.32, − 0.10
	Intercept	0.75	
Inhalants	Months—lower	0.17	0.06, 0.32
	Months—M–H	− 0.72	− 1.40, − 0.09
	Risk category	7.23	4.65, 10.16
	Month by risk	− 0.89	− 1.58, − 0.24
	Intercept	0.33	
Sedatives	Months—lower	0.09	− 0.01, 0.21
	Months—M–H	− 1.50	− 2.12, − 0.83
	Risk category	12.19	9.77, 14.96
	Month by risk	− 1.58	− 2.21, − 0.92
	Intercept	0.62	
Hallucinogens	Months—lower	0.16	0.05, 0.30
	Months—M–H	− 1.68	− 3.05, − 0.02
	Risk category	11.49	7.61, 15.86
	Month by risk	− 1.84	− 3.22, − 0.18
	Intercept	0.31	
Opioids	Months—lower	0.19	0.05, 0.35

Table 3 continued

Substance	Effect[a]	Coefficient[b]	95% BC CI[b, c] Lower, upper limit
	Months—M–H	− 1.13	− 1.93, − 0.17
	Risk category	13.68	10.87, 16.53
	Month by risk	− 1.31	− 2.13, − 0.36
	Intercept	0.72	

[a] Effects in each multilevel regression model. Months—lower is simple slope over time for lower risk category; months—M–H is simple slope over time for moderate–high risk category; reference group for risk category at baseline = 0 (lower risk); month by risk is the cross-level interaction (equivalent to the difference between the two simple slopes, with lower risk as the reference category; the display with only two decimals sometimes results in rounding errors in the table)

[b] The nonparametric, bootstrapped 95% bias-corrected confidence interval from 5000 repetitions

[c] The coefficient is significant if zero is not in the interval

[d] The test of the intercept against zero is not a hypothesis test of interest

While the levels of substance use self-reported among this cohort of PLHIV patients is higher than in the general U.S. national population [40], it can be difficult to make comparisons between studies because of the variability of substance use measures. For example, in a study with a safety-net primary care population, participants received an intervention based on reports of problem drug use via the Addiction Severity Index-Lite measure [43]. Because of differences between the Addiction Severity Index and the ASSIST, similar participants in each study may have been assessed at different levels of risk, and therefore may have differed in whether they qualified to receive an SBIRT intervention or not. Such differences make comparisons difficult.

Our study has several limitations. First, the data reported here were all self-reported, which could be biased due to participant recall or social desirability. Second, while these findings suggest that SBIRT delivery in HIV care settings may be associated with a decrease in the mean SSIS scores for moderate–high risk substance use, we do not have a good understanding of the clinical significance of these changes in mean scores. A decrease in the SSIS for any substance is a change in the right direction when our goal is to address substance use in HIV clinical settings. However, in the absence of a no-treatment control group it is possible that the decrease in SSIS scores across both arms of the study could be due to regression to the mean and not the intervention [48]. Third, for this analysis, which examined only those participants who received the intervention, our analytic sample may have been underpowered, despite the fact that we enrolled a sufficient number of participants into the study based on our a priori sample size calculations for a randomized trial. Notwithstanding the smaller analytic sample size, we did detect a statistically significant decrease on the moderate–high risk mean SSIS of those who received the SBIRT intervention when compared to those with lower risk scores. Fourth, while the ASSIST measure includes many drugs and does not solely capture the level of use for the substance of concern to the participant, the BI that was delivered by each modality was based on the substance of most concern to the patient. Nonetheless, our use of the ASSIST allowed us to gain a more expansive understanding of the number and types of substances used by this HIV primary care sample and this may be one benefit for using the ASSIST. Use of the ASSIST in clinical settings could have the advantage of giving providers screening and assessment information for multiple substances. Fifth, as part of our study procedures we did not adequately document the number of brief intervention visits either with a clinician or through the computer portal so we were unable to capture meaningful information about the dose of the exposure to the intervention to allow for dose–response analyses. Sixth, our findings may not be generalizable to PLHIV who are not engaged in primary care or to patients of HIV clinics that do not serve an urban safety-net population.

Further, while we collected baseline substance use and follow up data on 208 participants, and all participants were assigned to one of two SBIRT modalities, we observed a significant drop off between assessment and participation in the intervention; only 64% of participants who completed the baseline study visit actually received the intervention by either modality, leading to our decision to present an "as treated" analysis. This was particularly the case for those assigned to the computer group, which may indicate difficulties or discomfort with accessing computers and the Internet, or concern about the privacy of data entered into a computer linked to the Internet (a more detailed discussion of this phenomenon is available elsewhere [49]). In addition, very few of those referred to treatment actually met with the social worker as indicated, possibly indicating that they were not ready to take the initiative to seek out treatment for themselves, and that a more immediate and supported linkage might be needed. For participants assigned to the clinician group, this might take the form of a warm hand-off from the clinician conducting the screening to the social worker. For those using the web-based interface, a direct link in the portal to make an appointment, or some form of chat function could be useful. In addition, the 4 h per week may have occurred at a time when the participants could not participate and may have necessitated a follow-up or additional clinic visit to meet with the social worker.

Conclusions
Unhealthy substance use erodes PLHIV's progress at every step of the HIV continuum of care—from linkage to and retention in care, to antiretroviral adherence and viral suppression. This study suggests that among PLHIV presenting for care, HIV clinics have an opportunity to identify large numbers of patients that use multiple substances. While the study observed a significant decrease in mean self-reported risk to health and other problems among HIV clinic patients with moderate–high risk use who received a brief intervention, mean risk increased among lower risk patients. The model for offering BI or treatment in the clinic setting is important to understand, and integrated office-based addiction treatment is an important but underutilized alternative to referring patients elsewhere for specialty treatment [50, 51]. Additional research should examine whether the observed changes in ASSIST scores are clinically significant, elucidate what components of the intervention drive the reduction in moderate–high risk scores, and what other interventions might work for those at lower risk to maintain health and engagement along the HIV care continuum. This study suggests that among PLHIV presenting for care, HIV clinics have an opportunity to identify large numbers of patients that use multiple substances and to develop models for intervening.

Abbreviations
PLHIV: people living with HIV; SBIRT: screening, brief intervention, and referral to treatment; SSIS: Specific Substance Involvement Scores; SUD: substance use disorders; AUD: alcohol use disorder; UNAIDS: Jointed United Nations Programme on HIV and AIDS; ART: antiretroviral therapy; PHP: Positive Health Program; WHO: World Health Organization; UCSF: University of California, San Francisco; VL: viral load; CI: confidence interval; ASPIRE: Assessing Screening Plus brief Intervention's Resulting Efficacy; ED: emergency department; RCT: randomized controlled trial.

Authors' contributions
CDR and PL conceived the study and obtained funding. CDR, JD, YC, RZ and BC wrote the manuscript. JD, YC and BC analyzed the data. EH led data management and assisted in manuscript preparation. All authors read and approved the final manuscript.

Author details
[1] UCSF School of Nursing, 2 Koret Way, Box 0608, San Francisco, CA 94143-0608, USA. [2] Division of HIV, Infectious Diseases, and Global Medicine, UCSF Department of Medicine, San Francisco General Hospital, 1001 Potrero Ave, 307, Box 0874, San Francisco, CA 94110, USA. [3] Present Address: UC Davis Betty Irene Moore School of Nursing, 2450 48th Street, Suite 2600, Sacramento, CA 95817, USA.

Acknowledgements
The authors would like to acknowledge Shannon Eng, Emiko Kamitami, Guy Vandenberg, and Vanessa Blaz for their assistance with the study.

Competing interests
The authors declare that they have no competing interests.

Consent for publication
Not applicable.

Funding
This work was supported by Award No. 1RC1DA028224 from the National Institute of Drug Abuse and by Award No. 5T32 NR007081 from the National Institute of Nursing Research. The content is solely the responsibility of the authors and does not necessarily represent the official views of the National Institutes of Health.

References
1. CDC. HIV in the United States: at a Glance. 2016. http://www.cdc.gov/hiv/statistics/overview/ataglance.html. Accessed 29 Nov 2016.
2. Strathdee SA, Hallett TB, Bobrova N, Rhodes T, Booth R, Abdool R, et al. HIV and risk environment for injecting drug users: the past, present, and future. Lancet. 2010;376:268–84. https://doi.org/10.1016/s0140-6736(10)60743-x.
3. Williams EC, Hahn JA, Saitz R, Bryant K, Lira MC, Samet JH. Alcohol use and human immunodeficiency virus (HIV) infection: current knowledge, implications, and future directions. Alcohol Clin Exp Res. 2016;40:2056–72. https://doi.org/10.1111/acer.13204.
4. San Francisco Department of Public Health. HIV Epidemiology Annual Report 2015. 2015. https://www.sfdph.org/dph/comupg/oprograms/HIVepiSec/HIVepiSecReports.asp. Accessed 29 Nov 2016.
5. Westergaard RP, Hess T, Astemborski J, Mehta SH, Kirk GD. Longitudinal changes in engagement in care and viral suppression for HIV-infected injection drug users. AIDS. 2013;27:2559–66. https://doi.org/10.1097/QAD.0b013e328363bff2.
6. Christopoulos KA, Massey AD, Lopez AM, Geng EH, Johnson MO, Pilcher CD, et al. "Taking a half day at a time:" patient perspectives and the HIV engagement in care continuum. AIDS Patient Care STDs. 2013;27:223–30. https://doi.org/10.1089/apc.2012.0418.
7. Nicholas PK, Willard S, Thompson C, Dawson-Rose C, Corless IB, Wantland DJ, et al. Engagement with care, substance use, and adherence to therapy in HIV/AIDS. AIDS Res Treat. 2014. https://doi.org/10.1155/2014/675739.
8. Mimiaga MJ, Reisner SL, Grasso C, Crane HM, Safren SA, Kitahata MM, et al. Substance use among HIV-infected patients engaged in primary care in the United States: findings from the Centers for AIDS Research Network of Integrated Clinical Systems cohort. Am J Public Health. 2013;103:1457–67. https://doi.org/10.2105/AJPH.2012.301162.
9. Risher K, Mayer KH, Beyrer C. HIV treatment cascade in MSM, people who inject drugs, and sex workers. Curr Opin HIV AIDS. 2015;10:420–9. https://doi.org/10.1097/coh.0000000000000200.
10. Walley AY, Palmisano J, Sorensen-Alawad A, Chaisson C, Raj A, Samet JH, et al. Engagement and substance dependence in a primary care-based addiction treatment program for people infected with HIV and people at high-risk for HIV infection. J Subst Abuse Treat. 2015;59:59–66. https://doi.org/10.1016/j.jsat.2015.07.007.
11. Cohen SM, Hu X, Sweeney P, Johnson AS, Hall HI. HIV viral suppression among persons with varying levels of engagement in HIV medical care, 19 US jurisdictions. J Acquir Immune Defic Syndr. 2014;67:519–27. https://doi.org/10.1097/qai.0000000000000349.
12. Golin CE, Liu H, Hays RD, Miller LG, Beck CK, Ickovics J, et al. A prospective study of predictors of adherence to combination antiretroviral medication. J Gen Intern Med. 2002;17:756–65.
13. Volkow ND, Montaner J. Enhanced HIV testing, treatment, and support for HIV-infected substance users. JAMA. 2010;303:1423–4. https://doi.org/10.1001/jama.2010.421.
14. Dombrowski JC, Kitahata MM, Van Rompaey SE, Crane HM, Mugavero MJ, Eron JJ, et al. High levels of antiretroviral use and viral suppression among persons in HIV care in the United States, 2010. J Acquir Immune Defic Syndr. 2013;63:299–306. https://doi.org/10.1097/QAI.0b013e3182945bc7.
15. Substance Abuse and Mental Health Services Administration Center for Behavioral Health Statistics and Quality, "The NSDUH Report: HIV/AIDS and Substance Use," ed. Rockville; 2010.
16. U.S. Department of Health and Human Services (HHS) Office of the Surgeon General, "Facing Addiction in America: The Surgeon General's Report on Alcohol, Drugs, and Health," HHS, ed. Washington; 2016.
17. Williams EC, Lapham GT, Shortreed SM, Rubinsky AD, Bobb JF, Bensley KM, et al. Among patients with unhealthy alcohol use, those with HIV are less likely than those without to receive evidence-based alcohol-related care: a national VA study. Drug Alcohol Depend. 2017;174:113–20.
18. Mugavero MJ, Amico KR, Horn T, Thompson MA. The state of engagement in HIV care in the United States: from cascade to continuum to control. Clin Infect Dis. 2013;57:1164–71. https://doi.org/10.1093/cid/cit420.
19. Carroll K, Ball S, Martino S, Nich C, Babuscio T, Nuro K, et al. Computer-assisted delivery of cognitive-behavioral therapy for addiction: a randomized trial of CBT4CBT. Am J Psychiatry. 2008;165:881–8.
20. Madras BK, Compton WM, Avula D, Stegbauer T, Stein JB, Clark HW. Screening, brief interventions, referral to treatment (SBIRT) for illicit drug and alcohol use at multiple healthcare sites: comparison at intake and 6 months later. Drug Alcohol Depend. 2009;99:280–95. https://doi.org/10.1016/j.drugalcdep.2008.08.003.
21. Glass JE, Hamilton AM, Powell BJ, Perron BE, Brown RT, Ilgen MA. Revisiting our review of screening, brief intervention and referral to treatment (SBIRT): meta-analytical results still point to no efficacy in increasing the use of substance use disorder services. Addiction. 2016;111:181–3. https://doi.org/10.1111/add.13146.
22. Humeniuk R, Ali R, Babor T, Souza-Formigoni ML, de Lacerda RB, Ling W, et al. A randomized controlled trial of a brief intervention for illicit drugs linked to the Alcohol, Smoking and Substance Involvement Screening Test (ASSIST) in clients recruited from primary health-care settings in four countries. Addiction. 2012;107:957–66. https://doi.org/10.1111/j.1360-0443.2011.03740.x.
23. Glass JE, Hamilton AM, Powell BJ, Perron BE, Brown RT, Ilgen MA. Specialty substance use disorder services following brief alcohol intervention: a meta-analysis of randomized controlled trials. Addiction. 2015;110:1404–15. https://doi.org/10.1111/add.12950.
24. Williams EC, Lapham GT, Bobb JF, Rubinsky AD, Catz SL, Shortreed SM, et al. Documented brief intervention not associated with resolution of unhealthy alcohol use one year later among VA patients living with HIV. J Subst Abuse Treat. 2017;78:8–14.
25. Rahm AK, Boggs JM, Martin C, Price DW, Beck A, Backer TE, et al. Facilitators and barriers to implementing screening, brief intervention, and referral to treatment (SBIRT) in primary care in integrated health care settings. Subst Abuse. 2015;36:281–8. https://doi.org/10.1080/08897077.2014.951140.
26. WHO Assist Working Group. The Alcohol, Smoking and Substance Involvement Screening Test (ASSIST): development, reliability and feasibility. Addiction. 2002;97:1183–94.
27. McNeely J, Strauss SM, Wright S, Rotrosen J, Khan R, Lee JD, et al. Test–retest reliability of a self-administered Alcohol, Smoking and Substance Involvement Screening Test (ASSIST) in primary care patients. J Subst Abuse Treat. 2014;47:93–101.
28. Babor TF, McRee BG, Kassebaum PA, Grimaldi PL, Ahmed K, Bray J. Screening, brief intervention, and referral to treatment (SBIRT): toward a public health approach to the management of substance abuse. Subst Abus. 2007;28:7–30.
29. Humeniuk R, Ali R, Babor TF, Farrell M, Formigoni ML, Jittiwutikarn J, et al. Validation of the Alcohol, Smoking And Substance Involvement Screening Test (ASSIST). Addiction. 2008;103:1039–47. https://doi.org/10.1111/j.1360-0443.2007.02114.x.
30. Kahn JS, Hilton JF, Van Nunnery T, Leasure S, Bryant KM, Hare CB, et al. Personal health records in a public hospital: experience at the HIV/AIDS clinic at San Francisco General Hospital. J Am Med Inform Assoc. 2010;17:224–8.

31. StataCorp. Stata Statistical Software: Release 14. College Station: Stata-Corp LP; 2015.

32. Hox J. Multilevel analysis: techniques and applications. 2nd ed. New York: Routledge Academic, Taylor & Francis Group; 2010.

33. Rabe-Hesketh S, Skrondal A. Multilevel and longitudinal modeling using Stata. 3rd ed. College Station: Stata Press; 2012.

34. Singer JD, Willett JB. Applied longitudinal data analysis: modeling change and event occurrence. New York: Oxford University Press; 2003.

35. Carpenter J, Bithell J. Bootstrap confidence intervals: when, which, what? A practical guide for medical statisticians. Stat Med. 2000;19:1141–64.

36. Efron B. The bootstrap and modern statistics. J Am Stat Assoc. 2000;95:1293–6.

37. Wehrens R, Putter H, Buydens LM. The bootstrap: a tutorial. Chemom Intell Lab Syst. 2000;54:35–52. https://doi.org/10.1016/s0169-7439(00)00102-7.

38. Wood M. Bootstrapped confidence intervals as an approach to statistical inference. Organ Res Methods. 2005;8:454–70. https://doi.org/10.1177/1094428105280059.

39. Zhu WM. Making bootstrap statistical inferences: a tutorial. Res Q Exerc Sport. 1997;68:44–55.

40. Whiteford HA, Degenhardt L, Rehm J, Baxter AJ, Ferrari AJ, Erskine HE, et al. Global burden of disease attributable to mental and substance use disorders: findings from the Global Burden of Disease Study 2010. Lancet. 2013;382:1575–86. https://doi.org/10.1016/S0140-6736(13)61611-6.

41. Academic ED SBIRT Research Collaborative. The impact of screening, brief intervention, and referral for treatment on emergency department patients' alcohol use. Ann Emerg Med. 2007;50:699–710 (e6).

42. Saitz R, Palfai TP, Cheng DM, Alford DP, Bernstein JA, Lloyd-Travaglini CA, et al. Screening and brief intervention for drug use in primary care: the ASPIRE randomized clinical trial. JAMA. 2014;312:502–13. https://doi.org/10.1001/jama.2014.7862.

43. Roy-Byrne P, Bumgardner K, Krupski A, Dunn C, Ries R, Donovan D, et al. Brief intervention for problem drug use in safety-net primary care settings: a randomized clinical trial. JAMA. 2014;312:492–501. https://doi.org/10.1001/jama.2014.7860.

44. Bernstein J, Bernstein E, Tassiopoulos K, Heeren T, Levenson S, Hingson R. Brief motivational intervention at a clinic visit reduces cocaine and heroin use. Drug Alcohol Depend. 2005;77:49–59. https://doi.org/10.1016/j.drugalcdep.2004.07.006.

45. Cropsey KL, Hendricks PS, Jardin B, Clark CB, Katiyar N, Willig J, et al. A pilot study of screening, brief intervention, and referral for treatment (SBIRT) in non-treatment seeking smokers with HIV. Addict Behav. 2013;38:2541–6. https://doi.org/10.1016/j.addbeh.2013.05.003.

46. Manuel JK, Lum PJ, Hengl NS, Sorensen JL. Smoking cessation interventions with female smokers living with HIV/AIDS: a randomized pilot study of motivational interviewing. AIDS Care. 2013;25:820–7. https://doi.org/10.1080/09540121.2012.733331.

47. Whitlock EP, Polen MR, Green CA, Orleans T, Klein J, Force USPST. Behavioral counseling interventions in primary care to reduce risky/harmful alcohol use by adults: a summary of the evidence for the U.S. Preventive Services Task Force. Ann Intern Med. 2004;140:557–68.

48. Finney JW. Regression to the mean in substance use disorder treatment research. Addiction. 2008;103:42–52. https://doi.org/10.1111/j.1360-0443.2007.02032.x.

49. Dawson Rose C, Cuca YP, Kamitani E, Eng S, Zepf R, Draughon J, et al. Using interactive web-based screening, brief intervention and referral to treatment in an urban, safety-net HIV clinic. AIDS Behav. 2015;19(Suppl 2):186–93. https://doi.org/10.1007/s10461-015-1078-y.

50. Altice FL, Bruce RD, Lucas GM, Lum PJ, Korthuis PT, Flanigan TP, et al. HIV treatment outcomes among HIV-infected, opioid-dependent patients receiving buprenorphine/naloxone treatment within HIV clinical care settings: results from a multisite study. J Acquir Immune Defic Syndr. 1999;2011(56):S22.

51. Korthuis PT, Lum PJ, Vergara-Rodriguez P, Ahamad K, Wood E, Kunkel LE, et al. Feasibility and safety of extended-release naltrexone treatment of opioid and alcohol use disorder in HIV clinics: a pilot/feasibility randomized trial. Addiction. 2017;112:1036–44. https://doi.org/10.1111/add.13753.

16

Enhancing patient navigation to improve intervention session attendance and viral load suppression of persons with HIV and substance use

Maxine Stitzer[1]*, Tim Matheson[2], Colin Cunningham[1], James L. Sorensen[3], Daniel J. Feaster[4], Lauren Gooden[5], Alexis S. Hammond[1], Heather Fitzsimons[1] and Lisa R. Metsch[5]

Abstract

Background: Interventions are needed to improve viral suppression rates among persons with HIV and substance use. A 3-arm randomized multi-site study (Metsch et al. in JAMA 316:156–70, 2016) was conducted to evaluate the effect on HIV outcomes of usual care referral to HIV and substance use services (N = 253) versus patient navigation delivered alone (PN: N = 266) or together with contingency management (PN + CM; N = 271) that provided financial incentives targeting potential behavioral mediators of viral load suppression.

Aims: This secondary analysis evaluates the effects of financial incentives on attendance at PN sessions and the relationship between session attendance and viral load suppression at end of the intervention.

Methods: Frequency of sessions attended was analyzed over time and by distribution of individual session attendance frequency (PN vs PN + CM). Percent virally suppressed ($\leq$200 copies/mL) at 6 months was compared for low, medium and high rate attenders. In PN + CM a total of $220 could be earned for attendance at 11 PN sessions over the 6-month intervention with payments ranging from $10 to $30 under an escalating schedule.

Results: The majority (74%) of PN-only participants attended 6 or more sessions but only 28% attended 10 or more and 16% attended all eleven sessions. In contrast, 90% of PN + CM attended 6 or more visits, 69% attended 10 or more and 57% attended all eleven sessions (attendance distribution $\chi^2[11] = 105.81$; p < .0001). Overall (PN and PN + CM participants combined) percent with viral load suppression at 6-months was 15, 38 and 54% among those who attended 0–5, 6–9 and 10–11 visits, respectively ($\chi^2(2) = 39.07$, p < .001).

Conclusion: In this secondary post hoc analysis, contact with patient navigators was increased by attendance incentives. Higher rates of attendance at patient navigation sessions was associated with viral suppression at the 6-month follow-up assessment. Study results support use of attendance incentives to improve rates of contact between service providers and patients, particularly patients who are difficult to engage in care.

Trial Registration clinicaltrials.govIdentifier: NCT01612169.

Keywords: HIV health care, HIV substance users, Patient navigation, Contingent incentives, Session attendance, Vial suppression

*Correspondence: mstitzer@jhmi.edu
[1] Department of Psychiatry and Behavioral Sciences, Hopkins Bayview Medical Center, Johns Hopkins University School of Medicine, 5510 Nathan Shock Drive, Baltimore, MD 21224, USA
Full list of author information is available at the end of the article

Background

Inconsistent engagement with health care services is common among individuals with substance use disorders [2]. This is especially problematic for people living with HIV, due to the importance of ongoing engagement in care for optimal health outcomes. Because drug use can interfere with every step of the treatment cascade [3], there is evidence that HIV-infected drug users may have faster disease progression, higher risk of acquiring new AIDS-defining conditions [4] and higher rates of hospitalization [5] compared to non-drug users. Azar et al. [6] came to similar conclusions in a review of studies that addressed the associations among Alcohol Use Disorder (AUD), health care utilization, adherence to antiretroviral medications, and HIV treatment outcomes. These findings underscore the importance of focused engagement in care interventions for vulnerable populations with substance use.

Contingency management (CM) in the form of financial incentives for uptake and adherence to health care services has promising results in a variety of settings [7]. Examples of simple but effective attendance interventions include financial incentives for return to a test site to receive HIV [8] or tuberculosis [9, 10]) test results, completion of a 3-injection course of hepatitis B vaccine [11] return to a substance use disorders treatment program following intake to complete an individualized service plan [12] and persistence with substance use disorders treatment when modest financial incentives were offered for a return visit to the clinic following intake and for attendance on day 5 post-admission [13].

Studies targeting sustained attendance at therapy visits have also shown contingent financial incentives to be efficacious in improving engagement in HIV care among persons with substance use disorders [14, 15]. Other studies using a variety of specific incentive delivery methods report that incentives improve attendance at counseling sessions [16–22] or psychiatric services [23] in substance use disorders treatment programs. However, studies to date have not shown the effectiveness of contingency management in improving health-related outcomes including viral load suppression among HIV-positive substance users [1, 7, 15].

A recently completed 3-arm multi-site study conducted within the National Drug Abuse Treatment Clinical Trials Network (CTN 0049/Project HOPE: Hospital as Opportunity for Prevention and Engagement for HIV Infected Drug Users) provided an opportunity to examine the potential value of adding incentives to a behavioral intervention platform in improving HIV outcomes among substance users with uncontrolled HIV. CM was incorporated into a patient navigation (PN) intervention designed to improve engagement in HIV care and substance use treatment and adherence with HIV health care regimens among persons with HIV and substance use. Patient navigation is a clinical support intervention that uses motivational interviewing techniques and a flexible, problem-solving approach to overcoming barriers [24, 25] with the aim of promoting engagement in health care services. A navigation approach has been previously shown effective for improving linkage to [26] and retention in [27] HIV care. Outcomes for the navigation intervention with (PN + CM) and without (PN only) incentives was compared to a usual care referral group.

The primary outcome paper from the HOPE study [1] showed no difference among the 3 study arms at the primary 12-month endpoint, 6-months after the intervention ended. However, a secondary analysis showed that at 6 months, immediately after conclusion of the interventions, rates of viral load suppression were 38.2, 43.1 and 50.4% in usual care, PN-only and PN + CM, respectively with PN + CM rates being significantly (p = .03) higher compared to the usual care control. The present secondary post hoc analysis expands on these findings by analyzing attendance incentive effects over time during the intervention, differences in session attendance for PN versus PN + CM, and the relationship between PN contact and viral load suppression at the 6-month outcome time point.

Methods

The HOPE study enrolled and randomized 801 persons with HIV and substance use recruited from 11 hospitals across the US. More detail on study methods as well as participant characteristics can be found in the primary outcome manuscript [1]. The study was approved by local IRBs at each participating institution. Human subjects signed informed consent prior to participation. Eligibility criteria included having a detectable HIV viral load and evidence of (in medical records) any opioid, stimulant (cocaine, amphetamines, ecstasy) or heavy alcohol use within the past year. Participants were randomly assigned in a 3-arm design to receive standard of care which typically included referral to HIV and substance use services or one of two patient navigation interventions delivered with (PN + CM; N = 271) or without (PN only; N = 266) a multi-target incentive program. Participants in both PN conditions receive the same PN intervention lasting 6 months with 11 sessions specified in the protocol. During the sessions, navigators used motivational interviewing techniques to assist participants to draw on their own capabilities and resources while specifically encouraging them to engage in HIV care, initiate or reinstate antiretroviral therapy and take steps to reduce or stop their substance use, potentially including entry into substance use disorders treatment. Session schedules were flexible in both timing and location, with the intent that they be more frequent during early months of the intervention and less frequent in later months.

PN + CM participants could earn up to a total of $1160 during the 6-month intervention by meeting target goals on 8 different behaviors related to HIV treatment engagement and substance use abatement. Behavior targets included attending HIV care doctor visits, providing evidence of an active anti-retroviral medication prescription, entering substance abuse treatment and providing drug negative urine samples at PN visits. Details of the multi-target CM plan and rationale have been described [28]. For attendance at the 11 PN sessions, one of the components of the full multi-target incentive plan, a total of $220 (19% of total possible earnings) could be earned under an escalating schedule that increased by $2 for each successive session attended from $10 for session 1 to $30 for session 11. Payment was made for all sessions independent of when or where they occurred. Participants could receive earnings immediately or hold them in an account for receipt at a later time. Payment was made in cash (4 sites) or debit card transfer (1 site), in gift cards to local retail establishments (4 sites) or with a combination of cash and gift cards (2 sites; one using patient choice).

For this analysis, the PN + CM and CM conditions were compared on sessions attended over the 6-month intervention period and on HIV viral load suppression, at 6 months. The 6-month outcome time point was selected for this post hoc analysis because this outcome assessment occurred directly after completion of the intervention period. The Wilcoxon test for difference in medians is used to test between group (PN-only vs PN + CM) differences in attendance frequency due to the non-normal distribution of attendance frequency. We report the normal-approximation to the Wilcoxon test statistic due to the relatively large sample [29]. Categorical comparisons are tested using Chi square. Attendance frequency categories (0–5, 6–9, 10–11 sessions attended) used to analyze the association with viral suppression outcomes are based on empirical examination of obtained attendance frequency distributions.

Results

Figure 1 shows the significantly different distribution of session attendance frequency for PN only and PN + CM participants (χ^2 [11] = 105.81; p < .0001). There is a sharp peak of attendance in the PN + CM group where 56.5% of participants attended all eleven sessions, 69% attended 10 or more and 90% attended 6 or more sessions. The contrasting distribution in the PN only group shows that the majority (74.4%) attended 6 or more sessions but only 28.2% attended 10 or more and 16.2% attended all eleven sessions. Median number of sessions attended differed significantly between the two groups ($z = -9.8$, P < .0001). Median sessions attended was 7 (interquartile range [IQR], 5–10) for the PN-only group versus 11 (IQR, 8–11) in the PN + CM group.

Figure 2 shows how sessions were distributed over time (mean sessions per month) for the two groups. Between group differential was greatest in the first month when PN + CM participants attended nearly one whole visit more than navigation only participants (2.9 vs 2.1 visits). Frequency of visits declined over months 1–5 in both groups, but mean visits remained higher for the PN + CM than for PN only group throughout this time period (χ^2[5] = 24.03; p −.0002).

As shown in Fig. 3 with data combined for the two groups, there was a linear relationship between PN visit attendance and viral load suppression. Among those

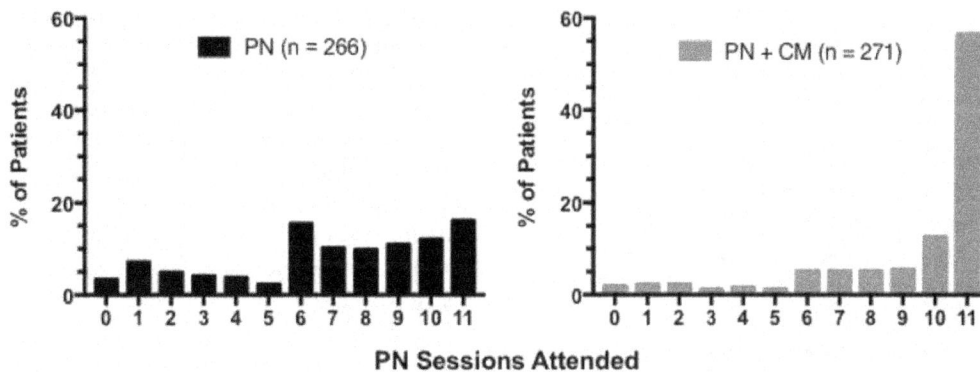

Fig. 1 The contrasting distribution of PN visit attendance for participants in the PN (N = 266) and PN + CM (N = 271) treatment groups. *Bars* indicate the percentage of participants in the designated treatment group who achieved each total number of PN visits from 0 to 11 during a 6-month intervention. Incentives were available on an escalating scale starting at $10 and increasing to $30 per visit; PN + CM could earn a total of $220 for attending all visits

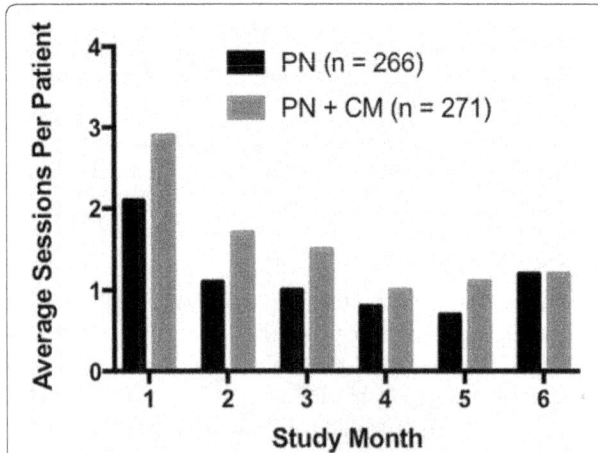

Fig. 2 shows mean number of PN visits attended per month during the 6-month intervention for PN (N = 266) and PN + CM (N = 271) participants

Table 1 Viral load outcomes at end of treatment (month 6) by number of PN visits attended

Visits attended	PN		PN + CM	
	N	% with viral suppression	N	% with viral suppression
0–5	57	19.3	21	4.8
6–9	116	40.5	53	32.1
10–11	75	52.0	186	54.8
Total	248		260	

Discussion

As previously reported [1], attendance incentives embedded in a multi-target contingency management program for persons with HIV and substance use increased contact between participants and their assigned navigators. Our analysis expanded on median differences previously reported. The most notable finding is in the number of patients attending all eleven of the possible scheduled sessions. Rates of full attendance were 3.5 times higher for PN + CM than for PN only participants. The increase in visit frequency for navigation only in month 6 is likely related to the opportunity to complete 6-month data collection for additional payment at that time.

The results are consistent with previous literature demonstrating that contingent financial incentives are effective for improving contact with services. Here, we also demonstrate a significant association between viral suppression and rates of attendance independent of whether incentives were used in the PN protocol. Specifically, in the combined groups, the more sessions attended, the more likely participants were to have viral suppression. This relationship suggests that the PN intervention was a useful part of the overall strategy for achieving the desired health outcome, with role of the incentives being to increase contact with the PN services. If the PN intervention accomplished it's aims, we would expect to see higher rates of engagement in HIV care and substance abuse treatment among PN + CM compared to PN only. This prediction will be examined in subsequent secondary analyses. The potential mediating influence of PN contact on viral load outcomes can also be further elucidated in multivariable analysis that takes into account other potential mediating and moderating variables including levels of on-going substance use. However, since multiple behaviors were incentivized in this protocol, it will not be possible to disentangle the independent mediating variable of PN contact, which could be done if PN contact were the only behavior incentivized.

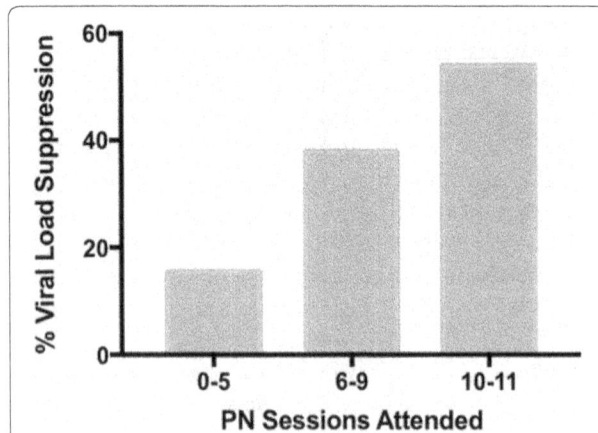

Fig. 3 The percent of all participants collapsed across PN and PN + CM (N = 508 due to missing viral load data) with suppressed viral load (≤200 copies/mL) at the 6-month assessment as a function of PN visits attended. Number of visits attended has been divided into 3 functional categories: low (0–5 visits; N = 78), moderate (6–9 visit; N = 169) and high (10–11 visits; N = 261)

attending 0-5 sessions, only 15.4% were virally suppressed at 6 months. Suppression rate more than doubled, rising to 37.9% among those attending an intermediate number of sessions (6–9). The highest rate of viral load suppression at 54% was seen in those who attended at least 10 of the 11 possible sessions (total sample $\chi^2(2) = 39.07$, p < .001). Table 1 shows that this relationship was apparent for the PN ($\chi^2(2) = 14.72$, p < .001) and PN + CM ($\chi^2(2) = 24.35$, p < .001) groups separately as well.

While the relationship between session attendance and HIV viral suppression was strong, it is also notable that nearly half the participants who attended 10 or 11 PN sessions were not virally suppressed at 6 months despite their high rate of contact with the PN intervention. This suggests that further examination of the project HOPE data is needed to identify areas where either the PN or CM intervention or both could be further improved. This could involve prolonging or intensifying the intervention, increasing incentive amounts or altering their distribution across target behaviors. New intervention features may also be useful such as in-hospital initiation of medication treatments for HIV and/or substance abuse.

Several features of the study may have affected outcomes. These include features of the appointment scheduling specified in the study protocol, the number and type of appointment reminders made by PNs to their participants, and details of the incentive program. For example, the difference between rates of attendance for PN versus PN + CM may have been even greater in a protocol where PN session number was not constrained. It is likely that providing the incentives immediately at PN sessions contributed to the effectiveness of the present intervention in promoting attendance at PN sessions. Further it is possible that the escalating schedule of reinforcement that provided higher incentives for attendance at later sessions played a role in supporting the full attendance observed in over half of the PN + CM participants., However, only a single set of attendance incentive parameters was tested (i.e. incentive amounts and method of delivery) and it is possible that rates of attendance could have been further improved with higher valued incentives, or that equivalent or better results could be obtained with use of other incentive delivery methods such as the prize draw method [30] or with fixed rather than escalating incentive values for successive attendance. More research on these parameters would be desirable.

This study showed that attendance incentives substantially improved rates of contact between persons with HIV and substance use and their patient navigators who delivered a strength-based intervention designed to encourage re-engagement into HIV health care and substance use services. The association between attendance and viral load suppression outcome is encouraging as it suggests that contact with the PN intervention was effective for improving this important health outcome. Study results support use of attendance incentives within the health care system to improve rates of contact between service providers delivering beneficial interventions and patients who need services, particularly patients who are difficult to engage in care due to untreated substance use.

Abbreviations
CM: contingency management; PN: patient navigation.

Authors' contributions
DJF analyzed the data, CC created the figures; LM had major editorial input. All authors read and approved the final manuscript.

Author details
[1] Department of Psychiatry and Behavioral Sciences, Hopkins Bayview Medical Center, Johns Hopkins University School of Medicine, 5510 Nathan Shock Drive, Baltimore, MD 21224, USA. [2] San Francisco Department of Public Health, 25 Van Ness Avenue Suite 500, San Francisco, CA 94102, USA. [3] UCSF Department of Psychiatry, Zuckerberg San Francisco General Hospital and Trauma Center, 1001 Potrero Avenue SFGH Building 20, Rm. 2117, San Francisco, CA 94110, USA. [4] Department of Public Health Sciences, University of Miami Miller School of Medicine, 1120 Northwest 14th Street, CRB 1059, Miami, FL 33136, USA. [5] Department of Sociomedical Sciences, Mailman School of Public Health, Columbia University, 722 West 168th Street, Room 918, New York, NY 10032, USA.

Acknowledgements
None.

Competing interests
Drs Stitzer, Metsch, Feaster, Gooden and Sorensen have received grants from the National Institute on Drug Abuse, National Institutes of Health (NIH). The authors declare that they have no other competing interests.

Funding
The project HOPE clinical trial and subsequent manuscript preparation activities were funded under NIDA Drug Abuse Treatment Clinical Trials Network cooperative agreements UG1DA013034, UG1DA015815 and UG1DA013720.

References
1. Metsch LR, Feaster DJ, Gooden L, Matheson T, Stitzer M, Das M, Nijhawan AE, et al. Effect of patient navigation with or without financial incentives on viral suppression among hospitalized patients with HIV infection and substance use: a randomized clinical trial. JAMA. 2016;316:156–70.
2. Milward J, Lynskey M, Strang J. Solving the problem of non-attendance in substance abuse services. Drug Alcohol Rev. 2014;33:625–36.
3. Lucas GM. Substance abuse, adherence with antiretroviral therapy, and clinical outcomes among HIV-infected individuals. Life Sci. 2011;88:948–52.
4. Lucas GM, Griswold M, Gebo KA, Keruly J, Chaisson RE, Moore RD. Illicit drug use and HIV-1 disease progression: a longitudinal study in the era of highly active antiretroviral therapy. Am J Epidemiol. 2006;163:412–20.
5. Buchacz K, Baker RK, Moorman AC, Richardson JT, Wood KC, Holmberg SD, Brooks JT. HIV Outpatient Study (HOPS) Investigators. Rates of hospitalizations and associated diagnoses in a large multisite cohort of HIV patients in the United States, 1994–2005. AIDS. 2008;2008(22):1345–54.
6. Azar MM, Springer SA, Meyer JP, Altice FL. A systematic review of the impact of alcohol use disorders on HIV treatment outcomes, adherence to antiretroviral therapy and health care utilization. Drug Alcohol Depend. 2010;112:178–93.
7. Bassett IV, Wilson D, Taaffe J, Freedberg KA. Financial incentives to improve progression through the HIV treatment cascade. HIV AIDS. 2015;10:451–63.
8. Thornton RL. The demand for, and impact of, learning HIV status. Am Econ Rev. 2008;98:1829–63.
9. Mallotte KC, Rhodes F, Mais KE. Tuberculosis screening and compliance with return for skin test reading among active drug users. Am J Public Health. 1998;88:792–6.
10. Mallotte KC, Hollingshead JR, Rhodes F. Monetary versus nonmonetary incentives for TB skin test reading among drug users. Am J Prev Med. 1999;16:182–8.

11. Weaver T, Metrebian N, Hellier J, Pilling S, Charles V, Little N, Poovendran D, Mitcheson L, Ryan F, Bowden-Jones O, Dunn J, Glasper A, Finch E, Strang J. Use of contingency management incentives to improve completion of hepatitis B vaccination in people undergoing treatment for heroin dependence: a cluster randomised trial. Lancet. 2014;384:153–63.
12. Corrigan JD, Bogner J, Lamb-Hart G, Heinemann AW, Moore D. Increasing substance abuse treatment compliance for persons with traumatic brain injury. Psychol Addict Behav. 2005;19:131–9.
13. Fitzsimons H, Tuten M, Borsuk C, Lookatch S, Hanks L. Clinician-delivered contingency management increases engagement and attendance in drug and alcohol treatment. Drug Alcohol Depend. 2015;152:62–7.
14. Petry NM, Martin B, Finocche C. Contingency management in group treatment: a demonstration project in an HIV drop-in center. J Subst Abuse Treat. 2001;21:89–96.
15. Solomon SS, Srikrishnan AK, Vasudevan CK, Anand S, Kumar MS, Balakrishnan P, Mehta SH, Solomon S, Lucas GM. Voucher incentives improve linkage to and retention in care among HIV-infected drug users in Chennai, India. Clin Infect Dis. 2014;59:589–95.
16. Branson CE, Barbuti AM, Clemmey P, Herman L, Bhutia P. A pilot study of low-cost contingency management to increase attendance in an adolescent substance abuse program. Am J Addict. 2012;21:126–9.
17. Jones HE, Haug N, Silverman K, Stitzer M, Svikis D. The effectiveness of incentives in enhancing treatment attendance and drug abstinence in methadone-maintained pregnant women. Drug Alcohol Depend. 2001;61:297–306.
18. Ledgerwood DM, Alessi SM, Hanson TH, Godley MD, Petry NM. Contingency management for attendance to group substance abuse treatment administered by clinicians in community clinics. J Appl Behav Anal. 2008;41:517–26.
19. Petry NM, Martin B, Simcic F. Prize reinforcement contingency management for cocaine dependence: integration with group therapy in a methadone clinic. J Consult Clin Psychol. 2005;2005(73):354–9.
20. Petry NM, Weinstock J, Alessi SM. A randomized trial of contingency management delivered in the context of group counseling. J Consult Clin Psychol. 2011;79:68–96.
21. Petry NM, Barry D, Alessi SM, Rounsaville BJ, Carroll KM. A randomized trial adapting contingency management targets based on initial abstinence status of cocaine-dependent patients. J Consult Clin Psychol. 2012;80:276–85.
22. Sigmon SC, Stitzer ML. Use of a low-cost incentive intervention to improve counseling attendance among methadone-maintained patients. J Subst Abuse Treat. 2005;29:253–8.
23. Kidorf M, Brooner RK, Gandotra N, Antoine D, King VL, Peirce J, Ghazarian S. Reinforcing integrated psychiatric service attendance in an opioid-agonist program: a randomized and controlled trial. Drug Alcohol Depend. 2013;133:30–6.
24. Bradford JB, Coleman S, Cunningham W. HIV system navigation: an emerging model to improve HIV care access. AIDS Patient Care STD. 2007;21(Suppl 1):49–58.
25. Dohan D, Schrag D. Using navigators to improve care of underserved patients. Cancer. 2005;104:848–55.
26. Gardner LI, Metsch LR, Anderson-Mahoney P, Loughlin AM, Del Rio C, Strathdee S, Holmberg SD. Efficacy of a brief case management intervention to link recently diagnosed HIV-infected persons to care. AIDS. 2005;19:423–31.
27. Cabral HJ, Tobias C, Rajabiun S, Sohler N, Cunningham C, Wong M, Cunningham W. Outreach program contacts: do they increase the likelihood of engagement and retention in HIV primary care for hard-to-reach patients? AIDS Patient Care STD. 2007;21(Suppl 1):59–67.
28. Stitzer M, Calsyn D, Matheson T, Sorensen J, Gooden L, Metsch L. Development of a multi-target contingency management intervention for HIV positive substance users. J Subst Abuse Treat. 2017;72:66–71.
29. Bellera CA, Julien M, Hanley JA. Normal approximations to the distribution of the Wilcoxon statistics: Accurate to what N? Graphical insights. J Stat Educ. 2010;18:1–17.
30. Petry NM. Contingency management for substance abuse treatment. A guide to implementing this evidence-based practice. NY, London: Routledge Taylor & Francis Group; 2012.

17

Substance use patterns and in-hospital care of adolescents and young adults attending music concerts

Stephanie M. Ruest[1*], Alexander M. Stephan[2], Peter T. Masiakos[3], Paul D. Biddinger[4], Carlos A. Camargo[4] and Sigmund Kharasch[4]

Abstract

Background: Few studies describe medical complaints and substance use patterns related to attending music concerts. As such, the objective of this study is to describe patient demographics, substance use and intoxication patterns, and medical interventions provided to adolescents and young adults assessed in an emergency department (ED) for complaints directly related to concert attendance.

Methods: A retrospective chart review of patients 13–30 years old who were transported to the ED directly from music concerts between January 2011 and December 2015 was conducted. Descriptive statistics and logistic regression were used to analyze patient demographic, intervention, and substance use data.

Results: There were 115 concerts identified, of which 48 (42%) were linked to 142 relevant ED visits; the total number of attendees at each concert is unknown. The mean age of the 142 described patients was 19.5 years (SD 3.3) with 72% < 21 and 33% < 18; 71% of patients were female and 96% of visits were substance-use related. Mean blood alcohol level was 242 mg/dL (range 104–412, SD 70). Glasgow Coma Scale (GCS) scores ranged from 3 to 15, with a mean of 14. Two patients required intubation and 61% of patients received interventions, including medications (47%), intravenous fluids (46%), specialty consultation (20%), restraints (14%), imaging (6%), and laceration repair (3%). Attendance at pop and electronic dance music concerts was associated with the widest ranges of GCS scores (8–15 and 6–14 respectively), mass casualty incident declarations, and among the highest mean blood alcohol levels (246 and 244 mg/dL, respectively).

Conclusions: Substance use is the predominant reason for music concert related ED visits and patients may have serious levels of intoxication, receiving multiple medical interventions. These data demonstrate the need for additional large-scale studies to confirm trends and increase awareness of this important public health problem.

Keywords: Music concerts, Substance use, Intoxication, Adolescents, Young adults

Background

Mass gathering events, such as sporting and political events, music concert events, visits by dignitaries, and others, have been defined as the presence of > 1000 people gathered at a specific location for a defined period of time [1]. Prior research has identified several attributes of mass gatherings that result in morbidity and mortality, including weather and environmental factors [2–6], alcohol and drug use [5–7], crowd attendance and density [8–10], and event type [6, 9, 10]. Music concerts are one unique type of mass gathering event that can occur in indoor or outdoor venues, are often associated with substance use, and are attended by individuals ranging in age from young children to the elderly depending upon the performer. As such, the morbidity and mortality associated with these events may be quite varied. While previous publications on mass gatherings have helped

*Correspondence: Stephanie.Ruest@gmail.com
[1] Section of Pediatric Emergency Medicine, Hasbro Children's Hospital, Alpert Medical School of Brown University, 593 Eddy St, Claverick 2, Providence, RI 02903, USA
Full list of author information is available at the end of the article

to advance our understanding of these event character-istics [9, 11, 12], only a handful of studies have uniquely addressed complaints directly related to music concert attendance, the majority of which have been cross-sectional event reports rather than longitudinal series, and are from outside of the United States [5–7, 13–18]. This may be because there is currently no universally standardized approach to data collection or large patient registries for reporting adverse outcomes at concerts or other mass gathering events [19].

Despite the limited number of publications on issues related to substance use patterns, levels of intoxication, and the need for medical care at concerts, in recent years there has been frequent media attention describing deaths and significant morbidity related to substance use at music concerts. Additionally, there have been multiple formal declarations of "mass casualty incidents" (MCIs) across the country when emergency medical services (EMS) and medical providers have been faced with large surges of patients, often adolescents and young adults, with significant levels of intoxication, dehydration, injuries, and other issues arising secondary to substance use at both indoor and outdoor concerts [20–30]. Previous publications have reported that adolescents and young adults below the age of 30 are more likely to present for medical care at concerts than older individuals [5–7, 18, 19]. Of note, a 2015 publication cited at least 68 concert-associated deaths that were reported by the press over 15 years [16]. In 2013–2014 alone, journalists reported at least 10 deaths of individuals under the age of 25 and > 650 hospital transports related to drug and alcohol use at concerts in cities throughout the United States, the vast majority of which occurred at electronic dance music (EDM) concerts or festivals [21, 26–29].

Although there is growing interest in these issues, there are no publications known to these authors that document in-hospital care, including patient demographics, substance use patterns, levels of intoxication, and toxicology results, provided to adolescents and young adults who attended shows across multiple music genres over a multi-year study period. The objective of this study was to identify adolescents and young adults evaluated in a large urban emergency department (ED) for complaints directly related to concert attendance over the course of 5 years and to describe these factors listed above based on the music genre of the concert attended.

Methods
Design, setting, and population
A retrospective chart review was performed on the identified case series of patients between the ages of 13 and 30 years old seen in the Massachusetts General Hospital (MGH) ED on nights coinciding with concerts at a large

nearby event venue between January 2011 and December 2015. This age range was chosen as prior publications have found that concert-goers below the age of 30 are more likely to present for medical evaluation [5, 6, 18]. MGH is a large urban academic medical center located within Boston, Massachusetts, approximately 0.75 miles from the concert venue of interest. The study was reviewed and approved by the MGH institutional review board.

The studied concert venue has a maximum patron capacity of over 19,000 people. Although the venue has on-site EMS, it does not have an on-site physician to evaluate and treat concert patrons. The total number of concert attendees and the number of patients treated and released at on-site first aid stations at each event are unknown to the authors. In part based on its geographic location, MGH is the primary hospital for transport of patients from this concert venue. All patients requiring medical evaluation, with the exception of those rerouted in MCI declarations based on EMS protocol, were directly transported from the venue to MGH (personal EMS communication, December 12, 2014). During the course of the study period, there were two MCI's resulting in the transport of approximately 30 patients to other area hospitals, although the exact number is unknown to the authors.

Concert dates were identified via publically available event schedules for the venue of interest and the performer and music genre for each concert were recorded. Music genre was designated based on the performer's official website or the Billboard™ music charts (e.g. pop, rock, electronic dance music, jazz, etc.). Patients seen on the day of the concert through 2 a.m. the following morning who had a chief complaint or discharge diagnosis related to ingestion, intoxication, alcohol or drug use, altered mental status, agitation, loss of consciousness, syncope, near syncope, headache, dizziness, dehydration, chest pain, shortness of breath, injury, trauma, wound, abrasion, or laceration underwent further chart review. Patient stated chief complaints and final ICD-9 primary and secondary discharge codes associated with the visits were provided by MGH health information services. This list of general complaints and diagnoses was chosen based on previous literature describing the most common presentations identified at music concerts [5, 7, 19]. The time frame up until 2 a.m. the following morning was chosen in an attempt to capture all concert-related patients, as concerts generally ended by 11 p.m. Patients were included in the study if they met the above criteria and their medical record included specific documented reference to concert attendance at the venue of interest. Patients were excluded if there was no mention of attending a concert at this venue or if it was not clearly specified in the available documentation.

Data collection and analysis

Age, sex, time of presentation, verbal report of drug or alcohol use, Glasgow Coma Scale (GCS) score by a triage nurse or first-contact physician on arrival and the lowest documented GCS score during the ED visit, medical intervention(s) (e.g. airway support, imaging, intravenous fluids, laceration repair, medications, restraints, etc.), serum and urine toxicology results, length of stay, final diagnosis, and disposition were abstracted by two physicians (AS and SR). AS performed the primary review of all charts (n = 698) and SR independently reviewed 25% of charts; 95% of re-reviewed charts yielded identical data. SR and AS discussed any discrepancies and came to a consensus for the final data analysis.

The study was mainly descriptive in nature. Data were transcribed into Microsoft Excel 2010 (Microsoft Corporation, Redmond, WA) and then exported into STATA 14.0 (StataCorp LP, College Station, TX) for analysis. Continuous variables were summarized using mean (standard deviation, SD) while categorical variables were summarized using frequency and percentage. Multivariable logistic regression analysis was performed to obtain odds ratios and 95% confidence intervals (CI). Odds ratios were adjusted for age and sex, consistent with a prior publication that controlled for the same covariates [5].

Results

Between January 2011 and December 2015, 115 concerts were identified via review of publically available schedules. Based on date and time of presentation, age, and chief complaint or discharge diagnoses, 698 patients met inclusion criteria for chart review. After more detailed chart review, 142 patients were eligible for data analysis. Five hundred and forty five patients' charts were reviewed and excluded because there was no specific reference to concert attendance, and an additional 11 patients were excluded because they came from concerts at venues that were not the main venue of interest.

Patients ranged in age from 13 to 30 years old with a mean age of 19.5 years (SD 3.3); 72% (n = 102) of patients were under the age of 21 and 33% (n = 47) were under age 18 (Fig. 1). When controlling for sex, individuals who attended rock concerts had 2.4 times the odds (95% CI 1.1–5.3, P = 0.027) of being aged 21 or older as compared with those who attended concerts of all other genres. There were no other statistically significant relationships found between age and the genre of the concert attended. Overall, 71% (n = 101) of patients were female. When controlling for age, individuals who attended pop concerts had 3.5 times the odds (95% CI 1.33–9.17, P = 0.01) of being female as compared with those who attended concerts of all other genres. There were no other statistically significant relationships found between sex and the genre of the concert attended.

Forty-eight (42%) of 115 concerts accounted for all identified ED concert-related patient visits (Table 1). Seven music genres were represented among these 48 concerts: country (n = 1), EDM (n = 3), heavy metal (n = 1), pop (n = 16), punk (n = 1), rap/hip hop (n = 7), and rock (n = 19). Overall, 31% of patients attended pop concerts, 29% rock, 19% rap/hip hop, 18% EDM, 2% punk, 1% country and 1% heavy metal (Fig. 2). There were no patients from jazz concerts.

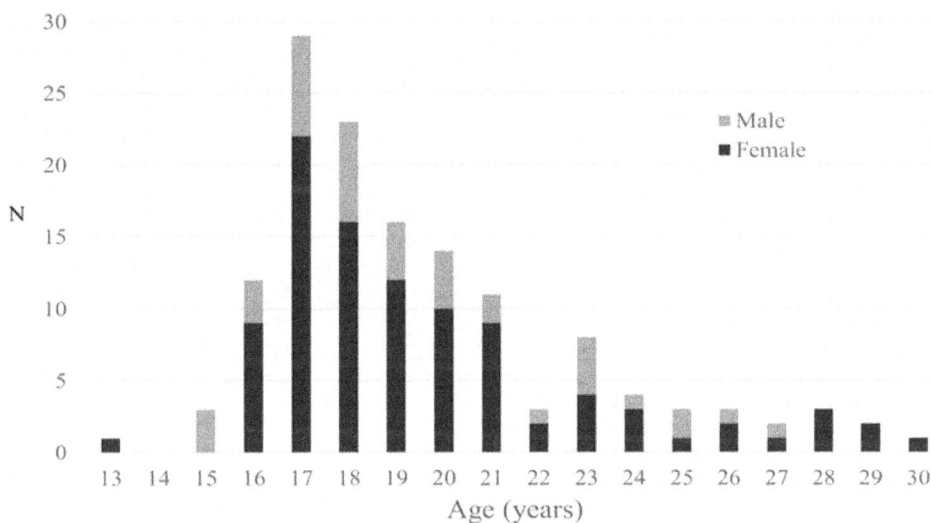

Fig. 1 Age and sex distribution of concert attendees seen in the emergency department. Mean age of all patients was 19.5 years (SD 3.3 years), with 72% less than age 21 and 33% less than age 18

Table 1 Concerts that resulted in ED visits

Genre[a]	Performer
Country	Lady Antebellum
Electronic dance music	Avicii[b,c], Pretty Lights
Heavy metal	Avenged Sevenfold
Pop	Beyonce[c,d], Britney Spears, Jingle Ball[c,e], Justin Beiber[c], Justin Timberlake, Lady Gaga, Madonna, Marc Anthony (Latin Pop), Miley Cyrus[b], New Kids on the Block, Rhianna[c,d], Stevie Wonder[d]
Punk	Dropkick Murphys
Rap/hip hop	Drake, Jay-Z, Kanye West, Mackelmore and Ryan Lewis, Monster Jam[c,g], The Throne Tour with Kanye West and Jay-Z
Rock	Avett Brothers, Black Keys, Bon Jovi, Boston Strong[f], Coldplay, Dave Matthews, Dispatch[h], Foo Fighters, Imagine Dragons, Kings of Leon, Mumford and Sons, Red Hot Chili Peppers, Tool, U2[h], Van Halen

[a] As per the artist's official website or Billboard™ music charts

[b] Concert resulted in an emergency medical services mass casualty incident (MCI) declaration

[c] Two separate concerts by the same performer resulted in ED visits

[d] Beyoncé, Rhianna, and Stevie Wonder are identified as both pop and rhythm and blues (R&B). For the purposes of this study, they were categorized as pop

[e] Multiple performer show, mostly pop performers

[f] Multiple performer show, mostly rock performers

[g] Multiple performer show, mostly rap/hip hop performers

[h] Three separate concerts by the same performer resulted in ED visits

Two specific concerts in the study period, one pop and one EDM, resulted in large volumes of patients requiring EMS transport, leading to a formal declaration of an MCI and distribution of patients to MGH and other local area hospitals according to the established Boston EMS MCI plan. The total number of patients transported from the pop concert is unknown to these authors, however, per press reports of the EDM concert, there were 50 patients who were treated and released on scene and an additional 36 patients transported to area hospitals, 13 of whom were seen at MGH [23].

Overall, 96% (n = 137) of all patient presentations involved alcohol or drug use based on patient report and/or clinician documentation. While the majority of patients did present with a chief complaint related to substance use, one patient with the complaint of chest pain, one with pre-syncope, one with migraine symptoms, two with agitation and three with injuries all were discharged with a primary or secondary diagnosis related to substance use. The five presentations that did not involve a primary or secondary diagnosis of intoxication or substance use included two complaints of chest pain, two lacerations, and one complaint of dizziness/pre-syncope.

All 142 patients were asked about alcohol use. Of those, 87% (n = 124) of patients reported using alcohol on the day of the ED visit. Of the 38 individuals who were

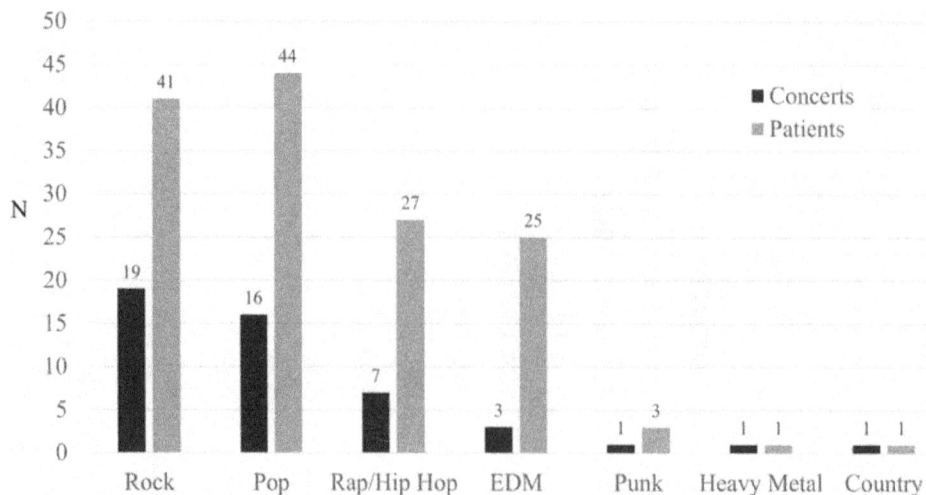

Fig. 2 Number of concerts resulting in ED visits compared to the number of patients, by music genre

specifically asked about whether or not they had consumed alcohol prior to entering the concert venue, 71% (n = 27) answered affirmatively, 21% (n = 8) denied this, and 8% (n = 3) refused to answer the question. Forty-three percent of individuals (n = 60) had serum toxicology screening sent at the discretion of the evaluating clinician to assist with medical decision-making and/or management and 98% of those screens were positive for alcohol, with an overall mean blood alcohol level (BAL) of 242 mg/dL (range 104–412, SD 70), which is equivalent to a blood alcohol content of 0.24% (SD 0.07%) (Fig. 3). Punk, pop and EDM shows had the highest mean BAL's of 311 mg/dL (SD 0), 246 mg/dL (SD 92) and 244 mg/dL (SD 48), respectively. Ten individuals who denied alcohol use had serum toxicology screens sent; all were positive with a mean BAL of 262 mg/dL (SD 36). Conversely, an additional 6 patients who denied alcohol use did not have screens sent; two were described as clinically intoxicated, two had lacerations, one each had dizziness, chest pain, and multiple injuries due to an assault.

Overall, 123 out of 142 individuals had documentation that they were asked about drug use. Of those, 18% (n = 22) reported drug use, 81% (n = 100) denied drug use, and < 1% (n = 1) refused to answer the question. Only 20 individuals had urine toxicology screening sent at the discretion of the clinician; screens were not necessarily sent on individuals who endorsed drug use. Of those sent, 50% were positive for one or more drugs, including opioids, marijuana, and amphetamines. Of note, one of the tested patients reported chronic opiate use for pain, one patient reported recreational ecstasy use, one reported prescribed methylphenidate use, and one reported recreational methylphenidate use.

The Glasgow Coma Scale (GCS) is a neurological scale used by medical providers to assess a patient's level of consciousness by evaluating an individual's eye, verbal, and motor responses to various stimuli. A low score of 3 denotes deep unconsciousness or coma whereas a high score of 15 denotes a fully awake and alert individual. The GCS score may be used to help guide medical decision making, such as determining the need for tracheal intubation in the setting of a low or precipitously declining score. In this study, scores were obtained via nursing or physician documentation. The mean GCS score on arrival for all patients was 14 (SD 1.8, range 6–15), and the mean lowest documented GCS for all patients was 13 (SD 2.5, range 3–15). Patients from EDM and pop concerts demonstrated the widest range of GCS scores on arrival, with means of 13 (SD 3, range 6–15) and 14 (SD 2, range 8–15), respectively. The lowest documented GCS score for all patients was 3, which was a subsequent GCS score recorded in a patient who attended an EDM show and who required intubation. Although 80% of patients did not have a difference between their arrival GCS and their lowest documented GCS score, 10% dropped 1–2 points, 5% dropped 3–4 points, and nearly 5% dropped ≥ 5 points. Of those with a decrease of ≥ 5 points, four were female and one was male, with ages ranging from 17 to 24 years, initial GCS scores of 12–15, and BAL's ranging 194–310 mg/dL.

While some patients only required clinical monitoring, 61% (n = 86) received interventions beyond clinical observation (Table 2). Two individuals required intubation for airway protection (1%), 1 had a nasopharyngeal airway placed (1%), 67 received medications (47%), 65 received intravenous fluids (46%), 19 required either physical restraints, chemical restraints, or both due to significant agitation (13%), 8 had imaging performed (6%), and 4 had laceration repairs (3%). There were 29 individuals (20%) who had specialty consultations, which included social work, plastic surgery, psychiatry, and pediatric intensive care.

The mean length of stay across all music genres was 4.3 h (SD 3.4), with a range of 0.4–18.6 h. The shortest mean length of stay was for individuals attending heavy metal concerts (2.9 h, SD 0), and the longest mean length of stay was for those who attended punk concerts (6.2 h, SD 4). Overall, 90% of patients were treated and released with an admission rate of less than 2%. The remainder of patients left without being seen or left without completing treatment.

Discussion

This study examined a series of 115 music concerts across multiple genres and described the presentations, demographics, substance use data, and interventions provided

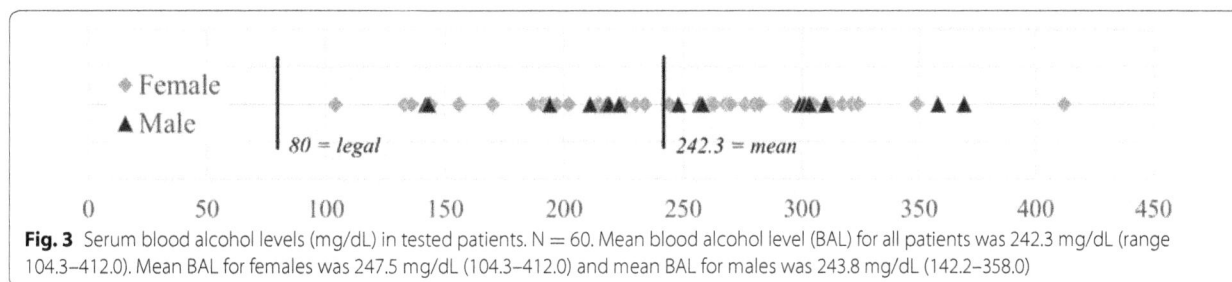

Fig. 3 Serum blood alcohol levels (mg/dL) in tested patients. N = 60. Mean blood alcohol level (BAL) for all patients was 242.3 mg/dL (range 104.3–412.0). Mean BAL for females was 247.5 mg/dL (104.3–412.0) and mean BAL for males was 243.8 mg/dL (142.2–358.0)

Table 2 Interventions, length of stay, and disposition of individuals seen in the ED (total patient n = 142)

	N (%)
Was any intervention received beyond clinical observation[a]	
Yes	86 (61)
Airway support	
Intubation	2 (1)
Nasopharyngeal airway	1 (< 1)
Imaging	8 (6)
Intravenous fluids	65 (46)
Laceration repair	4 (3)
Medications	
Antiemetics	49 (35)
Other[b]	30 (21)
Restraints	
Physical	17 (12)
Chemical	14 (10)
Both	12 (9)
Specialty consultations	
Any consult	29 (20)
Social work	22 (16)
Pediatric ICU	2 (1)
Plastic surgery	2 (1)
Psychiatry	3 (2)
	Mean (SD)
Overall mean length of stay (h)	
Min–Max 0.4–18.6	4.3 (3)
Mean ED length of stay, by musical genre	
Country (n = 1)	3.7 (–)
EDM (n = 25)	5.1 (3.0)
Heavy metal (n = 1)	2.9 (–)
Pop (n = 44)	4.0 (3.4)
Punk (n = 3)	6.2 (4.0)
Rap/hip hop (n = 27)	5.4 (4.7)
Rock (n = 41)	3.4 (2.2)
	N (%)
Patient disposition	
Treated and released	128 (90)
Left without being seen/without completing treatment	11 (8)
Admitted	2 (1)
Discharged to another hospital	1 (< 1)

[a] Interventions: airway support (nasopharyngeal airway or intubation), imaging, intravenous fluid administration, laceration repair, medication administration, restraints (chemical, physical, or both), and specialty consultation

[b] Other medications given: pain medications, antibiotics, anxiolytics, rapid sequence intubation medications, and electrolyte repletion

to individuals transported from a large music venue to an urban medical center for evaluation of complaints related to concert attendance. While there were no mortalities, 96% of visits involved substance use, the majority of patients were females under the age of 21, and > 60% of patients were provided with some type of intervention and/or treatment by medical providers.

Although prior studies have broadly evaluated the public health implications of mass gatherings, most of the concert-related literature to date has described the on-site care of single specific concerts or festivals and is based on non-U.S. populations. The lay-press reports of at least 10 deaths and over 650 hospital transports related to drug and alcohol use at concerts throughout the U.S. in 2013–2014 highlight the gap in our understanding of this important public health issue. Previous to this study, Chan et al. is the only study known to the authors that has addressed the in-hospital experience of patients who attended concerts (pop and rock only in their series) over an extended period of time; however, this study included patrons from events other than concerts and only 31% of their patients had alcohol or drug related complaints. Additionally, as their data was from over 15 years ago, it may not reflect the scope of substance use patterns and need for medical care by today's concert-going youth [18].

Prior studies have reported a sex disparity for patients who present for medical attention, with a published range of 57–69% females comprising the patient population [5, 6, 16, 31]. In this study population, there was also a female predominance, with females comprising 71% of patients. It has been hypothesized that this sex disparity may be related to a disproportionate number of young females attending some of the high patient-volume concerts, an increased likelihood of females becoming ill from substance use, and/or females presenting for care more often [5, 6]. Because the authors do not know the sex breakdown of concert attendees at each of the shows in the current sample, it is not possible to speak further to the possible causes of the female predominance in this study population.

Alcohol and drug use were a common reason for EMS transport from the concert venue to the MGH ED. While prior studies have reported a range of 11–48% of patients presenting from music concerts with substance use-related complaints, 87% of all patients in this study explicitly reported alcohol use and 98% of those tested had a positive serum toxicology screen, with a mean BAL over three times the legal limit for operation of a motor vehicle (80 mg/dL or 0.08%) [7, 18, 31]. Co-ingestions were also present in this series, identified by positive toxicology screens and/or patient verbal reports of tetrahydrocannabinol (THC) and amphetamine use (including methylenedioxy-methamphetamine, otherwise known as MDMA, "molly", or ecstasy). The proportion of substance-use related presentations in this series was more consistent with that of Lund et al's more recent population of EDM concert-goers, in which 79% of presentations involved substance use [16]. Over 70% of the patients in this series that were asked about when they consumed alcohol reported that they had used alcohol prior to entering the concert venue. A study by Chapman et al. highlighted the fact that many concertgoers will consume a large portion or all of their alcohol or drug supply before entering a venue to avoid confiscation, which is likely the case among this study population as well [32]. The mean BAL's were quite high in this patient population, possibly because patrons are often consuming large volumes of alcohol within a short period before entering the venues.

In this series, EDM, pop, rap/hip hop and rock concerts represented the genres with the highest patient volumes. Similar to prior studies, this data supports that rock and EDM are associated with higher rates of presentation, and EDM shows may result in higher acuity of presentations [16, 17, 33]. EDM represented only 6% of concerts in this series, yet resulted in 18% of the patient volume, an MCI declaration, one of the highest mean blood alcohol levels measured, and the lowest mean GCS of patients presenting to the MGH ED. Congruent with the New York City Department of Health and Mental Hygiene's publication investigating adverse health events from a local EDM festival in 2013, this series demonstrates that some patients who have attended concerts may arrive with significantly altered mental status and in need of close monitoring and more significant medical interventions [34].

The current publication adds a missing piece to the full spectrum of concert-related patient presentations by describing the in-hospital experience at a large Boston teaching hospital over 5 years and across multiple music genres. Lay-press articles and pre-hospital publications have demonstrated that attendance at music concerts may be associated with significant morbidity and mortality and that there is a need for on-site evaluation and treatment of patients by medical providers. This and other publications suggest that patrons attending EDM, pop and rock concerts and patrons who are female and under the age of 21 may be at greatest risk factors for needing medical assessment and care. When patrons present with higher acuity complaints, nearby hospitals must be prepared to care for these patients with significant intoxications and poly-substance ingestions. Medical providers should keep the various types of substances used at these concerts in mind, including timing to peak effects, when creating a treatment and disposition plan for patients, and local hospitals may consider increasing staffing on nights that could have higher patient volumes.

In Canada, harm reduction strategies, including free water, cool down stations, female-only break areas, pill/drug-checking stations, and on-site drug education programs and medical services have all been employed at EDM festivals with success. With these strategies in place at a 2014 seven day EDM festival with over 67,000 cumulative attendees, less than 1% of patrons who presented for care required transport to hospitals, there were no intubations, and no fatalities [17]. The acceptance and implementation of similar health and harm reduction strategies at large U.S. venues for concert-going patrons should be considered by venue owners as a means of decreasing the severity of substance related outcomes. Furthermore, increasing education and awareness for the patrons through public service announcements and on site education tables may also have a positive impact on outcomes. Adopting standardized data collection strategies at venues, including collecting patron demographics, presenting complaints, pertinent exam findings, and disposition plans may increase knowledge of substance use trends and lead to improved preparedness, both at the venue itself and by local EMS providers and hospitals.

Limitations

This study has some important limitations. The retrospective nature makes it dependent on publicly available information for concert date listings as well as on specific ED documentation of the patients' concert attendance. All patients without specific reference to concert attendance were excluded, so additional patients who were present at a concert and lacked this documentation may have been missed. Although the authors included a number of medical complaints and diagnoses in the initial medical chart retrieval based on the most common concert-related presentations described in previous publications, an exhaustive search of charts for all patients seen on the days of concerts was not done and, therefore, may have missed additional patients. If true, these data may under-represent the number of patients associated with concert attendance; the extent of the problem may well be greater.

Additionally, while concert date listings are public record and allowed for the targeted search of patients' hospital records analyzed in this study, both the total number of attendees present at each concert and the number who were evaluated and released by on-site first aid stations are proprietary data that were not made available by the operators of the private concert venue studied despite repeated attempts to obtain this information. Thus, the authors are unable to comment on the relative prevalence of concert-related morbidity between specific music genres. Furthermore, data obtained from the hospital records of those concert attendees who required transport to an ED by EMS is likely skewed towards younger patrons and those with greater levels of intoxication or more serious medical complaints.

While almost all toxicology testing obtained was positive, not all patients were screened; as such, all patients who used alcohol or other drugs prior to or during the concert may not have been identified. However, 87% of patients had laboratory-confirmed or verbal report of alcohol use. It is important to note that individuals who used marijuana in the preceding days to weeks may test positive for THC even if marijuana was not used on the day of the attended concert; nevertheless, the majority of patients either verbally endorsed use that day or showed signs of intoxication at the time of their ED visit, suggesting that positive screens in this study likely represented current use. Also, it should also be mentioned standard urine toxicology panels screen for phencyclidine, barbiturates, cannabinoids, amphetamines, benzodiazepines, opiates and cocaine metabolites, and some drugs, including synthetic marijuana and inhalants, are not detectable on routine toxicology screening, possibly resulting in false-negative screens.

Lastly, this single-venue study does not allow for larger scale predictions of substance use trends and in-hospital interventions and outcomes across all music genres at a variety of indoor and outdoor venues. The venue included was an indoor venue and did not host concerts of all genres. Outdoor country music concerts, for example, have been associated with large patient volumes in the lay press and were not represented in this series [28]. The authors encourage the design and implementation of multi-center, multi-venue studies that include venue-provided data on the total number of concert patrons and data from patrons treated and released by on-site medical providers combined with data on patrons transported to local hospitals.

Conclusions

The data from this study demonstrate that music concerts can result in the transport of adolescent and young adult patients to emergency departments, many of whom require a high level of medical care and receive significant interventions. In this retrospective case series, the preponderance of female patients, the frequency of alcohol intoxication and other drug use, the considerable number of patients with altered mental status, and the large number of interventions provided to this population, speaks to the substance use behavior among adolescents and young adults attending concerts. Although the sample size of this study limits the ability to predict large-scale trends, specific genres such as pop, EDM, and rock, as shown in this series, may be associated with higher risk as compared with other genres.

The present study provides in-hospital data, including toxicology, GCS, and medical intervention data, that

have not previously been reported in the mass casualty medicine literature. It supports the need for additional large-scale collaborative studies as well as universally standardized patient registries to identify patient volume and substance use trends at a national level, along with morbidity and mortality at music concerts. Such efforts may improve venue and local ED planning and preparedness on the days of these events and raise public awareness regarding the scope of adverse outcomes associated with substance use at concerts. Furthermore, the development of collaborative relationships among venues hosting concerts, EMS officials, police, lawmakers, and local hospitals may allow for improved interventions targeted around the well-known relationship between concert attendance and substance use.

Abbreviations
BAL: blood alcohol level; EDM: electronic dance music; ED: emergency department; EMS: emergency medical services; GCS: Glasgow Coma Scale; MCI: mass casualty incident; MGH: Massachusetts General Hospital; THC: tetrahydrocannabinol.

Authors' contributions
SMR conceptualized and designed the study, performed the patient chart review, carried out the analyses and drafted the manuscript. AMS performed patient chart review, assisted in the development of the study design and was a major contributor in writing the manuscript. PTM, PDB, and CAC assisted in the development of the study design and critically reviewed and revised the manuscript. SK co-conceptualized and designed the study and was a major contributor in revisions of the manuscript. All authors read and approved the final manuscript.

Author details
[1] Section of Pediatric Emergency Medicine, Hasbro Children's Hospital, Alpert Medical School of Brown University, 593 Eddy St, Claverick 2, Providence, RI 02903, USA. [2] Department of Pediatrics, Massachusetts General Hospital for Children, Harvard Medical School, 55 Fruit St, Boston, MA 02114, USA. [3] Division of Pediatric Surgery, Massachusetts General Hospital for Children, Harvard Medical School, 55 Fruit St, Boston, MA 02114, USA. [4] Department of Emergency Medicine, Massachusetts General Hospital, Harvard Medical School, 55 Fruit St, Boston, MA 02114, USA.

Acknowledgements
Not applicable.

Competing interests
The authors declare that they have no competing interests.

Consent for publication
Not applicable.

Funding sources
This research did not receive any specific grant from funding agencies in the public, commercial, or not-for-profit sectors.

References

1. Jaslow D, Yancey A, Milstein A. Mass gathering medical care. National Association of EMS Physicians Standards and Clinical Practice Committee. Prehosp Emerg Care. 2000;4(4):359–60.
2. Florida R, Goldfarb Z. Woodstock '94: peace, music, and EMS. J Emerg Med Serv. 1994;19(12):45–8.
3. Paul HM. Mass casualty: pope's Denver visit causes mega MCI (mass casualty incident). J Emerg Med Serv. 1993;18(11):64-8–72-5.
4. Baird MD, O'Connor RE, Williamson AL, et al. The impact of warm weather on mass event medical need: a review of the literature. Am J Emerg Med. 2010;28(2):224–9.
5. Hutton A, Ranse J, Verdonk N, et al. Understanding the characteristics of patient presentations of young people at outdoor music festivals. Prehosp Disaster Med. 2014;29(2):160–6.
6. Hutton A, Savage C, Ranse J, et al. The use of Haddon's matrix to plan for injury and illness prevention at outdoor music festivals. Prehosp Disaster Med. 2015;30(2):175–83.
7. Erickson TB, Aks SE, Koenigsberg M, et al. Drug use patterns at major rock concert events. Ann Emerg Med. 1996;28(1):22–6.
8. Serwylo P, Arbon, P, Rumantir, G. Predicting patient presentation rates at mass gatherings using machine learning. In: Proceedings of the 8th international ISCRAM conference, Lisbon, Portugal; 2011. p. 1–10.
9. Arbon P. Mass-gathering medicine: a review of the evidence and future directions for research. Prehosp Disaster Med. 2007;22(2):131–5.
10. Soomaroo L, Murray V. Disasters at mass gatherings: lessons from history. PLoS Curr. 2012;4:RRN301.
11. Milsten AM, Maguire BJ, Bissell RA, et al. Mass-gathering medical care: a review of the literature. Prehosp Disaster Med. 2002;17(3):151–62.
12. DeLorenzo R. Mass-gathering medicine: a review. Prehosp Disast Med. 1997;12(1):68–72.
13. Feldman MJ, Lukins JL, Verbeek RP, et al. Half-a million strong: the emergency services response to a single-day, mass-gathering event. Prehosp Disaster Med. 2004;9(4):287–96.
14. Janchar T, Samaddar C, Milzman D. The mosh pit experience: emergency medical care for concert injuries. Am J Emerg Med. 2000;18(1):62–3.
15. Yazawa K, Kamijo Y, Sakai R, et al. Medical care for a mass gathering: the Suwa Onbashira festival. Prehosp Disaster Med. 2007;22(5):431–5.
16. Lund A, Turris SA. Mass-gathering medicine: risks and patient presentations at a 2-day electronic dance music event. Prehosp Disaster Med. 2015;30(3):271–8.
17. Munn MB, Lund A, Golby R, et al. Observed benefits to on-site medical services during an annual 5-day electronic dance music event with harm reduction services. Prehosp Disaster Med. 2016;31(2):228–34.
18. Chan SB, Quinn JE. Outcomes in EMS-transported attendees from events at a large indoor arena. Prehosp Emerg Care. 2003;7(3):332–5.
19. Grange JT, Green SM, Downs W. Concert medicine: spectrum of medical problems encountered at 405 major concerts. Acad Emerg Med. 1998;6(3):202–7.
20. Molloy MS, Brady F, Maleady K. Impact of a single large mass gathering music event from a series of such events, on a receiving hospital's emergency department (ED). Prehosp Disaster Med. 2013;28(1):S186.
21. Sisario B, McKinley JC. Drug deaths threaten rising business of electronic music fests. The New York Times. 2013. http://www.nytimes.com/2013/09/10/arts/music/drugs-at-music-festivals-are-threat-to-investors-as-well-as-fans.html?pagewanted=all&_r=0. Accessed 16 May 2016.
22. Fox JC, Rocheleau M. More concert deaths linked to club drug: overdoses likely in Boston, New York. The Boston Globe. 2013. http://www.bostonglobe.com/metro/2013/09/01/more-local-overdoses-deaths-new-york-blamed-club-drug/I7KuCzoiugbZGdK4b4maZM/story.html. Accessed 16 May 2016.
23. Smith J, Feathers T, Sampson ZT, et al. EMS treat dozens at Avicii concert at TD Garden: 36 sent to hospital at techno show. The Boston Globe. 2014. http://www.bostonglobe.com/metro/2014/06/25/many-hospitalized-garden-concert/76Re9atwB1goSGELaC3oyL/story.html. Accessed 16 May 2016.
24. Schworm P, Andersen T. No sanctions for concert venues over drug overdoses. The Boston Globe. 2013. http://www.bostonglobe.com/metro/2013/10/10/boston-licensing-board-issues-sanctions-for-drug-overdoses/gX3DEBWcxyQRPhyeKhvK5I/story.html. Accessed 16 May 2016.
25. Blanding M. There's something about Molly: how a supposedly safe party drug turned lethal. The Boston Globe. 2014. http://www.bostonglobe.com/magazine/2014/01/26/what-drug-molly-and-how-turned-lethal/1x7T7p7IGlhxCaSUj3sUwI/story.html. Accessed 16 May 2016.
26. Wells C. One dead, 20 others hospitalized after apparent overdoses at Merriweather concert. The Baltimore Sun. 2014. http://articles.baltimoresun.com/2014-08-02/news/bs-md-ho-concert-drug-overdoses-20140802_1_apparent-overdoses-drug-overdoses-concert. Accessed 16 May 2016.
27. Rogers P. More than a dozen hospitalized during navy pier Skrillex show. NBC Chicago. 2014. http://www.nbcchicago.com/entertainment/the-scene/navy-pier-skrillex-280211782.html. Accessed 16 May 2016.
28. Allen P, Carter L. Officials place 50 in protective custody, treat 46 for alcohol-related illnesses during Keith Urban concert at Xfinity Center. 2014. The Sun Chronicle. http://www.thesunchronicle.com/news/local_news/officials-place-in-protective-custody-treat-for-alcohol-related-illnesses/article%2036b6c956-15cf-11e4-93df-001a4bcf887a.html. Accessed 16 May 2016.
29. Slattery G. Concert subculture under scrutiny after dozens hospitalized at Avicii concert. The Christian Science Monitor. 2014. http://www.csmonitor.com/USA/USA-Update/2014/0626/Concert-subculture-under-scrutiny-after-dozens-hospitalized-at-Avicii-concert. Accessed 16 May 2016.
30. Associated Press. 'Molly' death at Paradiso Festival, more than 100 overdoses at Gorge Ampitheatre in Washington. WPTV. 2013. http://www.wptv.com/news/national/molly-death-at-paradiso-festival-more-than-100-overdoses-at-gorge-amphitheatre-in-washington. Accessed 16 May 2016.
31. Blistein J. Electric Zoo deaths confirmed as drug overdoses. Rolling Stone. 2013. http://www.rollingstone.com/music/news/electric-zoo-deaths-confirmed-as-drug-overdoses-20130913. Accessed 16 May 2016.
32. Ridpath A, Driver CR, Nolan ML, et al. Illnesses and deaths among persons attending an electronic dance-music festival—New York City, 2013. CDC MMWR Morb Mortal Wkly Rep. 2014;63(50):1195–8.
33. Lund A, Turris SA, Amiri N, et al. Mass-gathering medicine: creation of an online event and patient registry. Prehosp Disaster Med. 2012;27(6):601–11.
34. Chapman KR, Carmichael FJ, Goode JE. Medical services for outdoor rock music festivals. Can Med Assoc J. 1982;126(8):935–8.

18

Role of substance use in HIV care cascade outcomes among people who inject drugs in Russia

Bulat Idrisov[1,10], Karsten Lunze[1,2], Debbie M. Cheng[3], Elena Blokhina[4], Natalia Gnatienko[2], Emily Quinn[5], Carly Bridden[2], Alexander Y. Walley[1], Kendall J. Bryant[6], Dmitry Lioznov[4,7], Evgeny Krupitsky[4,8] and Jeffrey H. Samet[1,9*]

Abstract

Background: Engaging people who drink alcohol or inject drugs in HIV care can be challenging, particularly in Eastern Europe. Healthcare facilities in Russia are organized by specialty; therefore linking patients from addiction care to HIV hospitals has been difficult. The HIV care cascade outlines stages of HIV care (e.g., linkage to care, prescribed antiretroviral therapy [ART], and achieving HIV viral suppression). We hypothesized that unhealthy alcohol use, injection drug use, and opioid craving are associated with unfavorable HIV care cascade outcomes.

Methods: We analyzed data from a cohort (n = 249) of HIV-positive Russians who have been in addiction hospital treatment in the past year and had a lifetime history of injection drug use (IDU). We evaluated the association between unhealthy alcohol use (AUDIT score > 7 [both hazardous drinking and dependence]), past-month injection drug use (IDU), and opioid craving (visual analogue scale from 1 to 100) with HIV care cascade outcomes. The primary outcome was linkage to HIV care within 12 months. Other outcomes were prescription of ART (secondary) and achievement of undetectable HIV viral load (HVL < 500 copies/mL) within 12 months (exploratory); the latter was analyzed on a subset in which HVL was measured (n = 48). We assessed outcomes via medical record review (linkage, ART) and serum tests (HVL). To examine the primary outcome, we used multiple logistic regression models controlling for potential confounders.

Results: Among 249 study participants, unhealthy alcohol use (n = 148 [59%]) and past-month IDU (n = 130 [52%]) were common. The mean opioid craving score was 49 (SD: 38). We were unable to detect significant associations between the independent variables (i.e., unhealthy alcohol use, IDU and opioid craving) and any HIV care cascade outcomes in unadjusted and adjusted analyses.

Conclusion: In this cohort of HIV-positive Russians with a history of IDU, individual substance use factors were not significantly associated with achieving HIV care cascade milestones (i.e., linkage to HIV care; prescription for ART; or suppressed viral load). Given no detection of an association of cascade outcomes with recent unhealthy use of alcohol or injection drugs in this cohort, examining systemic factors to understand determinants of HIV care engagement for people with drug use would be important.

Keywords: HIV care cascade, Russia, Injection drug use, Unhealthy alcohol use, Opioid craving, Linkage to care, ART, Suppressed viral load

*Correspondence: jsamet@bu.edu
[1] Clinical Addiction Research and Education Unit, Section of General Internal Medicine, Department of Medicine, Boston University School of Medicine/Boston Medical Center, 801 Massachusetts Avenue, 2nd Floor, Boston, MA 02118, USA
Full list of author information is available at the end of the article

Background

HIV elimination is a major health target in the United Nations' (UN) global Sustainable Development Goals, which call for additional resources to effectively address the expanded scope of the HIV epidemic by 2030 [1, 2]. Given that it is challenging to diagnose, link to care, retain, and achieve viral suppression among people with substance use, examining the association of substance use with effective engagement in HIV care is of great interest [3–5].

The HIV care cascade is a framework of consecutive stages of HIV care (i.e., diagnosed, linked to care, retained in care, prescribed ART, and achieved viral suppression) [6, 7]. The HIV care cascade framework is useful for identifying gaps and areas to target HIV interventions [6]. It has been shown that for some HIV-positive individuals, substance use is associated with poor HIV outcomes, even when care is provided free of charge [8–11]. For example, people with unhealthy alcohol or opioid use frequently have reduced adherence to ART medications [12, 13]. As such, people with unhealthy alcohol use and people who inject drugs (PWID) face greater barriers in the path to optimal HIV care and have more rapid HIV disease progression [12, 13]. Understanding the factors that contribute to better HIV care cascade outcomes in a cohort of people who use substances could help to inform strategies to achieve the ambitious UN objectives addressing HIV infection.

Achieving optimal HIV care cascade outcomes is particularly challenging in Eastern Europe. As healthcare services in Russia are organized by specialty [14], linking patients from addiction hospitals to HIV facilities can be a challenging transition [15]. This is mainly important since in the region, the overlapping prevalence of alcohol use, injection opioid use, and HIV infection is very high [16, 17]. The HIV epidemic in Russia has been driven largely by injection drug use, predominantly opioids [18, 19]. In 2015, 17–29% of HIV-positive Russians were estimated to be receiving ART, lower than the global 2015 coverage estimate of 40% and the coverage in the USA and France (70% and 63%, respectively) [20, 21]. The combination of high rates of new HIV infections and low ART coverage contributed to 27,564 HIV-related deaths officially reported in Russia in 2015 [21]. Government statistics put the number of HIV-positive people in Russia over one million [21]. Among those newly diagnosed with HIV in 2015, almost 54% of individuals were infected via injection drug use [21]. People with HIV and substance use comorbidity are a vulnerable population, as their engagement in specialty care remains low [22].

In Russia, healthcare, including addiction and ART, is provided free of charge at governmental facilities, such as addiction (i.e., narcology) or HIV clinics [15]. Opioid agonist therapy with methadone or buprenorphine is not available in Russia [22]. Naltrexone is available for treatment of opioid and alcohol use disorder, but rarely administered due to its cost [23]. The standard of care at Russian inpatient addiction hospitals consists of diagnostic procedures, detoxification for 10–14 days and rehabilitation for an additional 30 days for selected patients. In the first week of hospitalization, patients are detoxified with possible use of tramadol, non-opiate analgesics, clonidine and benzodiazepines [15, 24]. Patients receive drug counselling and treatment for comorbid psychiatric conditions within addiction hospitals, but integration to other treatment modalities such as HIV care is very limited.

The Russian HIV epidemic is a major public health challenge intertwined with substance use, creating a need to better understand barriers to HIV treatment among populations with substance use. Substance use has not been a major focus of previous analyses of the HIV care cascade in Russia. In order to understand whether unhealthy alcohol use, injection drug use (IDU), and opioid craving are associated with HIV care cascade outcomes, we conducted a secondary analysis of prospectively collected observational data about HIV-positive Russians who have been in addiction hospital treatment in the past year and had a lifetime history of IDU. We hypothesized that unhealthy alcohol use, IDU, and opioid craving are associated with unfavorable HIV care cascade outcomes, specifically linkage to HIV care, prescribed ART, and viral load suppression.

Methods
Datasets
We conducted a secondary data analysis based on participants from the LINC (Linking Infectious and Narcology Care) study, a randomized controlled trial (RCT) conducted in St. Petersburg, Russia, to assess the effectiveness of a behavioral and structural intervention designed to support and motivate HIV-positive PWID to engage in HIV medical care and ultimately improve their HIV outcomes [25]. LINC participants (n = 349) were recruited from inpatient wards at the City Addiction Hospital in St. Petersburg, Russia between July 2012 and May 2014. Lifetime history of IDU and documented HIV infection were entry criteria. Other inclusion requirements were: (1) aged 18–70 years; (2) hospitalized at the addiction hospital; (3) agree to CD4 cell count testing; (4) having a phone; (5) sharing 2 contacts to assist with follow-up; and (5) residing at a stable address within 100 kilometers of St. Petersburg. Participants were excluded from the study for the following: (1) currently receiving ART; (2) not fluent in Russian; or (3) cognitive impairment precluding informed consent.

The LINC study did not measure HIV viral load (HVL). However, a subset of LINC participants (n = 48) were co-enrolled in another study (Russia ARCH [Alcohol Research Collaboration on HIV/AIDS]) in which the outcome HVL was available. Russia ARCH is an observational cohort of HIV-positive people examining alcohol use and HIV outcomes [26]. Russia ARCH participants were recruited between November 2012 and June 2015 from clinical HIV and addiction sites, non-clinical sites, and via snowball recruitment in St. Petersburg, Russia. Study inclusion criteria were: (1) documented HIV infection; (2) ART-naive at baseline; (3) aged 18–70 years; (4) stable address within 100 km of St. Petersburg; (5) having a phone and; (6) sharing 2 contacts to assist with follow-up. Exclusion criteria were the same as for LINC.

All study participants provided written informed consent and both studies were approved by Institutional Review Boards of Boston University Medical Campus and First St. Petersburg Pavlov State Medical University. Co-enrolled participants provided consent to link their data from the two studies.

Variable selection
Outcomes
The primary outcome of interest was linkage to HIV care. The linkage to care variable was a dichotomous outcome defined as at least one HIV physician appointment within 12 months of study enrollment as all patients were not on ART; this information was obtained from the participants' medical records [25]. Such an appointment would be made initially at one of two St. Petersburg hospitals serving HIV-positive patients.

The secondary outcomes were prescription of ART (yes or no) and achievement of viral control (exploratory). We defined prescription of ART as being prescribed ART within 12 months following the baseline assessment. This variable was obtained via medical records. We considered achievement of viral control, any HVL < 500 copies/mL within a year of study enrollment. HIV viral load data was obtained via serum tests. This variable was only assessed among LINC participants who were co-enrolled in Russia ARCH.

Main independent variables
We assessed 3 key substance use variables at 6 months post-baseline: unhealthy alcohol use, past-month IDU, and opioid craving. Alcohol use was measured via the Alcohol Use Disorder Identification Test (AUDIT, score ranging from 0 to 40) and divided into 3 categories (scores of 0–7; scores of 8–19; and scores > 19) [27]. The AUDIT is a screening tool that helps providers to assess patients' alcohol related risks; a score of 7 and below suggests that person abstains or has lower-risk

drinking. Individuals who score between 8 and 19 are at risk for consequences. A score of above 19 is suggestive of alcohol dependence [27, 28]. We defined an AUDIT score > 7 as unhealthy alcohol use.

We defined injection drug use as self-report of any past 30-day IDU (yes or no). Opioid craving was measured via a visual analogue scale ranging from 0 to 100, modeled using tertiles. The opioid craving measure was validated and used in prior studies [29, 30]. We did not model craving as a continuous variable in order to avoid assumptions of linearity.

Covariates
In the analysis of the primary outcome (linkage to care), the following potential confounders were included based on the literature and our clinical knowledge: age, gender, education, marital status, income, social support [31], depressive symptoms (Center for Epidemiologic Studies Depression Scale [CES-D]), [32, 33] homelessness, and HIV stigma (Berger HIV stigma scale) [34]. As LINC is an RCT, we also considered the study arm as a covariate.

Statistical analyses
Descriptive statistics were used to characterize study participants overall and stratified separately by each of the 3 main independent variables. For each of the 3 main independent variables, we presented baseline characteristics by each category of the particular substance use variable (e.g., as shown in Table 1, for the AUDIT score that measured alcohol use, baseline characteristics were presented for the following three categories: scores of 0–7; scores of 8–19; and scores > 19). We compared exposure groups for descriptive purposes using Chi square and Student's t tests or Wilcoxon rank-sum tests, as appropriate. Spearman correlations were calculated to assess correlations between independent variables and covariates and no pair of variables included in the same regression model was highly correlated (r < 0.40 in all cases). Separate multiple logistic regression models were used to evaluate associations between each independent variable with each outcome adjusting for potential confounders. We reported adjusted odds ratios (aOR) and 95% confidence intervals (CI) from the regression models. For the secondary outcome, prescribed ART, due to a limited number of events (i.e., 31 prescribed ART within 12 months), we limited the adjusted analyses to the following covariates: age, gender, and stigma. As only 5 events for the undetectable viral load outcome were identified, we present only an unadjusted model for this outcome. Confirmatory analyses were conducted additionally adjusting for randomization to the LINC intervention in analyses of the primary outcome of linkage to HIV care and the secondary outcome of being prescribed

Table 1 Characteristics of HIV-positive Russians with opioid use, overall and by AUDIT score (n = 249)

Characteristic	Total N = 249	AUDIT[a] score 0–7 n = 101	AUDIT[a] score 8–19 n = 81	AUDIT[a] score 20–40 n = 67	p value
Age: mean (SD)	34.3 (4.8)	34.6 (4.9)	34 (5.1)	34.2 (4.2)	0.70
Male	184 (74%)	72 (71%)	64 (79%)	48 (72%)	0.44
Married or partnered	84 (34%)	32 (32%)	30 (37%)	22 (33%)	0.52
Education (less than 9 grades)	67 (27%)	24 (24%)	24 (30%)	19 (28%)	0.36
Depressive symptoms CES-D $\geq$ 16	208 (88%)	79 (84%)	67 (88%)	62 (95%)	0.06
Social support: mean (SD)	19 (5)	19 (5)	19 (5)	19 (5)	0.85
Stigma score: mean (SD)[a]	2 (1)	2 (1)	2 (1)	2 (1)	0.62
Injection drug use, past-month[a]	130 (52%)	41 (41%)	51 (63%)	38 (57%)	< 0.001
Opioid craving: mean (SD)[a]	49 (38)	41 (37)	54 (36)	53 (41)	0.04
Linked to care	119 (48%)	48 (48%)	39 (48%)	32 (48%)	1.00
ART initiation	31 (12%)	13 (13%)	11 (14%)	7 (10%)	0.85

[a] Collected at 6 months from baseline

ART within 12 months. We conducted analyses using 2-sided tests and an alpha level of 0.05. All statistical analyses were conducted using SAS version 9.3 (SAS Institute, Inc., NC, USA).

Results

Participant characteristics

Participants in the primary analysis of linkage to HIV care and the secondary analysis of prescription of ART (N = 249) are described in Tables 1 and 2. The subset of these participants with HIV viral load results (n = 48) were examined in the exploratory analysis of the cascade outcome, HVL suppression. Characteristics of this Russian HIV-positive cohort are the following: mean age 34 years (SD: 4.8); 74% men; 34% married, 24% separated and 42% never married; 27% completed 9 years or less of school, 62% completed 12 years of schooling, and 10% reported some higher education. Only 3% were homeless. Mean CD4 cell count at baseline was 365 cells/mm³ (SD: 260). The median monthly individual income of participants was 25,000 rubles (USD 775 [2013 exchange rate]). We used the median split approach [35] to dichotomize participants into 2 groups: lower than median income (0–25,000 rubles) or higher than median income (> 25,000 rubles). Of note, the minimum necessary income for an individual to meet basic needs (living

Table 2 Characteristics of HIV-positive Russians with opioid use, overall and by past-month IDU status (n = 249)

Characteristic	Total N = 249	IDU past month[a] n = 130	No IDU past month[a] n = 119	p value
Age: mean (SD)	34.3 (4.8)	33.6 (5.1)	35.1 (4.3)	0.01
Male	184 (74%)	89 (69%)	95 (80%)	0.04
Married or partnered	83 (33%)	45 (35%)	38 (32%)	0.23
Education (less than 9 grades)	68 (27%)	39 (30%)	29 (24%)	0.06
Depressive symptoms CES-D $\geq$ 16	208 (88%)	113 (92%)	95 (85%)	0.10
Social support: mean (SD)	19 (5)	19 (5)	19 (5)	0.25
Stigma score: mean (SD)[a]	2 (1)	2 (1)	2 (1)	0.85
AUDIT[a]				
Score 0–7	100 (40%)	41 (31%)	59 (50%)	0.009
Score 8–19	81 (33%)	51 (39%)	30 (25%)	
Score 20–40	67 (27%)	38 (29%)	29 (25%)	
Opioid craving: mean (SD)[a]	49 (38)	71 (31)	24 (29)	< 0.001
Linked to care	119 (48%)	57 (43.8%)	62 (52%)	0.21
ART initiation	31 (12%)	15 (11%)	16 (13%)	0.70
CD4 cell count: mean (SD)	365 (260)	340 (256)	393 (264)	0.11

[a] Collected at 6 months from baseline

wage) in St. Petersburg in 2013 was 6900 rubles (USD 214) [36]. Depressive symptoms were common, with 88% scoring above 16 on the CES-D [32].

Unhealthy alcohol use was common, with a majority (59%) having an AUDIT score of 8 or higher. Past-month IDU was also common (52%). Unhealthy alcohol use occurred among 68% of those with past-month IDU (89/130). The mean opioid craving score was 49 (SD: 38). Variables indicative of the HIV care cascade were as follows: 119/249 participants (48%) were linked to HIV care; 31/249 (12%) were prescribed ART; 5/48 (10%) achieved viral suppression (HVL < 500 cells/mm^3) within a year of study enrollment.

Regression analyses
Linkage to HIV care
We were unable to detect significant associations between the linkage to care outcome and the independent variables (i.e., unhealthy alcohol use, IDU, and opioid craving) in unadjusted and adjusted analyses (Table 3). Adjusted odds ratio (aOR) for unhealthy alcohol use and linkage to care were as follows: 1.14 for AUDIT score of 20–40 (95% CI 0.57–2.29, p = 0.71) and 1.26 for AUDIT

score of 8–19 (95% CI 0.65–2.24, p = 0.49) compared with people with lower-risk drinking and abstainers (AUDIT scores 0–7). Similarly, in both unadjusted and adjusted analyses, past-month IDU was not significantly associated with linkage to HIV care (aOR 0.79 [95% CI 0.45–1.38, p = 0.39]).

We found no significant association between opioid craving and linkage to HIV care outcome in unadjusted or adjusted regression models (aOR 0.84, [95% CI 0.43–1.64, p = 0.61), highest (71–100) versus lowest (0–29) tertile; (aOR 0.78, [95% CI 0.39–1.57, p = 0.48]), middle (30–70) versus lowest tertile.

Married or partnered status was associated with significantly lower odds of linkage to care in alcohol use (0.46 [0.24, 0.89]), and other models, see Table 3. Stigma—another covariate in our analyses—was not significantly associated with HIV care cascade outcomes (p > 0.05 for all linkage to care models). However, more education, appeared to be positively associated with linkage to care in all models, for example aOR for education in the alcohol use and linkage to care model was 1.97 (95%CI 1.02, 3.78), p = 0.04. Our main findings were consistent after

Table 3 Separate logistic regression models evaluating the association between substance use (unhealthy alcohol use, past-month IDU, opioid craving) and linkage to care (n = 249)

Variable	Outcome					
	Linkage to care and unhealthy alcohol use n = 249		Linkage to care and IDU n = 249		Linkage to care and opioid craving n = 250	
	Adjusted odds ratio (95% CI)	p value	Adjusted odds ratio (95% CI)	p value	Adjusted odds ratio (95% CI)	p value
AUDIT 20–40 Alcohol dependence	1.14 (0.57, 2.29)	0.72	–	–	–	–
AUDIT 8–19 Hazardous drinking	1.26 (0.65, 2.44)	0.49	–	–	–	–
IDU	–	–	0.79 (0.45, 1.38)	0.40	–	–
Opioid craving 30–70	–	–	–	–	0.78 (0.39, 1.57)	0.49
Opioid craving 71–100	–	–	–	–	0.84 (0.43, 1.64)	0.61
Gender (female vs. male)	1.45 (0.74, 2.84)	0.27	1.45 (0.74, 2.82)	0.27	1.39 (0.72, 2.71)	0.33
Age	1.00 (0.94, 1.07)	0.90	1.00 (0.93, 1.07)	0.93	1.00 (0.94, 1.07)	0.97
Stigma (continuous)	0.71 (0.44, 1.14)	0.16	0.71 (0.44, 1.14)	0.15	0.71 (0.44, 1.15)	0.16
Social support (continuous)	1.00 (0.94, 1.06)	0.95	1.00 (0.95, 1.07)	0.88	1.00 (0.94, 1.07)	0.91
Married or partnered	0.46 (0.24, 0.89)	0.02	0.45 (0.23, 0.87)	0.01	0.47 (0.24, 0.91)	0.02
Separated, divorced, or widowed	1.05 (0.49, 2.28)	0.89	1.09 (0.51, 2.32)	0.82	1.07 (0.50, 2.29)	0.85
Education	1.97 (1.02, 3.78)	0.04	1.91 (0.99, 3.68)	0.05	1.99 (1.03, 3.84)	0.04
Depressive symptoms (past-week symptoms)	0.83 (0.34, 2.00)	0.67	0.87 (0.36, 2.08)	0.74	0.90 (0.37, 2.19)	0.82
Income (high vs. low)	1.04 (0.55, 1.96)	0.91	1.09 (0.58, 2.02)	0.79	1.09 (0.58, 2.04)	0.78
Homeless	1.70 (0.30, 9.57)	0.54	1.75 (0.31, 9.93)	0.52	1.87 (0.33, 10.59)	0.48

adjustment for randomization to the LINC intervention group (data not shown).

ART and suppressed HIV viral load

We did not find significant associations between the main independent variables (i.e., unhealthy alcohol use, IDU, and opioid craving) and secondary (prescription of ART) or exploratory (achievement of viral control) outcomes (Tables 4, 5). In fact, the estimated effects did not even suggest an association in the hypothesized direction that substance use factors examined were associated with worse HIV care cascade outcomes.

Discussion

Substance use is not associated with the examined stages in the HIV care cascade in this cohort

Alcohol and drug use have been implicated in HIV disease transmission and progression, but the role of these behaviors in each step of the HIV care cascade is less explored, especially in Eastern Europe. In this cohort of HIV-positive Russians who have been in addiction hospital treatment in the past year and had a lifetime history of injection drug use, we did not find a major role of individual substance use characteristics in the HIV care cascade milestones. Given the high prevalence of substance

Table 4 Separate logistic regression models evaluating the association between substance use (unhealthy alcohol use, past-month IDU, opioid craving) and ART (n = 249)

Variable	Outcome					
	ART and unhealthy alcohol use n = 249 use		ART and IDU n = 249		ART and opioid craving n = 250	
	Adjusted odds ratio (95% CI)	p value	Adjusted odds ratio (95% CI)	p value	Adjusted odds ratio (95% CI)	p value
AUDIT 20-40 Alcohol dependence	0.98 (0.37, 2.57)	0.97	–	–	–	–
AUDIT 8–19 Hazardous drinking	1.24 (0.52, 2.95)	0.62	–	–	–	–
IDU	–	–	0.89 (0.41, 1.90)	0.76	–	–
Opioid Craving 30–70	–	–	–	–	1.34 (0.53, 3.37)	0.53
Opioid Craving 71–100	–	–	–	–	1.16 (0.46, 2.92)	0.76
Gender (female vs. male)	1.25 (0.52, 2.97)	0.61	1.23 (0.51, 2.93)	0.64	1.22 (0.51, 2.90)	0.65
Age	1.04 (0.97, 1.13)	0.28	1.04 (0.96, 1.13)	0.31	1.05 (0.97, 1.13)	0.27
Stigma	0.74 (0.39, 1.40)	0.35	0.73 (0.39, 1.40)	0.35	0.74 (0.39, 1.40)	0.35

Table 5 Separate logistic regression models evaluating associations between substance use (unhealthy alcohol use, past-month IDU, opioid craving) and HVL suppression (n = 49)

Variable	Outcome					
	Suppressed HVL and AUDIT		Suppressed HVL and IDU		Suppressed HVL and opioid craving	
	Odds ratio (95% CI)	p value	Odds ratio (95% CI)	p value	Odds ratio (95% CI)	p value
AUDIT 20–40 Alcohol dependence	3.07 (0.32, 29.06)	0.33	–	–	–	–
AUDIT 8–19 Hazardous drinking	1.77 (0.20, 15.82)	0.61	–	–	–	–
IDU	–	–	0.90 (0.15, 5.25)	0.90	–	–
Opioid craving 30–70	–	–	–	–	0.96 (0.16, 5.86)	0.97
Opioid craving 71–100	–	–	–	–	0.27 (0.01, 6.48)	0.42

use and HIV infection in Russia, examining such associations is important.

The impact of alcohol use on HIV outcomes has been examined in other settings, and while areas of uncertainty exist, collective evidence suggests that there are possible mechanisms by which alcohol may be related to HIV disease progression, via low medication adherence and suboptimal retention in care [13, 37–39]. Research suggests that heavy drinkers are less likely to receive a prescription for ART [40–42]. However, it is unknown which stages of the HIV care cascade are most affected by unhealthy alcohol use. Our analysis attempted to examine this question by looking at alcohol's effect on different steps of the HIV care cascade. Similar to alcohol use, opioid use is a known barrier to HIV care [43]. Specific effects of opioids on HIV disease progression are not fully understood, although some insights have been gained [44–46]. For example, studies have demonstrated a negative effect on CD4 count with heroin withdrawal in Russia [44]. A recent cross-sectional study among PWID in St. Petersburg and Kohtla-Järve, Estonia demonstrated that high alcohol consumption and injection frequency are significantly associated with missing HIV care cascade steps [47].

Systemic factors merit further investigation

In some countries, access to HIV care among people who inject drugs (PWID) is disproportionately low due to system level characteristics. Systemic factors such as provider discrimination and stigmatization of affected people, low quality of care, criminalization of drug use, or detention in camps without effective treatment [22, 48, 49] might play a more important role resulting in poor HIV cascade outcomes. An example of a system level barrier to HIV care is providers' negative attitudes about PWID in France in the early 2000s, when people with active injection use were threefold more likely not to receive ART because physicians doubted their ability to adhere to the regimen [50]. In contrast, evidence suggests that systemic factors associated with successful HIV treatment outcomes include provision of quality alcohol and/or drug addiction treatment, having a regular source of primary care, and provider expertise with HIV care [11].

Contrary to our hypotheses, individual determinants of people's substance use do not appear to be key factors driving HIV care in this study population of Russians discharged in the previous year from an addiction hospital. It is possible that in Russia, systemic factors (e.g., related to access to HIV treatment and receipt of quality services) were major determinants of the HIV care cascade.

Infrastructural challenges

These findings from Russia suggest that individual substance use factors were not significantly associated with achieving HIV care cascade milestones. This was unexpected and raises the possibility that alternative systemic barriers may dominate over individual substance use specific issues. One such possibility is that the infrastructure for delivery of HIV care is inadequate. Although HIV clinics have in recent years been increasingly distributed across city neighborhoods, availability of HIV facilities may still have been limited at the time of the study, making accessing these sites difficult for those who do not live in close proximity. The relationship of such structural issues can be tested with access to appropriate geographical data and if demonstrated as a substantial burden to HIV care, could be addressed by further expansion of accessible facilities. However, at this time, this is a hypothesis that merits further investigation. There are also barriers to adequate addiction care for example opioid agonist therapy does not exist in Russia, and alcohol treatment guidelines are far from evidence-based. It is therefore challenging for providers to offer high-quality addiction treatment, which has been shown to improve HIV outcomes [11, 15, 24].

A substantial body of literature exists on the protective effects of education on HIV care; this seems to be the case in this cohort, as education was positively associated with achievement of HIV care cascade outcomes [51, 52]. Married or partnered status was associated with significantly lower odds of linkage to care, suggesting that participants who were single had more progress with this HIV cascade outcome. This finding is surprising, given that partnered status usually has beneficial effects on overall health outcomes and HIV care [53, 54]. It is possible that single participants in this Russian cohort lived with their parents, and were therefore more motivated and financially better positioned to receive HIV care. This hypothesis merits further investigation.

Limitations

The results of this study should be interpreted with caution and several limitations should be considered. This is a secondary data analysis and there may be lack of power to detect the relationships of interest. Given that all participants in the study were hospitalized for a substance use disorder, one could posit that the association of substance use with HIV care cascade outcomes could have been significant if the sample included participants without a substance use disorder (i.e., abstainers) as a comparison group. Initiation of ART had a limited number of events which precluded analysis with regression models controlling for the full set of desired covariates. Also, for the same outcome, due to limited sample size, we did not conduct analyses restricting the sample to only those who were eligible for ART, based on the Russian Federation guidelines for the initiation of pharmacotherapy at the time of the study (i.e., CD4 < 350 cells/mm^3) [55], but rather included all participants, regardless of their CD4 status. In addition, due to limited sample size, HVL suppression could not be examined in multivariate analyses.

Conclusion

Unhealthy alcohol use, past-month injection drug use, and opioid craving do not appear to play a major role in achieving the HIV care cascade milestones (i.e., linkage to HIV care; prescribed ART; and achievement of suppressed viral load) among a cohort of HIV-positive Russians with history of IDU. Continuing to pursue an understanding of the systemic factors that contribute to successful HIV care cascade outcomes in populations of PWID will be key to meeting an ambitious United Nations' goal of global elimination of HIV infection.

Abbreviations
ART: antiretroviral therapy; PWID: people who inject drugs; UN: United Nations; IDU: injection drug use; LINC: Linking Infectious and Narcology Care study; RCT: randomized controlled trial; ARCH: Alcohol Research Collaboration on HIV/AIDS; HVL: HIV viral load; AUDIT: alcohol use disorder identification test; CES-D: Center for Epidemiologic Studies Depression Scale; AOR: adjusted odds ratio; CI: confidence intervals; SD: standard deviation; OAT: opioid agonist therapy.

Authors' contributions
BI, AW, KB, DC, KL and JHS conceived and refined the study question. BI led the analytic planning with support from DC and wrote the first draft of the manuscript with KL and NG. EQ conducted analyses. NG, CB, and EB coordinated study activities. In Russia, EB and EK oversaw acquisition of data and monitored study activities in the field. EK led the Russian team as the local principal investigator with co-investigator DL. JHS was the principal investigator of the parent study. All authors contributed to developing the analytic plan, reviewed, revised, and approved the submitted manuscript. All authors read and approved the final manuscript.

Author details
[1] Clinical Addiction Research and Education Unit, Section of General Internal Medicine, Department of Medicine, Boston University School of Medicine/Boston Medical Center, 801 Massachusetts Avenue, 2nd Floor, Boston, MA 02118, USA. [2] Clinical Addiction Research and Education Unit, Section of General Internal Medicine, Department of Medicine, Boston Medical Center, 801 Massachusetts Avenue, 2nd Floor, Boston, MA 02118, USA. [3] Department of Biostatistics, Boston University School of Public Health, 801 Massachusetts Avenue, 3rd Floor, Boston, MA 02118, USA. [4] First St. Petersburg Pavlov State Medical University, Lev Tolstoy St. 6/8, St. Petersburg, Russian Federation 197022. [5] Data Coordinating Center, Boston University School of Public Health, 85 E Newton St M921, Boston, MA 02118, USA. [6] HIV/AIDS Research, National Institute on Alcohol Abuse and Alcoholism, National Institute of Health, 5365 Fishers Lane, Bethesda, MD 20892, USA. [7] Pasteur Research Institute of Epidemiology and Microbiology, Mira St. 14, St. Petersburg, Russian Federation 197101. [8] St. Petersburg Bekhterev Research Psychoneurological Institute, Bekhtereva St., 3, St. Petersburg, Russian Federation 192019. [9] Department of Community Health Sciences, Boston University School of Public Health, 801 Massachusetts Avenue, Boston, MA 02118, USA. [10] Department of Infectious Diseases, Bashkir State Medical University, 3 Lenina St., Ufa, Bashkortostan Republic, Russian Federation 450000.

Acknowledgements
The idea for this study was conceived and fostered by the Fellow Immersion Training (FIT) Program in Addiction Medicine (R25 DA013582). Authors would like to acknowledge Katherine Calver and Sally Bendiks for their assistance with manuscript preparation.

Competing interests
The authors declare that they have no competing interests.

Funding
The study was supported by the following NIH Grant funding: NIDA INVEST, U01AA020780, U24AA020778, U24AA020779, U01AA021989, R01DA032082, and R25DA013582. KL was supported by K99DA041245.

References
1. UNAIDS. 90–90–90—an ambitious treatment target to help end the AIDS epidemic. 2014; http://www.unaids.org/en/resources/documents/2014/90-90-90. Accessed 23 Jan 2017.
2. Global Burden of Diseases 2015 SDG collaborators. Measuring the health-related Sustainable Development Goals in 188 countries: a baseline analysis from the Global Burden of Disease Study 2015. Lancet. 2016;388:1813–50.
3. HIV/AIDS. Together we will end AIDS. Geneva: UNAIDS; 2012.
4. Beyrer C, Malinowska-Sempruch K, Kamarulzaman A, Kazatchkine M, Sidibe M, Strathdee SA. Time to act: a call for comprehensive responses to HIV in people who use drugs. Lancet. 2010;376(9740):551–63.
5. Kamarulzaman A, Altice FL. Challenges in managing HIV in people who use drugs. Curr Opin Infect Dis. 2015;28(1):10–6.
6. Gardner EM, McLees MP, Steiner JF, Del Rio C, Burman WJ. The spectrum of engagement in HIV care and its relevance to test-and-treat strategies for prevention of HIV infection. Clin Infect Dis. 2011;52(6):793–800.
7. Kay ES, Batey DS, Mugavero MJ. The HIV treatment cascade and care continuum: updates, goals, and recommendations for the future. AIDS Res Ther. 2016;13:35.
8. Lucas GM, Cheever LW, Chaisson RE, Moore RD. Detrimental effects of continued illicit drug use on the treatment of HIV-1 infection. J Acquir Immune Defic Syndr. 2001;27(3):251–9.
9. Carrico AW. Substance use and HIV disease progression in the HAART era: implications for the primary prevention of HIV. Life Sci. 2011;88:940–7.
10. Strathdee SA, Palepu A, Cornelisse PG, Yip B, O'Shaughnessy MV, Montaner JS, Schechter MT, Hogg RS. Barriers to use of free antiretroviral therapy in injection drug users. JAMA. 1998;280(6):547–9.
11. Malta M, Ralil da Costa M, Bastos FI. The paradigm of universal access to HIV-treatment and human rights violation: how do we treat HIV-positive people who use drugs? Curr HIV/AIDS Rep. 2014;11(1):52–62.
12. Moore RD, Keruly JC, Chaisson RE. Differences in HIV disease progression by injecting drug use in HIV-infected persons in care. J Acquir Immune Defic Syndr. 2004;35(1):46–51.
13. Williams EC, Hahn JA, Saitz R, Bryant K, Lira MC, Samet JH. Alcohol Use and human immunodeficiency virus (HIV) infection: current knowledge, implications, and future directions. Alcohol Clin Exp Res. 2016;40(10):2056–72.
14. Popovich L, Potapchik E, Shishkin S, Richardson E, Vacroux A, Mathivet B. Russian Federation: Health system review. Health Systems in Transition. 2011; 13:1–190. http://www.euro.who.int/__data/assets/pdf_file/0006/157092/HiT-Russia_EN_web-with-links.pdf.
15. Idrisov B, Murphy SM, Morrill T, Saadoun M, Lunze K, Shepard D. Implementation of methadone therapy for opioid use disorder in Russia—a modeled cost-effectiveness analysis. Subst Abuse Treat Prev Policy. 2017;12(1):4.

16. Rhodes T, Platt L, Maximova S, Koshkina E, Latishevskaya N, Hickman M, Renton A, Bobrova N, McDonald T, Parry JV. Prevalence of HIV, hepatitis C and syphilis among injecting drug users in Russia: a multi-city study. Addiction. 2006;101(2):252–66.

17. Krupitsky EM, Horton NJ, Williams EC, Lioznov D, Kuznetsova M, Zvartau E, Samet JH. Alcohol use and HIV risk behaviors among HIV-infected hospitalized patients in St. Petersburg, Russia. Drug Alcohol Depend. 2005;79(2):251–6.

18. Cepeda JA, Odinokova VA, Heimer R, Grau LE, Lyubimova A, Safiullina L, et al. Drug network characteristics and HIV risk among injection drug users in Russia: the roles of trust, size, and stability. AIDS Behav. 2011;15:1003–10.

19. Goliusov AT, Dementyeva LA, Ladnaya NN, Pshenichnaya VA. Country progress report of the Russian Federation on the implementation of the declaration of commitment on HIV/AIDS. Ministry of Health and Social Development of the Russian Federation: Federal service for surveillance of consumer rights protection and human well-being of the Russian Federation; 2010.

20. Wang H, Wolock TM, Carter A, Nguyen G, Kyu HH, Gakidou E, Hay SI, Mills EJ, Trickey A, Msemburi W, et al. Estimates of global, regional, and national incidence, prevalence, and mortality of HIV, 1980–2015: the Global Burden of Disease Study 2015. Lancet HIV. 2016;3(8):e361–87.

21. Ministry of Health. HIV infection in Russia. In: Federal Research Center for HIV/AIDS Prevention and Treatment; Russian Ministry of Health. http://aids-centr.perm.ru/%D0%A1%D1%82%D0%B0%D1%82%D0%B8%D1%81%D1%82%D0%B8%D0%BA%D0%B0/%D0%92%D0%98%D0%A7/%D0%A1%D0%9F%D0%98%D0%94-%D0%B2-%D0%A0%D0%BE%D1%81%D1%81%D0%B8%D0%B8; 2015.

22. Lunze K, Idrisov B, Golichenko M, Kamarulzaman A. Mandatory addiction treatment for people who use drugs: global health and human rights analysis. BMJ (Clin Res Ed). 2016;353:i2943.

23. Krupitsky E, Woody GE, Zvartau E, O'Brien CP. Addiction treatment in Russia. Lancet. 2010;376(9747):1145.

24. Mendelevich VD, Zalmunin KY. Paradoxes of evidence in Russian addiction medicine. Int J Risk Saf Med. 2015;27(Suppl 1):S102–3.

25. Gnatienko N, Han SC, Krupitsky E, Blokhina E, Bridden C, Chaisson CE, Cheng DM, Walley AY, Raj A, Samet JH. Linking Infectious and Narcology Care (LINC) in Russia: design, intervention and implementation protocol. Addict Sci Clin Pract. 2016;11(1):10.

26. So-Armah K, Cheng DM, Freiberg M, et al. Longitudional association between alcohol use and inflammatory biomarkers. In: Poster presentation at 2017 conference on retroviruses and opportunistic infections (CROI). 2017.

27. Babor TF, Higgins-Biddle JC, Saunders JB, Monteiro MG. AUDIT. The alcohol use disorders identification Test (AUDIT): guidelines for use in primary care 2001.

28. Friedmann PD. Clinical practice. Alcohol use in adults. N Engl J Med. 2013;368(4):365–73.

29. Franken IH, Hendriksa VM, van den Brink W. Initial validation of two opiate craving questionnaires the obsessive compulsive drug use scale and the desires for drug questionnaire. Addict Behav. 2002;27(5):675–85.

30. Krupitsky E, Nunes EV, Ling W, Illeperuma A, Gastfriend DR, Silverman BL. Injectable extended-release naltrexone for opioid dependence: a double-blind, placebo-controlled, multicentre randomised trial. Lancet. 2011;377(9776):1506–13.

31. Chesney MA, Ickovics JR, Chambers DB, Gifford AL, Neidig J, Zwickl B, Wu AW. Self-reported adherence to antiretroviral medications among participants in HIV clinical trials: the AACTG adherence instruments. Patient Care Committee & Adherence Working Group of the Outcomes Committee of the Adult AIDS Clinical Trials Group (AACTG). AIDS Care. 2000;12(3):255–66.

32. Radloff LS. The CES-D scale a self-report depression scale for research in the general population. Appl Psychol Meas. 1977;1(3):385–401.

33. Chishinga N, Kinyanda E, Weiss HA, Patel V, Ayles H, Seedat S. Validation of brief screening tools for depressive and alcohol use disorders among TB and HIV patients in primary care in Zambia. BMC Psychiatry. 2011;11(1):1.

34. Berger BE, Ferrans CE, Lashley FR. Measuring stigma in people with HIV: psychometric assessment of the HIV stigma scale. Res Nurs Health. 2001;24(6):518–29.

35. Iacobucci D, Posavac SS, Kardes FR, Schneider M, Popovich DL. The median split: robust, refined, and revived. J Consum Psychol. 2015;25:690–704.

36. Petersburg legal portal. Living wage in St. Petersburg. (2017). Retrieved January 18, 2017, from http://ppt.ru/info/5 In: Petersburg legal portal [Rus: Гетербургский правовой портал Прожиточный минимум в Санкт-Петербурге) 2017.

37. Hahn JA, Samet JH. Alcohol and HIV disease progression: weighing the evidence. Curr HIV/AIDS Rep. 2010;7(4):226–33.

38. Samet JH, Horton NJ, Meli S, Freedberg KA, Palepu A. Alcohol consumption and antiretroviral adherence among HIV-infected persons with alcohol problems. Alcohol Clin Exp Res. 2004;28(4):572–7.

39. Shuper PA, Neuman M, Kanteres F, Baliunas D, Joharchi N, Rehm J. Causal considerations on alcohol and HIV/AIDS—a systematic review. Alcohol Alcohol. 2010;45(2):159–66.

40. Conen A, Fehr J, Glass TR, Furrer H, Weber R, Vernazza P, Hirschel B, Cavassini M, Bernasconi E, Bucher HC, et al. Self-reported alcohol consumption and its association with adherence and outcome of antiretroviral therapy in the Swiss HIV Cohort Study. Antivir Ther. 2009;14(3):349–57.

41. Martinez P, Andia I, Emenyonu N, Hahn JA, Hauff E, Pepper L, Bangsberg DR. Alcohol use, depressive symptoms and the receipt of antiretroviral therapy in southwest Uganda. AIDS Behav. 2008;12(4):605–12.

42. Chander G, Lau B, Moore RD. Hazardous alcohol use: a risk factor for non-adherence and lack of suppression in HIV infection. J Acquir Immune Defic Syndr. 2006;43(4):411–7.

43. Centers for Disease Control and Prevention. Incorporating HIV prevention into the medical care of persons living with HIV. Recommendations of CDC, the Health Resources and Services Administration, the National Institutes of Health, and the HIV Medicine Association of the Infectious Diseases Society of America. MMWR Recomm Rep. 2003;52:1–24.

44. Edelman EJ, Cheng DM, Krupitsky EM, Bridden C, Quinn E, Walley AY, Lioznov DA, Blokhina E, Zvartau E, Samet JH. Heroin use and HIV disease progression: results from a pilot study of a russian cohort. AIDS Behav. 2015;19(6):1089–97.

45. Kipp AM, Desruisseau AJ, Qian HZ. Non-injection drug use and HIV disease progression in the era of combination antiretroviral therapy. J Subst Abuse Treat. 2011;40(4):386–96.

46. Cabral GA. Drugs of abuse, immune modulation, and AIDS. J Neuroimmune Pharmacol. 2006;1(3):280–95.

47. Heimer R, Usacheva N, Barbour R, Niccolai LM, Uuskula A, Levina OS. Engagement in HIV care and its correlates among people who inject drugs in St Petersburg, Russian Federation and Kohtla-Jarve, Estonia. Addiction. 2017;112(8):1421–31.

48. Gerbert B, Maguire BT, Bleecker T, Coates TJ, McPhee SJ. Primary care physicians and aids: attitudinal and structural barriers to care. JAMA. 1991;266(20):2837–42.

49. Wolfe D, Carrieri MP, Shepard D. Treatment and care for injecting drug users with HIV infection: a review of barriers and ways forward. Lancet. 2010;376(9738):355–66.

50. Carrieri MP, Moatti JP, Vlahov D, Obadia Y, Reynaud-Maurupt C, Chesney M. Access to antiretroviral treatment among French HIV infected injection drug users: the influence of continued drug use. MANIF 2000 Study Group. J Epidemiol Community Health. 1999;53(1):4–8.

51. Kelly M. Preventing HIV transmission through education: HIV/AIDS and education. Perspect Educ. 2002;20(1):1–12.

52. Iorio D, Santaeulalia-Llopis R. Education, HIV status and risky sexual behavior: how much does the stage of the HIV epidemic matter? 2016.

53. Iwashyna TJ, Christakis NA. Marriage, widowhood, and health-care use. Soc Sci Med. 2003;57(11):2137–47.

54. Stein JA, Nyamathi A, Ullman JB, Bentler PM. Impact of marriage on HIV/AIDS risk behaviors among impoverished, at-risk couples: a multilevel latent variable approach. AIDS Behav. 2006;11(1):87.

55. Degenhardt L, Charlson F, Stanaway J, Larney S, Alexander LT, Hickman M, Cowie B, Hall WD, Strang J, Whiteford H, et al. Estimating the burden of disease attributable to injecting drug use as a risk factor for HIV, hepatitis C, and hepatitis B: findings from the Global Burden of Disease Study 2013. Lancet Infect Dis. 2016;2016(16):1385–98.

19

Evaluation of the effect of methamphetamine on traumatic injury complications and outcomes

Michael M. Neeki[1,5]*, Fanglong Dong[2], Lidia Liang[2], Jake Toy[2]●, Braeden Carrico[1], Nina Jabourian[1], Arnold Sin[1,5], Farabi Hussain[3,5], Sharon Brown[1], Keyvan Safdari[4,5], Rodney Borger[1,5] and David Wong[3,5]

Abstract

Background: This study investigates the impact of methamphetamine use on trauma patient outcomes.

Methods: This retrospective study analyzed patients between 18 and 55 years old presenting to a single trauma center in San Bernardino County, CA who sustained traumatic injury during the 10-year study period (January 1st, 2005 to December 31st, 2015). Routine serum ethanol levels and urine drug screens (UDS) were completed on all trauma patients. Exclusion criteria included patients with an elevated serum ethanol level (>0 mg/dL). Those who screened positive on UDS for only methamphetamine and negative for cocaine and cannabis (MA(+)) were compared to those with a triple negative UDS for methamphetamine, cocaine, and cannabis (MA(−)). The primary outcome studied was the impact of a methamphetamine positive drug screen on hospital mortality. Secondary outcomes included length of stay (LOS), heart rate, systolic and diastolic blood pressure (SBP and DBP, respectively), and total amount of blood products utilized during hospitalization. To analyze the effect of methamphetamine, age, gender, injury severity score, and mechanism of injury (blunt vs. penetrating) were matched between MA(−) and MA(+) through a propensity matching algorithm.

Results: After exclusion, 2538 patients were included in the final analysis; 449 were patients in the MA(+) group and 2089 patients in the MA(−) group. A selection of 449 MA(−) patients were matched with the MA(+) group based on age, gender, injury severity score, and mechanism of injury. This led to a final sample size of 898 patients with 449 patients in each group. No statistically significant change was observed in hospital mortality. Notably, a methamphetamine positive drug screen was associated with a longer LOS (median of 4 vs. 3 days in MA(+) and MA(−), respectively, $p < 0.0001$), an increased heart rate at the scene (103 vs. 94 bpm for MA(+) and MA(−), respectively, $p = 0.0016$), and an increased heart rate upon arrival to the trauma center (100 vs. 94 bpm for MA(+) and MA(−), respectively, $p < 0.0001$). Moreover, the MA(+) group had decreased SBP at the scene compared to the MA(−) group (127 vs. 132 bpm for MA(+) and MA(−), respectively, $p = 0.0149$), but SBP was no longer statistically different when patients arrived at the trauma center ($p = 0.3823$). There was no significant difference in DBP or in blood products used.

Conclusion: Methamphetamine positive drug screens in trauma patients were not associated with an increase in hospital mortality; however, a methamphetamine positive drug screen was associated with a longer LOS and an increased heart rate.

Keywords: Methamphetamine, Trauma, Length of stay, Hospital mortality, Traumatic outcome

---

*Correspondence: michaelneeki@gmail.com
[1] Department of Emergency Medicine, Arrowhead Regional Medical Center, Medical Office Building, Suite 7, 400 N Pepper Ave, Colton, CA 92324, USA
Full list of author information is available at the end of the article

Background

Methamphetamine is a potent stimulant that affects the central nervous system. Use of methamphetamine results in immediate effects that often include euphoria, aggression, erratic behavior, increased libido, emotional lability, and psychosis lasting on average for 6 to 12 h [1–4]. In 2015, an increasing trend of methamphetamine use in the United States among individuals 12 years and older was noted with an estimated 5.4% of the population having tried methamphetamine in their lifetime [5]. Geographically, methamphetamine use is most predominant on the West Coast and in the Midwest; however, the prevalence of use is rapidly spreading east across the United States [1, 5, 6]. This increase in methamphetamine use has been reflected in emergency departments (ED) around the country [1, 7–10]. The economic impact has also been significant [9, 11]. In 2005, the economic burden of methamphetamine use in the United States was estimated to be $23.4 billion [11].

There are extensive published reports on the deleterious cardiovascular and neurological effects of methamphetamine; however, there is a paucity of evidence pertaining to the impact of methamphetamine in the context of traumatic injury [6, 12–16]. Previous studies have demonstrated an association between methamphetamine use and an increased risk of traumatic injury [10, 17]. Yet studies assessing the rate of ambulance transport, percentage of hospital admissions, length of stay (LOS), and need for emergent surgery amongst this demographic are varied and infrequent [1, 6, 10, 17–19]. Additionally, positive methamphetamine screens amongst trauma patients in the ED have been associated with inconsistent findings concerning the impact of methamphetamine on mortality outcomes in a limited number of studies [17–19]. Though trauma patients often receive urine drug screening for methamphetamine upon admission at many centers, the value of this laboratory marker is poorly understood.

We seek to assess the impact of methamphetamine use in the context of traumatic injury and the impact of methamphetamine use on hospital mortality outcomes, LOS, and acute physiologic profile. A greater understanding of these variables may aid in improving clinical management and allocation of hospital resources.

Methods

This retrospective chart review was undertaken at Arrowhead Regional Medical Center (ARMC). ARMC is a 456-bed acute care teaching facility and the only American College of Surgeons certified level II trauma center located in San Bernardino County, CA with over 92,000 visits annually. San Bernardino County is the largest county by area in the contiguous United States with a population of over two million.

Data were gathered from the trauma registry at ARMC. Trauma patients between 18 and 55 years old who were admitted between January 1st, 2005 and December 31st, 2015 were assessed for inclusion. During the study period, all trauma patients seen at our center underwent routine urine drug screening (UDS) and measurement of a serum ethanol level in the ED prior to admission. Exclusion criteria included patients with an elevated serum ethanol level (greater than 0 mg/dL) and UDS positive for any drug other than methamphetamine (including cocaine and cannabis). For trauma patients presenting to the trauma center with multiple visits, only the most recent visit was included in the analysis.

Patients were divided into two groups based on the presence of methamphetamine on urine drug screen (MA(+) vs. MA(−)). The MA(+) group included patients with a positive UDS for methamphetamine, negative UDS for cocaine and cannabis, and serum ethanol level less than 0 mg/dL. The MA(−) group was defined as patients with a triple negative UDS for methamphetamine, cocaine, and cannabis, and serum ethanol level less than 0 mg/dL. Routine UDS and serum ethanol level were performed using the Cobas 6000 analyzer series (Roche Diagnostics USA, Indianapolis, Indiana, USA). Though urine opiate levels were included in the UDS at our center, this data was not included in the study. The threshold to detect urine amphetamine concentrations was set at greater than 1000 ng/ml. Additional patient data collected included age, gender, injury severity score (ISS), mechanism of injury (blunt vs. penetrating), transfusion need during hospital stay, LOS, hospital mortality, and heart rate (normal adult resting heart rate is 60–100) and blood pressure (normal adult resting diastolic blood pressure [DBP] is less than 80 mmhg and systolic blood pressure [SBP] less than 120 mmhg) taken by first responders after arrival at the scene and by ED staff upon arrival to the trauma center. The ISS is derived from a validated scoring system used to describe overall injury severity based on the anatomic regions involved [20]. Major trauma (polytrauma) has been defined as ISS greater than 15 and a higher ISS has been correlated with an increase in morbidity and mortality [21].

The primary outcome was mortality during hospital stay. Other outcomes included hospital LOS, total amount of blood products utilized during the hospital stay, heart rate taken at the scene and upon arrival to the trauma center, and SBP and DBP at the scene and upon arrival to the trauma center.

All statistical analyses were conducted using the SAS software for Windows version 9.3 (SAS Institute, Cary, North Carolina, USA). Descriptive statistics were presented as means and standard deviations for continuous variables, and frequencies and proportions for categorical variables. Chi square crosstab analysis was conducted to identify whether the proportion of penetrating trauma was comparable between the MA(+) and MA(−). If the proportions of penetrating trauma were statistically different between the MA(+) and MA(−) group, a propensity score 1–1 matching was conducted to select the same number of participants from the MA(−) to match the participants from the MA(+) group based on age, gender, ISS, and mechanism of injury (blunt vs. penetrating) using the package "MatchIt" in R. The choice of these four matching variables for the matching process was to eliminate the confounding effect on primary and secondary outcomes. After data were matched, comparison of continuous variables was conducted using the independent T test between the MA(+) and MA(−) groups. Comparison of categorical variables was conducted using the Chi square test. All statistical analyses were two-sided. p values < 0.05 were considered to be statistically significant. This study was approved by the Institutional Review Board at ARMC.

Results

Among the 6898 patients included in the original database, 3900 patients were excluded due to elevated serum ethanol levels, 349 patients were excluded due to positive cocaine on UDS, and 111 patients were excluded due to positive cannabis on UDS, which led to a cohort of 2538 patients. A total of 449 patients were positive for MA(+) and 2089 patients were MA(−) (see Fig. 1). A selection of 449 patients in the MA(−) group was matched with MA(+) group based on age, gender, ISS, and mechanism of injury. This led to a final sample size of 898 patients with 449 patients in each group.

No difference in hospital mortality was noted between the two groups (3.3 vs. 2.7% for MA(+) and MA(−), respectively, $p = 0.5577$). Patients in the MA(+) group, however, had a longer hospital LOS (a median of 4 vs. 3 days for MA(+) and MA(−), respectively, $p = 0.0001$). MA(+) patients also utilized less blood products (2054 ml vs. 2481 ml for MA(+) and MA(−), respectively, $p = 0.3547$), though blood product utilization was not statistically different.

A comparison between the MA(+) and MA(−) groups was conducted to assess their acute physiologic profile (Table 1). Patients in the MA(+) group had a statistically significant increase in pulse taken both on scene (103 vs. 94 beats per minute for MA(+) and MA(−), respectively, $p < 0.0001$) and upon arrival to the trauma center (100 vs. 94 beats per minute for MA(+) and MA(−), respectively, $p = 0.0063$). Moreover, patients in the MA(+) group had a statistically significant decrease in SBP at the scene

than patients in the MA(−) group (127 vs. 132 beats per minute for MA(+) and MA(−), respectively, $p = 0.0149$), however, SBP was no longer statistically different when patients arrived at the trauma center ($p = 0.3823$). There was no difference on DBP regardless whether at the scene or upon arrival to the trauma center (both p values > 0.05).

Discussion

Although it has been widely established that methamphetamine use results in toxic effects on the body and increases the likelihood of sustaining a traumatic injury, the effects of methamphetamine on traumatic injury outcomes in the post-injury period remain unclear. The current study suggests no change in hospital mortality outcomes and a longer hospital LOS in trauma patients with positive methamphetamine drug screens. With respect to the association between a positive methamphetamine drug screen and trauma patient mortality, Yegiyants et al. [18] demonstrated a conflicting trend toward reduced mortality among trauma patients who had a positive methamphetamine drug screen. However, Hadjizacharia et al. [19] noted no significant correlation. Taken together, it appears that a positive methamphetamine drug screen does not correlate with trauma patient mortality. With regards to hospital LOS, the findings of the current study are consistent with select prior reports suggesting that minimally injured trauma patients with positive methamphetamine drug screens have a significantly longer hospital LOS [6, 17]. Yet other studies have reported that trauma patients with positive methamphetamine drug screens did not have an increased LOS in the intensive care unit (ICU) or the hospital, but may be more likely to be admitted to the ICU [17, 19].

We further assessed the acute physiologic profile of the trauma patients studied. Given the known impact of methamphetamine on an individual's physiologic status (i.e. tachycardia, vasoconstriction, vasospasm) [22], we hypothesized that tachycardia and an elevated blood pressure among patients with methamphetamine positive drug screens may offer an explanation to the observed mortality outcomes noted in the aforementioned studies [18, 19]. An unstable acute physiologic profile may have elicited a higher level of care from clinicians providing a possible explanation for the reduced and unchanged mortality outcomes previously observed in patients with positive methamphetamine screens. Though a significant difference in pulse rate was found amongst trauma patients with positive methamphetamine screens in this study, this difference was minimal and likely clinically insignificant. A significant difference in blood pressure was also noted at the scene amongst trauma patients with positive methamphetamine

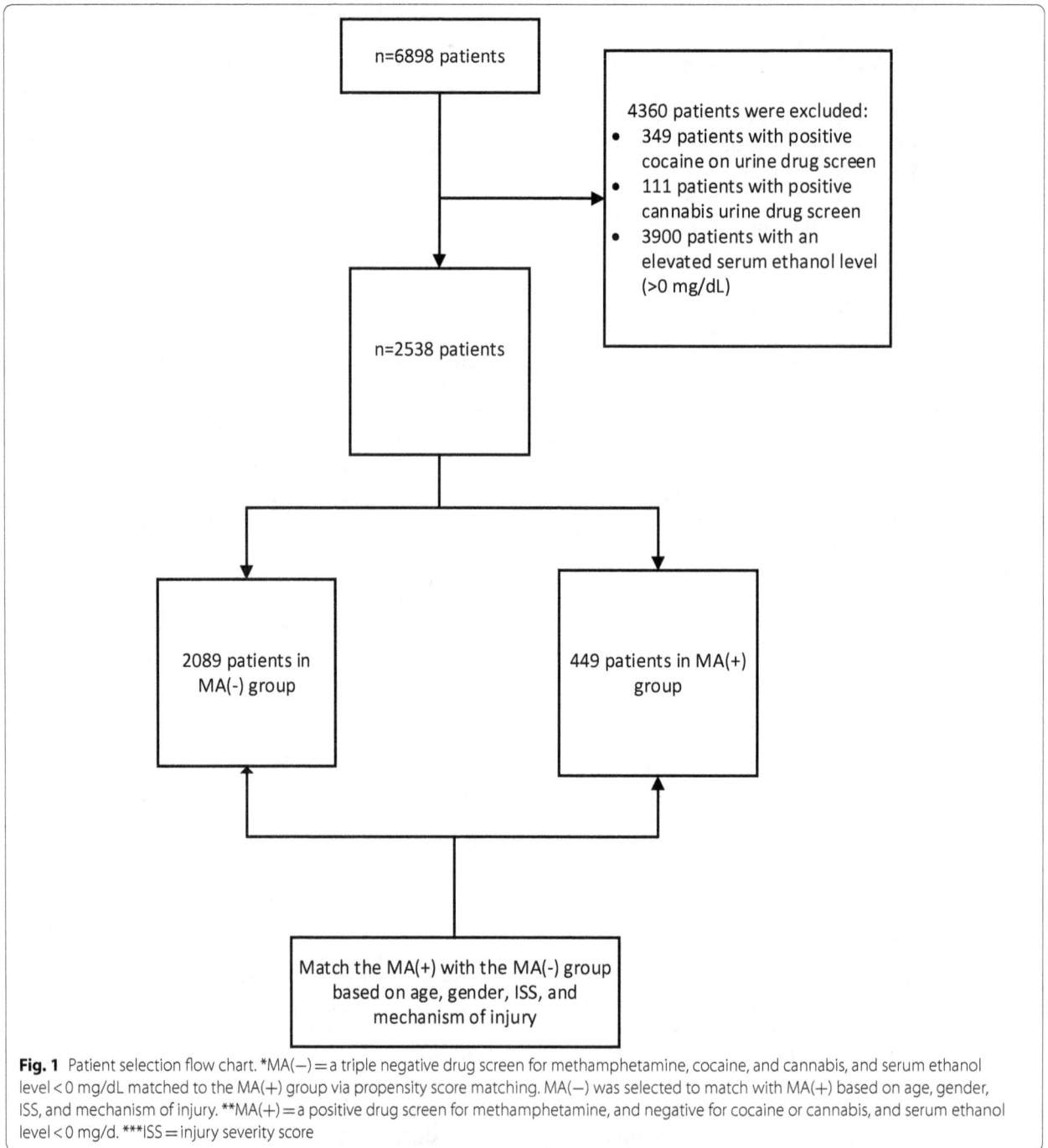

Fig. 1 Patient selection flow chart. *MA(−) = a triple negative drug screen for methamphetamine, cocaine, and cannabis, and serum ethanol level < 0 mg/dL matched to the MA(+) group via propensity score matching. MA(−) was selected to match with MA(+) based on age, gender, ISS, and mechanism of injury. **MA(+) = a positive drug screen for methamphetamine, and negative for cocaine or cannabis, and serum ethanol level < 0 mg/d. ***ISS = injury severity score

drug screens; however, this difference was also minimal and likely clinically insignificant. Of note, given that methamphetamine metabolites may be present on UDS for approximately two to five days after last use without substantial lasting physiologic effects, it may be difficult to attribute all of the observed findings to methamphetamine. To our knowledge, no previous study has assessed

the impact of positive methamphetamine drug screens on the acute physiological profile in trauma patients.

Reasons for the increased hospital LOS observed among trauma patients with methamphetamine positive drug screens in this study were likely multifactorial. One contributing factor may be a delay in surgical care due to a positive methamphetamine drug screen upon admission. Based on our hospital anesthesiology

Table 1 Comparison between positive (MA(+)) and negative (MA(−)) methamphetamine drug screens

	MA(+) n = 449	MA(−) n = 449	p value
Age	34.18 ± 10.75	34.23 ± 11.1	0.9367
Gender			0.6736
Female	90 (20%)	85 (18.9%)	
Male	359 (80%)	364 (81.1%)	
Mechanism of Injury			0.6116
Blunt	309 (68.8%)	316 (70.4%)	
Penetrating	140 (31.2%)	133 (29.6%)	
Injury severity score	14.76 ± 10.86	14.72 ± 10.7	0.9548
Hospital Mortality			0.5577
Alive	434 (96.7%)	437 (97.3%)	
Dead	15 (3.3%)	12 (2.7%)	
Blood product			0.2452
No blood product received (n)	351 (78.2%)	365 (81.3%)	
Any Blood product received (n)	98 (21.8%)	84 (18.7%)	
Units of Total amount of blood product received (mL)	2053.65 ± 2824.25	2480.64 ± 3383.46	0.3547
Median Hospital LOS in days (Q1, Q3)	4 (2, 8)	3 (1, 7)	0.0001
Pulse on scene	102.6 ± 22.06	94.31 ± 20.97	< 0.0001
SBP on scene	126.89 ± 26.9	131.52 ± 24.34	0.0149
DBP on scene	83.31 ± 18.29	85.23 ± 19.73	0.2537
Pulse on arrival to the trauma center	99.96 ± 22.76	94 ± 20.61	< 0.0001
SBP on arrival to the trauma center	139.78 ± 25.92	141.25 ± 24.46	0.3823
DBP on arrival to the trauma center	86.59 ± 20.19	87.03 ± 19.48	0.7449

* MA(−) = a triple negative urine drug screen for methamphetamine, cocaine, and cannabis as well as serum ethanol level < 0 mg/dL matched to the MA(+) group via propensity score matching. MA(+) = a positive urine drug screen for methamphetamine, and negative for cocaine or cannabis as well as serum ethanol level < 0 mg/dL

** All continuous values were presented as mean ± SD or median (Q1, Q3) for hospital LOS. Categorical variables were presented as frequency with column percentages inside the parenthesis

*** LOS length of stay, SBP systolic blood pressure, DBP diastolic blood pressure

protocols, patients suffering from open fractures or other injuries requiring emergent procedures will undergo surgery regardless of drug screen results upon admission; however, patients who have positive methamphetamine drug screens and require non-emergent surgeries may wait up to five days for a subsequently negative methamphetamine drug screen on repeat toxicology testing. As a potent sympathomimetic, methamphetamine and its metabolites have been shown to change the minimum alveolar concentration of inhaled anesthetics as well as both increase and decrease the required dose of anesthetic agents [23–25]. By altering anesthetic requirements, amphetamines have been implicated in cases of cardiac arrest, severe intraoperative intracranial hypertension, and reflex hypotension during general anesthesia [26–29]. Nonetheless, the impact of anesthesiology protocols on LOS may be institution dependent.

An additional and widely generalizable contributory factor to the increased LOS observed may have been an unreliable patient exam secondary to acute methamphetamine intoxication. This may have contributed to an extended observation period and extra diagnostic studies, potentially leading to an increased LOS. Alternatively, a higher frequency of comorbidities seen in chronic methamphetamine users, complications associated with methamphetamine withdrawal, or issues concerning placement after discharge may have contributed to the observed difference in LOS [13]. Future studies are warranted to assess the impact of these factors on LOS among patients with positive methamphetamine screens.

Irrespective of the root cause, the potential downstream effects resulting from added hospital days are numerous. With an average inpatient hospital day costing over $7000 at our center, an additional hospital day for patients with a positive methamphetamine screen places significant financial burden on the patient, hospital, and healthcare system. Increased costs associated with the hospitalization of trauma patients with positive methamphetamine screens have been consistently demonstrated in previous literature [6, 9, 17]. Other consequences include the diversion of trauma care resources away from other patients and increased risk of hospital-acquired infections due to an extended LOS.

Limitations

This study has several limitations. First, patients seen at our center suffering from traumatic injury during the study period underwent routine drug and alcohol screening prior to admission; however, those directly admitted or who require emergent surgery for life-threatening injuries may not have undergone drug screening. Though a small subset of patients with methamphetamine positive drugs screens may not have been included, the impact on our results was likely minimal given our matching algorthim.

Second, this study did not assess rates of ICU admission or ICU LOS. However, analysis of hospital mortality, injury severity, and transfusion need yielded no significant differences. Together, these findings suggest similar hospital courses for trauma patients with positive or negative methamphetamine screens in our study. The study also did not assess the need for surgical intervention amongst our patient sample. Combined, these two aspects significantly limit our understanding of the exact etiology leading to the observed increase in LOS.

Third, this study did not exclude patients with urine drug screens that were positive for opiates. Our sample included patients suffering from acute traumatic injuries, many of whom received analgesic drugs including opioid derived drugs in both the prehospital setting and upon arrival to the trauma center. Approximately 33% of patients in the MA(+) group screened positive for opiates on urine drug screen and 17% of patients in the MA(−) group screened positive for opiates. Unfortunately, we could not differentiate between opiate positive urine drugs screens that were due to analgesic cause versus illicit use. However, given the differing mechanism of action of methamphetamines and opioids, we feel that study outcomes were minimally affected.

A final limitation includes both the potential for false positive and false negative drug screens. Amphetamine and methamphetamine have been documented as the most commonly reported illicit drugs with a false-positive UDS due to their cross-reactivity with many commonly prescribed drugs like bupropion, trazodone, chlorpromazine, promethazine, ranitidine, and various antihistamines and decongestants [30]. Additionally, false negative results arise because toxicology screening for popular amphetamine analogues such as cathinone, a beta-ketone amphetamine moiety that has physiologic properties remarkably similar to that of methamphetamine, are underdeveloped due to the novelty of such analogues [31–33].

Conclusion

The current study suggests that trauma patients with positive methamphetamine drug screens do not have a significant difference in hospital mortality outcomes when compared to those with negative methamphetamine drug screens. Despite these findings, routine urine toxicology screening and measurement of serum ethanol level amongst trauma patients may still be warranted as these findings could assist in medical decision making throughout a patient's hospital course and disposition. Future studies are warranted to further assess the factors that contribute to an increased LOS for trauma patients with positive methamphetamine screens and to develop a greater insight into the clinical value of urine drug testing for trauma patients upon admission.

Abbreviations
ED: emergency department; LOS: length of stay; ARMC: Arrowhead Regional Medical Center; UDS: urine drug screening; MA(+): methamphetamine positive; MA(−): methamphetamine negative; ISS: injury severity score; SBP: systolic blood pressure; DBP: diastolic blood pressure.

Authors' contributions
This project was originally conceived by MMN, FH, AS Literature search was completed by LL, JT, BC, NJ IRB application was written by MMN, BC, NJ Data collection and database compilation was completed by FD, NJ, SB Statistics completed by FD Initial manuscript was written by MMN, FD, LL, JT and revised by all listed authors. MMN supervised all aspects of this study. All authors read and approved the final manuscript.

Author details
[1] Department of Emergency Medicine, Arrowhead Regional Medical Center, Medical Office Building, Suite 7, 400 N Pepper Ave, Colton, CA 92324, USA. [2] Western University of Health Sciences, College of Osteopathic Medicine of the Pacific, 309 E 2nd St., Pomona, CA 91766, USA. [3] Department of General Surgery, Arrowhead Regional Medical Center, 400 N Pepper Ave, Colton, CA 92324, USA. [4] Department of Anesthesiology, Arrowhead Regional Medical Center, 400 N Pepper Ave, Colton, CA 92324, USA. [5] California University of Sciences and Medicine, 1405 W Valley Boulevard, Suite 101, Colton, CA 92321, USA.

Acknowledgements
We would like to acknowledge Sahar Nikdel, MD, Richard Vara, RN, and Tyler Jacks for data collection and database compilation; Michelle Burgett-Moreno, BA, Michelle McBride, BA, and Carlos Peace, RN, for manuscript editing.

Competing interests
The authors declare that they have no competing interests.

Consent for publication
Not applicable.

Declarations
This original research project was presented at the American College of Emergency Physicians Scientific Assembly, October 29th, 2017; Washington, D.C, and the abstract is published in the conference proceedings in the *Annals of Emergency Medicine*. This original research manuscript is not currently under consideration with any other journal.

Funding
No funding was received for this original research study.

References

1. Schermer CR, Wisner DH. Methamphetamine use in trauma patients: a population-based study. J Am Coll Surg. 1999;189(5):442–9.
2. Murray JB. Psychophysiological aspects of amphetamine-methamphetamine abuse. J Psychol. 1998;132(2):227–37.
3. National Center for Injury Prevention and Control. CDC injury fact book. Atlanta: Center for Disease Control; 2006.
4. Russell K, Dryden D, Liang Y, et al. Risk factors for methamphetamine use in youth: a systematic review. BCM Pediatr. 2008;8:48. https://doi.org/10.1186/1471-2431-8-48.
5. Gruenewald PJ, Ponicki WR, Remer LG, et al. Mapping the spread of methamphetamine abuse in California From 1995 to 2008. Am J Public Health. 2013;103(7):1262–70.
6. Tominaga GT, Garcia G, Dzierba A, et al. Toll of methamphetamine on the trauma system. Arch Surg. 2004;139(8):844–7.
7. National estimates of drug-related emergency department visits. DAWN Series D-39 2011; Publication No. SMA 13-4760. http://www.samhsa.gov/data/2k13/DAWN2k11ED/DAWN2k11ED.htm. Accessed 1 Aug 2016.
8. Mattson ME. Emergency Department Visits Involving Methamphetamine: 2007 to 2011. Rockville, MD2014.
9. Hendrickson RG, Cloutier R, McConnell KJ. Methamphetamine-related emergency department utilization and cost. Acad Emerg Med. 2008;15(1):23–31.
10. Richards JR, Bretz SW, Johnson EB, et al. Methamphetamine abuse and emergency department utilization. West J Med. 1999;170(4):198–202.
11. Nicosia N, Pacula RL, Kilmer B, et al. The economic cost of methamphetamine use in the United States, 2005. Santa Monica: RAND Corporation; 2009.
12. Lee C, Walters E, Borger R, et al. The San Bernardino, California, terror attack: two emergency departments' response. West J Emerg Med. 2016;17(1):1–7.
13. Neeki MM, Kulczycki M, Toy J, et al. Frequency of methamphetamine use as a major contributor toward the severity of cardiomyopathy in adults ≤ 50 years. Am J Cardiol. 2016;118(4):585–9.
14. Gawin FH, Ellinwood EH Jr. Cocaine and other stimulants: actions, abuse, and treatment. N Engl J Med. 1988;318(18):1173–82.
15. Furst SR, Fallon SP, Reznik GN, Shah PK. Myocardial Infarction after Inhalation of Methamphetamine. New Engl J Med. 1990;323(16):1147–8.
16. Albertson TE, Derlet RW, Van Hoozen BE. Methamphetamine and the expanding complications of amphetamines. West J Med. 1999;170(4):214–9.
17. London JA, Utter GH, Battistella F, et al. Methamphetamine use is associated with increased hospital resource consumption among minimally injured trauma patients. J Trauma. 2009;66(2):485–90.
18. Yegiyants S, Abraham J, Taylor E. The effects of methamphetamine use on trauma patient outcome. Am Surg. 2007;73(10):1044–6.
19. Hadjizacharia P, Green DJ, Plurad D, et al. Methamphetamines in trauma: effect on injury patterns and outcome. J Trauma. 2009;66(3):895–8.
20. Baker SP, O'Neill B, Haddon W Jr, et al. The injury severity score: a method for describing patients with multiple injuries and evaluating emergency care. J Trauma. 1974;14(3):187–96.
21. Copes WS, Champion HR, Sacco WJ, et al. The Injury Severity Score revisited. J Trauma. 1988;28(1):69–77.
22. Kaye S, McKetin R, Duflou J, et al. Methamphetamine and cardiovascular pathology: a review of the evidence. Addiction. 2007;102(8):1204–11.
23. Johnston RR, Way WL, Miller RD. Alteration of anesthetic requirement by amphetamine. Anesthesiology. 1972;36(4):357–63.
24. Foex P, Prys-Roberts C. Anaesthesia and the hypertensive patient. Br J Anaesth. 1974;46(8):575–88.
25. Hatch RC. Experiments on antagonism of barbiturate anesthesia with adrenergic, serotonergic, and cholinergic stimulants given alone and in combination. Am J Vet Res. 1973;34(10):1321–31.
26. Samuels SI, Maze A, Albright G. Cardiac arrest during cesarean section in a chronic amphetamine abuser. Anesth Analg. 1979;58(6):528–30.
27. Michel R, Adams AP. Acute amphetamine abuse: problems during general anaesthesia for neurosurgery. Anaesthesia. 1979;34(10):1016–9.
28. Brunton LL, Chabner B, Goodman LS, Knollmann BC. Goodman & Gilman's the pharmacological basis of therapeutics, 12th edn. New York: McGraw-Hill Education LLC.; 2011. pp. 297–299.
29. Stibolt O, Wachowiak-Andersen G. Altered response to intravenous thiopental and succinylcholine in acute amphetamine abuse. Acta Anaesthesiol Scand. 2002;46(5):609–10.
30. Brahm NC, Yeager LL, Fox MD, et al. Commonly prescribed medications and potential false-positive urine drug screens. Am J Health Syst Pharm. 2010;67(16):1344–50.
31. Prosser JM, Nelson LS. The toxicology of bath salts: a review of synthetic cathinones. J Med Toxicol. 2012;8(1):33–42.
32. Blum K, Foster Olive M, Wang KK, et al. Hypothesizing that designer drugs containing cathinones ("bath salts") have profound neuro-inflammatory effects and dangerous neurotoxic response following human consumption. Med Hypotheses. 2013;81(3):450–5.
33. Capriola M. Synthetic cathinone abuse. Clin Pharmacol. 2013;5:109–15.

20

Barriers and facilitators to implementing addiction medicine fellowships: a qualitative study with fellows, medical students, residents and preceptors

J. Klimas[1,4] (ID), W. Small[1,5], K. Ahamad[1,2,3], W. Cullen[4], A. Mead[1,2,3], L. Rieb[1,2,3], E. Wood[1,4] and R. McNeil[1*]

Abstract

Background: Although progress in science has driven advances in addiction medicine, this subject has not been adequately taught to medical trainees and physicians. As a result, there has been poor integration of evidence-based practices in addiction medicine into physician training which has impeded addiction treatment and care. Recently, a number of training initiatives have emerged internationally, including the addiction medicine fellowships in Vancouver, Canada. This study was undertaken to examine barriers and facilitators of implementing addiction medicine fellowships.

Methods: We interviewed trainees and faculty from clinical and research training programmes in addiction medicine at St Paul's Hospital in Vancouver, Canada (N = 26) about barriers and facilitators to implementation of physician training in addiction medicine. We included medical students, residents, fellows and supervising physicians from a variety of specialities. We analysed interview transcripts thematically by using NVivo software.

Results: We identified six domains relating to training implementation: (1) organisational, (2) structural, (3) teacher, (4) learner, (5) patient and (6) community related variables either hindered or fostered addiction medicine education, depending on context. Human resources, variety of rotations, peer support and mentoring fostered implementation of addiction training. Money, time and space limitations hindered implementation. Participant accounts underscored how faculty and staff facilitated the implementation of both the clinical and the research training.

Conclusions: Implementation of addiction medicine fellowships appears feasible, although a number of barriers exist. Research into factors within the local/practice environment that shape delivery of education to ensure consistent and quality education scale-up is a priority.

Keywords: Addiction, Substance-related disorders, Medical education, Qualitative research

Background

Around the globe, harms stemming from substance use represent a significant social, health, and economic burden [1]. The associated mortality and morbidity stemming from substance use (e.g., HIV, hepatitis C) place considerable demands on healthcare systems [2, 3] and represent an urgent public health priority. Advances in addiction science have helped to identify effective treatments for substance use disorders (e.g. opioid agonist therapies, contingency management) [4, 5]. These treatments are often delivered in general medical settings and are associated with significant improvements in health and social outcomes of people with substance use disorders (SUD) [6, 7], including physical and mental health functioning [8].

The important role of physicians in the management of SUD is well documented [9, 10]. Specifically,

*Correspondence: rmcneil@cfenet.ubc.ca
[1] Department of Medicine, B.C. Centre on Substance Use, St. Paul's Hospital, University of British Columbia, 608-1081 Burrard Street, Vancouver, BC V6Z 1Y6, Canada
Full list of author information is available at the end of the article

evidence-based therapeutic interventions delivered by trained physicians, including pharmacological and psychosocial interventions, can increase motivation for and enrolment in specialised treatment programmes [11]. For example, people receiving opioid agonist treatment in primary care are twice as likely to stay in treatment compared with those who attend a specialist site [12]. However, the impact of physicians in SUD-related care is often diminished due to the widespread underutilisation of evidence-based treatments for SUDs [13].

Adequate diagnosis and treatment of SUDs by physicians often does not occur due to a lack of knowledge and accredited training in addiction medicine [14, 15]. Historically, undergraduate medical education and postgraduate clinical training programs have not invested in the implementation of addiction medicine training for health care providers, and, when they have, it has mostly been for psychiatrists trained in small programmes [13, 16]. As a result, many physicians feel unprepared to treat people with SUDs, most of whom receive care from non-medical professionals without formal substance-related training [13, 17]. Recently, a number of diverse initiatives to address this shortcoming have emerged internationally. For instance, the Addiction Medicine Foundation (AMF) has established fellowships in addiction medicine and accredited 27 of these programmes (63 total slots annually) to date, including four programmes (16 slots) in Canada [18]. This limited number of training opportunities falls far short of the demand for specialised addiction treatment services due to the high number of people with SUDs who need such treatment [1]. Countries like Australia or Netherlands have developed substantial training programmes and Masters in Addiction Medicine, respectively [19]. Other governments (e.g., Norway) have recognised the increasing interest in addiction medicine among doctors and created addiction medicine diplomas or specialties [19, 20]. Focusing on the new generation of doctors, the UK's project on 'Substance Use in the Undergraduate Medical Education' improved the addiction medicine knowledge of medical students [21], while the importance of addiction medicine training for clinicians has also been recently highlighted in Ireland [22]. Unfortunately, although these programmes teach addiction medicine to physicians, their content and intensity varies significantly from country to country.

To overcome the deficits in training locally, two fellowship training programmes have been established in Vancouver, Canada: (1) the interdisciplinary St. Paul's Hospital Goldcorp Addiction Medicine Fellowship, and (2) the Canadian Addiction Medicine Research Fellowship [23]. Of note, Vancouver has Canada's largest drug scene, which has been a significant driver of local HIV and hepatitis C epidemics [24]. As a result, this has led to

an environment in which drug policies and programmes have been launched as pragmatic responses to the local drug use epidemic (requiring comprehensive responses) and their successful evaluation has led some to be adopted or pursued elsewhere [25]. The two fellowships are examples of such pragmatic responses.

First, within this environment operates the St. Paul's Hospital Goldcorp Addiction Medicine Fellowship that provides 12 months of funded training to 12 trainees from Psychiatry, Internal Medicine, Family Medicine, Social Work and Nursing. The physician component is accredited by the AMF and includes specialty training in in-patient and outpatient addiction management, as well as concurrent disorders [26]. There are nine core mandatory blocks of four weeks' duration each, and three elective blocks. The core blocks are: (1) the St. Paul's Hospital Addiction Medicine Consultation Service; (2) inpatient and outpatient chemical dependency detox; (3) outpatient chemical dependency; (4) women's recovery; (5) pain management; (6) management of concurrent disorders; (7) inner city youth mental health programme; (8) longitudinal outpatient continuity of care experience, and (9) research. Fellows' salary is funded through a private donation and the B.C. Ministry of Health. For further description of how the programme is delivered, please refer to previous publication [27].

Second, a new research fellowship for addiction specialists was launched in 2014. The Canada Addiction Medicine Research Fellowship trains physicians to develop the skills required for a career as clinician-scientists in substance use research. This training occurs through: (1) immersion in SUDs research training programme (i.e., British Columbia Centre on Substance use and B.C. node of the Canadian Research Initiative in Substance Misuse); (2) training in diverse research methodologies (e.g., cohort studies, qualitative studies) through didactic lectures, workshops, and monthly journal clubs; (3) mentorship in the development of manuscripts for submission to peer reviewed journals using data from two prospective cohorts of people who use drugs [28–30]. Each year, four part-time, one-year fellowships of $50,000 CDN each are available thanks to funding from the National Institute of Drug Abuse. The content and delivery methods of the fellowship have been described elsewhere [31].

Finally, the Addiction Medicine Consult Team (AMCT) at St. Paul's Hospital supports the fellowship programmes and is a distinct clinical service consisting [26]. AMCT provides inpatient Addiction Medicine consultations to general inpatient and psychiatry wards in the hospital. Patients come often from the Downtown Eastside area of Vancouver, BC, where AMCT's colleagues from the B.C. Centre on Substance Use conduct longitudinal cohort studies of people who inject drugs or who live with HIV/

AIDS. The overlap between research and clinical care informs research agendas and fosters the uptake of novel research findings in practice [26, 32]. In sum, the integration of both research and clinical training in addiction medicine at the under- and post-graduate level, which has been developed within a single academic centre, is unique and has not been described previously. We sought to develop a more complete description of the implementation process to aid educators and administrators in the development of similar programmes elsewhere [33].

We, therefore, conducted a qualitative evaluation of this rare combination of clinical plus research training courses, focusing on barriers and facilitators of implementing physician training in addiction medicine.

Methods

We conducted qualitative interviews to explore implementation of the St. Paul's Hospital Goldcorp Addiction Medicine Fellowship and the Canada Addiction Medicine Research Fellowship, as well as barriers and facilitators to the implementation of these fellowship programmes. We selected the qualitative design specifically because of its capacity to elucidate participants' experiencing during the implementation of these fellowship programmes and thus deepen understandings of contextual influences on their uptake [34, 35].

We sought to recruit individuals who: had competed a clinical fellowship, research fellowship, or enhanced skills training; were staff of the AMCT; and, had completed a 1-month research rotation with the training programme as part of their undergraduate medical training or residency. We also sought to recruit (4) teaching faculty for the fellowship (including nurse, social worker and fellowship director). We sent an email to all potential participants explaining the study and inviting them to participate. Two email reminders followed if they did not respond between March and July 2015. We based our interview guide on a scoping literature review about addiction medicine education and a qualitative study on a similar topic that piloted the questions [36, 37]. The first author conducted and audio-recorded the interviews in the hospital, or in a location convenient for participants; external staff transcribed the recordings. All participants were informed of the study purposes, voluntary and confidential participation, before they signed informed consents.

Data were imported into NVivo (version 10), a qualitative data analysis software programme, to facilitate coding. We analysed the data according to Braun and Clarke's five-step process, including: (1) data preparation, transcription and familiarization; (2) generation of initial codes; (3) theme assessment; (4) theme review; and, (5) theme finalization [38, 39]. Furthermore, our analysis was informed by Damschroder et al.'s [40] Consolidated Framework for Advancing Implementation Science Research (CFIR). This meta-framework attempts to unify all published implementation theories based on the robustness of the evidence behind them. As such, its generic nature allows studying underlying concepts to overcome artificial barriers and to transcend beyond the limitations of individual "labels". The framework has five major domains: intervention characteristics, outer setting, inner setting, characteristics of the individuals involved, and the process of implementation [40]. The first author analysed the data, and two team members reviewed data and provided feedback on the analysis and themes.

Results

Participant demographics

In total, 26 learners from the 2013–15 training cohorts (84% of 31 potential participants) participated in this study, including 14 women and 12 men. All participants were involved in the fellowship programmes as learners (n = 23) or staff (n = 3). Participants included: (a) clinical fellows (*n* = 8); (b) research fellows (*n* = 4); (c) enhanced skills learners (*n* = 2); (d) students and residents who had completed a 1-month rotation and prepared a case report or other publication (*n* = 11); and, (e) staff of the AMCT and teaching faculty for the fellowship (including nurse, social worker and fellowship ex-director; *n* = 4).

We organised the data in relation to Damschroder et al.'s consolidated framework into six major types of barriers and facilitators of the implementation: (1) structural, (2) organisational, (3) mentor, (4) learner, (5) patient and (6) community concerns. As shown in Fig. 1, at the heart of the training implementation was the learner-mentor-patient triad set in the organisational and structural context. We operationalized the outer setting as structural, community and organisational concerns, the inner setting as learner concerns, and the individuals involved were teachers and patients.

Structural concerns

Funding for the training helps "get rid of the fire" but not completely

Although funding for the fellowship programmes was welcomed, it was perceived as a partial solution in efforts to address the underlying conditions affecting people with SUDs. For example, SUDs were characterised by one of the participating physicians as "the smoke from a fire, and the fire is burning really strongly right now, and the fellowship is a way to train fire people, although you need more than just a fire person to put out a fire. [Participant #24]" She further emphasized that the training

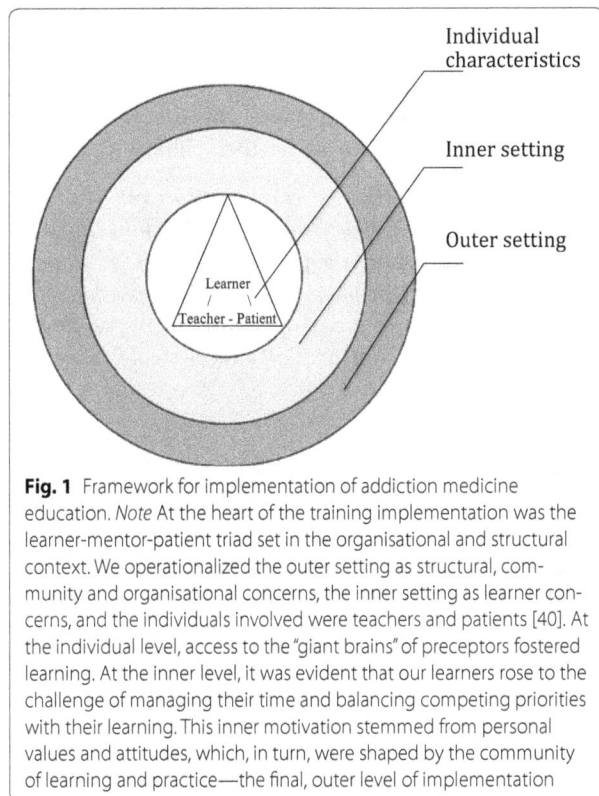

Fig. 1 Framework for implementation of addiction medicine education. *Note* At the heart of the training implementation was the learner-mentor-patient triad set in the organisational and structural context. We operationalized the outer setting as structural, community and organisational concerns, the inner setting as learner concerns, and the individuals involved were teachers and patients [40]. At the individual level, access to the "giant brains" of preceptors fostered learning. At the inner level, it was evident that our learners rose to the challenge of managing their time and balancing competing priorities with their learning. This inner motivation stemmed from personal values and attitudes, which, in turn, were shaped by the community of learning and practice—the final, outer level of implementation

is an important aspect of solving SUDs. However, as she explained, it is not the ultimate answer:

"It's [fellowship] just going to make a dent in getting rid of that fire [SUD], and it's an important aspect of it, and it's great that people are getting opportunities to grow and change and focus on this and learn about all the different nuances of addiction medicine etc., but it's not [the answer]." [Participant #24, clinical fellow]

Most of the patients treated by study participants in the St Paul's Hospital were extremely marginalised people with multiple chronic diseases, were despised by the mainstream society and engaged in shunned income-generation activities that included scavenging and stealing. While quality health care provided by qualified professionals can improve health of people with SUDs, it cannot in and of itself fully address the underlying issues of poverty, displacement, colonisation, homelessness, and unemployment.

Faculty and administrative staff perceived the funded fellowship programmes (full or partial) favourably because it secured protected time to build the educational infrastructure of the Addiction Medicine Fellowship (e.g., clinical sites for rotations, didactic sessions and materials). From the learners' perspective, the funding

allowed them to engage in learning activities and limit clinical duties:

"It was an opportunity where you could be funded part-time to step away, a little bit away, from clinical responsibilities." [Participant #1, research fellow]

The funding also accelerated the fellowship establishment by providing financial stability and allowing the accreditation of the fellowship, giving fellows the opportunity to apply for the license from the AFM, and thus supporting the growth of the SUD specialist workforce. For example:

"Then, funding came in the summer of 2012 which really again boosted us a lot cause we knew it could be a reality, and then we applied for [accreditation]." [Participant #11, faculty]

Implementation of knowledge and practice environment and patient population

The learners recognised that the fellowship "really was geared to teaching the science behind addiction." However, the 'knowledge' learned through the fellowship was not always perceived as transferable to daily practice because of the nature of practice environment and patient population. Therefore, it was necessary to adapt practices to the specifics of the environment and population, as well as broader social-structural determinants of health (e.g., insurance, employment). Some participants saw potential financial constraints as a barrier to treatment provision, especially among low-income populations. As one participant explained:

"I had difficulty because I knew that none of the patients that I would end working with would be able to even afford [these specific medications]." [Participant #10, clinical fellow]

The preceptors applied best-practice guidelines in their decisions intuitively without talking to learners about the evidence, or specific trials, explicitly. The following quote illustrates barriers encountered by the participants when implementing new knowledge and the iterative process of seeking new evidence and applying it in practice:

"I don't [think] it's always verbalized that we're choosing this medication because this is the evidence-based medication, it's just kind of get [it] done and then you sort of have to figure out later whether that was the most correct decision..." [Participant #16, resident]

She continued to describe financial and social barriers to implementing the learning on evidence-based medicine in disadvantaged populations:

"There are limitations, we always say there's no typical patient, especially on the [hospital] addiction service, because there are so many limitations around finances, around social issues that influence people's [...] results, treatment and you can't always do what might be the best possible thing, because it's not safe in that situation, or it's not feasible..." [Participant #16, resident]

She further describes how the patient in question experienced multiple methadone and antiretroviral treatment interruptions and re-initiations due to drug use and social instability. The participant described that the most evidence-based approach in this situation would be to start the patient on an opioid agonist and an antiretroviral treatment, and to keep her on them "forever," but felt that it might not be "doable" or given the underlying social-structural inequities.

Organisational concerns
Organisational and staffing support as the 'backbone' of implementation
Participant accounts underscored how faculty and staff facilitated the implementation of both the clinical and the research training. They included not only mentors and administrators, but also attending physicians, statisticians, senior researchers and other centre staff. Senior researchers met with the learners to formulate their research questions, draft analysis plans and refine the manuscripts. Centre staff helped with other tasks, such as, admission, clinical rotations or organisation of meetings. Statisticians analysed the data for the learners' manuscripts. As one participant spoke about his relationships with the clinical team:

"I've actually established nice long-standing relationships with almost everyone who I worked with on the [hospital] addiction service which is fantastic." [Participant #3, resident]

Participants from both streams—clinical and research—emphasized the utility of the overlap between faculties of both streams that ensured continuity of their learning process. Some learners did the clinical fellowship and then the research fellowship and were then in the programme for two years, maximizing opportunities for learning.

First-year hurdles—infrastructure and resources
Time constraints and limited availability of research or clinical space were the main barriers in the organisational domain. The learners pointed to the newness of the fellowship that was lacking infrastructure in some rotations (e.g., financial, technical and bureaucratic infrastructure). One or two rotation clinics did not have a learning space with a desk for participants. This prevented people from performing tasks learned in their clinical training:

"[The clinical rotation] was quite disorganised and they didn't really have much of a teaching infrastructure developed when I went through, so there was a lot of independent work at that rotation. It was ok but there's areas of improvement for that rotation, for sure." [Participant #26, clinical fellow]

Mentorship concerns
Mentors' responses
There was considerable overlap between mentors for the clinical rotations, research projects and fellowships that fostered development of working relationships between faculty and learners. It allowed participants to continue their professional growth and move between different educational programmes. Some learners suggested that mentors needed to supervise their work more closely, especially for research projects. Therefore, the main issues within this domain were interpersonal. If mentors met with the learners regularly, learners were able to track their progress better:

"I think if there's set blocks maybe even just once a month where you have like a half an hour sit-down with the mentors, which should be mandatory, where you can go over the month, the progress, the struggles, what works, what didn't work - I think that would be helpful." [Participant #26, clinical fellow]

Educators looked up to as 'role models'
Teaching made clinician teachers "better doctors" and their characteristics were paramount in clinical learning through role modelling: "I'm a better doctor because I'm a teacher at the fellowship [Participant #12, faculty]." If the teacher was from the same medical discipline, learners perceived it as being especially helpful. Furthermore, non-physician mentors sometimes induced stress in learners by requesting too many updates. Learners felt better understood by physicians because they "went through the medical school" and saw clinical mentors as role models:

"I think also having him [mentor] who's done internal medicine residency and we had the same training, so from the clinical aspect, I looked up to him." [Participant #10, clinical fellow]

Learner concerns
Tough balance

Learners' concerns included barriers and facilitators of programme implementation from the perspective of trainees. The lack of previous background in research among clinicians was perceived as a barrier to training in addiction medicine research. At times, learners coming from more clinical backgrounds felt frustrated, isolated, and anxious about the future, especially in cases where their previous research training was limited. By extension, physicians on clinical rotations struggled with the prevailing stigma associated with drug use. Although they recognised that their peers did not generally see medically managing SUDs as a "super popular thing to do," they thought that training SUD specialists, and creating jobs for them in health care, could help establish addiction medicine as a respected specialty and counter existing stigma.

For most learners, training in addiction medicine and research was something performed in addition to their already busy schedules, which included seeing patients and running clinics. Providers with high clinical workloads struggled in the clinical and research training activities and some clinical rotations were busier than others. The tension between training and competing priorities is well illustrated in this participant's quote:

"The one thing that I'm struggling a little bit with is that I'm busier this year than I was last year, and the project to me is a bit bigger as well, so this time, I feel like I'm the one slowing the project down cause I'm not always able to get back to the researchers." [Participant #8, student]

Learners prioritise writing papers over "twiddling their thumbs"

Demanding workloads put an increased strain on the participants. However, learners sought to take steps to manage their time effectively and efficiently, such as rotating their tasks or finding some extra time in their schedules. As one learner explained:

"I think always trying to have a challenge on the side so that's why I was so happy to engage in so many different research projects that year because if there was a couple of hours of down time, I made sure that I had something that I could be doing [Writing papers] yeah exactly, or editing, or whatever as opposed to just sort of sitting here twiddling my thumbs or going for coffee." [Participant #10, clinical fellow]

Other facilitators of clinical-research training were mainly related to the personal characteristics of learners,

such as previous background and training in research and motivation to learn from the experience. Those who were capable of self-directed learning benefitted from the training the most because of the experiential nature of learning. For example:

I feel like I'm able to provide better care, and talk to patients, and educate them around their disease, and I'm more comfortable teaching, once I've personally had a bit of experience in it. [...] the more cases I see, and the more teaching I do, the more I like it." [Participant #14, research fellow]

Patient concerns
Becoming 'sensitised' to learning from patients

Our analysis demonstrated that patients "taught" learners lessons regarding addiction medicine, and thus facilitated learning implementation. Physicians learned that trust in the therapeutic relationship was critical to patient engagement and treatment success. Subsequently, patients' engagement increased the potential for success of treatment. The physicians became sensitised to learning from patients:

"So, I really learned more and more, just from my participants and the patients that I see." [Participant #9, nursing fellow]

Having both research and clinical interactions with patients, due to the fluidity between the clinical and science programmes, helped to solidify the new learning:

"It was nice to see that progression where you have an incident and then you can write about it and then let people know that [...] It really helped me to appreciate the research." [Participant #18, student]

However, barriers related mainly to the practice environment and patient population, described above, thwarted this learning. Patients in hospitals had severe SUDs with many concurrent social and mental health problems that rendered them unstable and the complexity of their conditions precipitated numerous challenges related to their care.

Patients' struggles

The learners recognised that the patient population in the hospital was more complex than in other settings due to housing issues, mental health comorbidities and polysubstance use disorder that required specialised treatments. The faculty also recognised this dynamic and highlighted the need to de-centralise housing and diversify treatment modalities. Sometimes, the learning was difficult and confrontational, probably varying as a result of setting—inpatient versus outpatient—and help seeking:

"I was verbally assaulted by patients. I had trays hurled at me and I had people who didn't want to talk about their addictions issues, or receive any sort of care, so that, as the predominant population [in hospital], I found very difficult, whereas an out-patient setting, people are dying to see a doctor for this, and they really wish to get into it, and talk about it, and focus on treatment options." [Participant #25, clinical fellow]

This experience resonated with the perceived need for outpatient clinical rotation that would give the clinical learners different perspectives. Similarly, the research learners felt their "hands were a bit tied" due to the restrictions integral to the nature of the researcher-participant relationship. Within addiction medicine research, the study restrictions could be difficult to navigate for the clinician-researcher because of other co-morbid diseases and social circumstances that make it hard to just focus on study protocol. As one participant observed during the research interview with a patient:

"I have the best interests of the participant [patient with SUD treated by the service] in mind but within the constraints of a study protocol." [Participant #16, resident]

Community concerns
Gains of the community of practice
The wider context of implementing addiction medicine and best practice was the community of practice [41]. It consisted of colleagues within the healthcare system that were not part of the training, preceptors and staff in the clinical rotations, as well as the prevention and harm reduction organisations not involved in the rotations. This community of practice provided support and mentoring to junior learners, as well as linkages between the senior clinicians and staff. The hospital team was perceived as a group of innovators who sought to provide improved or enhanced care to patients:

"...because I've had this contact with them and all so lovely, it's so easy to have access to these giant brains [...] it's about connection and about creating that web of people that you can use as resources." [Participant #19, enhanced skills learner]

Although this community was a source of peer support and mentorship, providing many gains for the fellows (e.g., access to experts and expertise or teamwork), being part of it was not without risks.

Risks of the community of practice
However, some negative attitudes of this closely woven "web of people" could be detrimental to the growth of

an early-career addiction specialist. Some learners were challenged to advocate on behalf of addiction medicine as a discipline because it was seldom considered to be "sexy area of medicine" by colleagues in other disciplines. However, having those conversations forced them to be certain that this was a suitable career path. Other inter-professional challenges within addiction medicine, such as entrenched attitudes and clinical practices, made implementation of new learning difficult:

"I think when people are very set about the way that they should do things. Either because they side with a certain side of the evidence, or if they choose to not follow the evidence, that can make things very difficult because it not only makes the learning difficult, but it also makes discussion and solidification of ideas much more difficult." [Participant #20, clinical fellow]

Discussion
Our qualitative analysis of interviews explored how structural, personal and organisational barriers shape the implementation of provider training in addiction medicine. Money, time and space limitations inhibited implementation. Human resources, variety of rotations, peer support and mentoring facilitated training. In summary, our results yield further support for using the Damschroder et al.'s Consolidated Framework for Advancing Implementation Science Research (CFIR) [40] to operationalise and analyse barriers and facilitators of implementing addiction medicine fellowships.

Our participants recalled several formative experiences when their attitude to working with people who have SUDs has been challenged by community members. Although difficult, our findings suggest that having to defend one's positive regard to working in the SUD field can solidify the resolve of being an SUD specialist [42, 43]. The other CFIR domains of our implementation strategy—intervention characteristics and process of implementation—have been described elsewhere [23, 26].

Several narrative reviews have focused on undergraduate and postgraduate education regarding SUDs [22, 44–46], noting how it is hindered by inflexibility of training programmes and a lack of hands-on training [47–50]. Mentoring in balancing the competing needs of clinical and research careers is inadequate and career guidance is minimal to non-existent [51, 52]. Such an unsupportive training environment can allow physicians to be distracted by other competing interests [49, 53, 54]. Additionally, there seems to be few mechanisms for addiction physicians to pursue formal training in research as clinician-scientists. Programmes, such as the one described in this article, have the potential to overcome these barriers, in addition to integrating addiction medicine into graduate medical education [55]. In particular, the integration should address the two identified major barriers to practicing addiction medicine: (1) insufficient knowledge, training and experience working with patients with SUDs; and, (2) a lack of specialist support [56].

Our results are consistent with previous literature that has endorsed a combined didactic and interactive learning strategy for SUD education [45, 57–59]. Physicians in our study suggested several improvements to the outer level of implementation, especially the structure and organisation of the addiction medicine education. Some suggestions for improvement appeared to reflect the "newness" of the fellowship and that some rotations were having learners present for the first time. This can be overcome by continued funding for the programme and refinement of activities, and subsequent expansion of the SUD-specialist workforce coming out of the fellowship. Indeed, funding current programmes is not enough; new programmes should be established and other comprehensive responses, such as increased profile of SUD and of those who treat it, are needed to meet the needs of people with SUDs. Promoting SUD education among generalist physicians can heighten the chances of screening, early diagnosis and treatment [60]. Although training alone will not solve the SUD problem, it is a *conditio sine qua non* for successful treatment.

There are several limitations to this study. The small sample comprising clinical fellows, residents, students and staff from a single Canadian programme limits potential generalizability. Our participants were not selected randomly, although we invited everybody who was involved in the training and obtained an excellent response rate. We met the threshold of data saturation as recommended for non-probabilistic sample sizes [61]. It is likely that physicians, who seek specialised training, are more likely to have positive attitudes towards, and more clinical experience with, people who have SUD [62]. Nevertheless, the key strength of our study is examination of the unique combination of physician training in addiction medicine and research that provided a rare opportunity to explore the implementation of clinical and academic training in this field. Future studies should truly differentiate the barriers to each type of fellowship program. Though such programs often have common goals, it will be beneficial to more fully understand the challenges experienced by individual programs to further optimize their implementation and impact on learning.

Conclusion

Training in addiction medicine is feasible and acceptable for healthcare providers. Learners experience the training favourably. Its implementation faces barriers

like any other innovation. We must understand the barriers and facilitators specific to these types of programmes if we want to develop stronger local implementation strategies and quality standards. These findings can inspire set up, scale up and standardisation of addiction medicine programmes in other countries.

Authors' contributions
JK contributed substantially to the conception and design of the work and analysed the data for the work. RM contributed substantially to the analysis of data for the work. WS, KA, AM, LR, EW and WC contributed substantially to the conception and design and interpretation of the data of the work. All authors read and approved the final manuscript.

Author details
[1] Department of Medicine, B.C. Centre on Substance Use, St. Paul's Hospital, University of British Columbia, 608-1081 Burrard Street, Vancouver, BC V6Z 1Y6, Canada. [2] Department of Family Practice, University of British Columbia, 1081 Burrard St., Vancouver, BC V6Z 1Y6, Canada. [3] Department of Family and Community Medicine, St. Paul's Hospital, 1081 Burrard St., Vancouver, BC V6Z 1Y6, Canada. [4] School of Medicine, Coombe Healthcare Centre, University College Dublin, Dolphins Barn, Dublin 8, Ireland. [5] Faculty of Health Sciences, Simon Fraser University, Blusson Hall, 8888 University Drive, Burnaby, BC V5A 1S6, Canada.

Acknowledgements
We thank the study participants for their contribution to the research, as well as current and past researchers and staff.

Competing interests
The authors declare that they have no competing interests.

Funding
The Canadian Institutes of Health Research (MOP–81171) and the US National Institutes of Health (R01DA033147) supported the study. This research was also undertaken, in part, by funding from the Canada Research Chairs program through a Tier 1 Canada Research Chair in Inner City Medicine, and by the US National Institutes of Health (R25DA037756) that supports Dr. Evan Wood. The ELEVATE grant: Irish Research Council International Career Development Fellowship—co-funded by Marie Cure Actions (ELEVATEPD/2014/6); and a European Commission (701698) grants—supported Dr. Jan Klimas. The European Commission (HepCare) grant supports Dr. Walter Cullen. Drs Ryan McNeil and Will Small are supported by the Michael Smith Foundation for Health Research. Ryan McNeil is also supported by the Canadian Institutes of Health Research. The funders had no role in the design and conduct of the study; the collection, analysis, and interpretation of the data; the preparation of the manuscript; or the decision to submit the manuscript for publication.

References
1.	Degenhardt L, Hall W. Extent of illicit drug use and dependence, and their contribution to the global burden of disease. Lancet. 2012;379:55–70.
2.	European Drug Report (2014). http://www.emcdda.europa.eu/edr2014.
3.	US Burden of Disease Collaborators. The state of US health, 1990–2010: burden of diseases, injuries, and risk factors. JAMA. 2013;310:591–608.
4.	Kaner E, Bland M, Cassidy P, Coulton S, Deluca P, Drummond C, Gilvarry E, Godfrey C, Heather N, Myles J, et al. Screening and brief interventions for hazardous and harmful alcohol use in primary care: a cluster randomised controlled trial protocol. BMC Public Health. 2009;9:287.
5.	Mattick RP, Breen C, Kimber J, Davoli M. Buprenorphine maintenance versus placebo or methadone maintenance for opioid dependence. Cochrane Database Syst Rev. 2014;2:CD002207.
6.	Bowman S, Eiserman J, Beletsky L, Stancliff S, Bruce RD. Reducing the health consequences of opioid addiction in primary care. Am J Med. 2013;126:565–71.
7.	Fiellin DA, O'Connor PG, Chawarski M, Pakes JP, Pantalon MV, Schottenfeld RS. Methadone maintenance in primary care: a randomized controlled trial. JAMA. 2001;286:1724–31.

8. Kaner EFS, Brown N, Jackson K. A systematic review of the impact of brief interventions on substance use and co-morbid physical and mental health conditions. Mental Health Subst Use. 2011;4:38–61.

9. Kaner E, Bland M, Cassidy P, Coulton S, Dale V, Deluca P, Gilvarry E, Godfrey C, Heather N, Myles J, et al. Effectiveness of screening and brief alcohol intervention in primary care (SIPS trial): pragmatic cluster randomised controlled trial. Br Med J. 2013;346:e8501.

10. Cullen W, Stanley J, Langton D, Kelly Y, Staines A, Bury G. Hepatitis C infection among injecting drug users in general practice: a cluster randomised controlled trial of clinical guidelines' implementation. Br J Gen Pract. 2006;56:848–56.

11. Ries RK, Miller SC, Fiellin DA. Principles of addiction medicine. Philadelphia: Lippincott Williams & Wilkins; 2009.

12. Mullen L, Barry J, Long J, Keenan E, Mulholland D, Grogan L, Delargy I. A national study of the retention of irish opiate users in methadone substitution treatment. Am J Drug Alcohol Abuse. 2012;38:551–8.

13. Miller NS, Sheppard LM, Colenda CC, Magen J. Why physicians are unprepared to treat patients who have alcohol- and drug-related disorders. Acad Med. 2001;76:410–8.

14. National Center on Addiction and Substance Abuse at Columbia University. Missed opportunity: CASA national survey of primary care physicians and patients on substance abuse. Columbia: National Center on Addiction and Substance Abuse at Columbia University; 2000.

15. The National Centre on Addiction and Substance Abuse at Columbia University: Addiction medicine: closing the gap between science and practice. New York: CASA; 2012. https://www.centeronaddiction.org/addiction-research/reports/addiction-medicine-closing-gap-between-science-and-practice

16. Tontchev GV, Housel TR, Callahan JF, Kunz KB, Miller MM, Blondell RD. Specialized training on addictions for physicians in the United States. Subst Abuse. 2011;32:84–92.

17. Columbia C. Addiction medicine: closing the gap between science and practice. New York: The National Center on Addiction and Substance Abuse (CASA) at Columbia University; 2012. p. 1–573.

18. Wood E, Samet JH, Volkow ND. Physician education in addiction medicine. JAMA. 2013;310:1673–4.

19. Haber PS. International Perspectives in postgraduate medical training in addiction medicine. Subst Abuse. 2011;32:75–6.

20. el-Guebaly N, Violato C. The international certification of addiction medicine: validating clinical knowledge across borders. Subst Abuse. 2011;32:77–83.

21. Carroll J, Goodair C, Chayor A, Notley C, Ghodse H, Kopelman P. Substance misuse teaching in undergraduate medical education. BMC Med Educ. 2014;14:34.

22. O'Brien S, Cullen W. Undergraduate medical education in substance use in Ireland: a review of the literature and discussion paper. Ir J Med Sci. 2011;180:787–92.

23. Wood E, Sakakibara T, McIver G, McLean M. A UBC, Vancouver Coastal Health and St. Paul s hospital strategy for education in addiction medicine. UBC Med J. 2013;5:5–7.

24. Small W, Rhodes T, Wood E, Kerr T. Public injection settings in Vancouver: physical environment, social context and risk. Int J Drug Policy. 2007;18:27–36.

25. McCann E, Temenos C. Mobilizing drug consumption rooms: inter-place networks and harm reduction drug policy. Health Place. 2015;31:216–23.

26. Rieb L, Wood E. The evolution of addiction medicine education in British Columbia. Can J Addict. 2014;5:17–20.

27. Klimas J, McNeil R, Ahamad K, Mead A, Rieb L, Cullen W, Wood E, Small W. Two birds with one stone: experiences of combining clinical and research training in addiction medicine. BMC Med Educ. 2017;17:22.

28. Strathdee SA, Palepu A, Cornelisse PG, Yip B, O'Shaughnessy MV, Montaner JS, Schechter MT, Hogg RS. Barriers to use of free antiretroviral therapy in injection drug users. JAMA. 1998;280:547–9.

29. Wood E, Hogg RS, Bonner S, Kerr T, Li K, Palepu A, Guillemi S, Schechter MT, Montaner JS. Staging for antiretroviral therapy among HIV-infected drug users. JAMA. 2004;292:1175–7.

30. Kerr T, Small W, Johnston C, Li K, Montaner JS, Wood E. Characteristics of injection drug users who participate in drug dealing: implications for drug policy. J Psychoact Drugs. 2008;40:147–52.

31. Klimas J, Fernandes E, deBeck K, Hayashi K, Milloy M-J, Kerr T, Cullen W, Wood E. Preliminary results and publication impact of a dedicated addiction clinician scientist research fellowship. J Addict Med. 2017;11:80–1.

32. Klimas J, Ahamad K, Fairgrieve K, McLean M, Mead A, Nolan S, Wood E. Impact of a brief addiction medicine training experience on knowledge self-assessment among medical learners. Subst Abuse. 2017;38:141–4.

33. Tavakol M, Sandars J. Quantitative and qualitative methods in medical education research: AMEE Guide No 90: Part II. Med Teach. 2014;36:838–48.

34. Morse JM. What is qualitative health research. Chapter 24. In: Denzin NK, Lincoln YS, editors. The SAGE handbook of qualitative research. 2011. p. 401–14.

35. Neale J, Hunt G, Lankenau S, Mayock P, Miller P, Sheridan J, Small W, Treloar C. Addiction journal is committed to publishing qualitative research. Addiction. 2013;108:447–9.

36. Klimas J. Training in addiction medicine should be standardised and scaled up. BMJ. 2015;351:h4027.

37. Klimas J, Muench J, Wiest K, Croff R, Rieckman T, McCarty D. Alcohol screening among opioid agonist patients in a primary care clinic and an opioid treatment program. J Psychoact Drugs. 2015;47:65–70.

38. Braun V, Clarke V. Using thematic analysis in psychology. Qual Res Psychol. 2006;3:77–101.

39. Elliott R, Timulák L. Descriptive and interpretative approaches to qualitative research. In: Miles J, Gilbert P, editors. A handbook of research methods in clinical and health psychology. Oxford: Oxford University Press; 2005.

40. Damschroder LJ, Aron DC, Keith RE, Kirsh SR, Alexander JA, Lowery JC. Fostering implementation of health services research findings into practice: a consolidated framework for advancing implementation science. Implement Sci. 2009;4:50.

41. Li L, Grimshaw J, Nielsen C, Judd M, Coyte P, Graham I. Evolution of Wenger's concept of community of practice. Implement Sci. 2009;4:11.

42. Geller G, Levine DM, Mamon JA, Moore RD, Bone LR, Stokes EJ. knowledge, attitudes, and reported practices of medical students and house staff regarding the diagnosis and treatment of alcoholism. JAMA. 1989;261:3115–20.

43. Roche AM. Drug and alcohol medical education: evaluation of a national programme. Br J Addict. 1992;87:1041–8.

44. Ewan CE, Whaite A. Training health professionals in substance abuse: a review. Int J Addict. 1982;17:1211–29.

45. El-Guebaly N, Toews J, Lockyer J, Armstrong S, Hodgins D. Medical education in substance-related disorders: components and outcome. Addiction. 2000;95:949–57.

46. Rasyidi E, Wilkins JN, Danovitch I. Training the next generation of providers in addiction medicine. Psychiatr Clin North Am. 2012;35:461–80.

47. Kashiwagi DT, Varkey P, Cook DA. Mentoring programs for physicians in academic medicine: a systematic review. Acad Med. 2013;88:1029–37.

48. Kusurkar RA, Croiset G. Autonomy support for autonomous motivation in medical education. Med Educ Online. 2015;20:27951.

49. Tooke J, Wass J. Nurturing tomorrow's clinician scientists. Lancet. 2013;381(Suppl 1):S1–2.

50. The Standards of Reporting Trials Group. A proposal for structured reporting of randomized controlled trials. JAMA. 1994;272:1926–31.

51. Rosier RN. Institutional barriers to the orthopaedic clinician-scientist. Clin Orthop Relat Res. 2006;449:159–64.

52. Berk M, Hallam K, Lucas N, Hasty M, McNeil CA, Conus P, Kader L, McGorry PD. Early intervention in bipolar disorders: opportunities and pitfalls. Med J Aust. 2007;187:S11–4.

53. Lander B, Hanley GE, Atkinson-Grosjean J: Clinician-scientists in Canada: barriers to career entry and progress. PLoS One. 2010;5(10):e13168. doi:10.1371/journal.pone.0013168.

54. Hauser SL, McArthur JC. Saving the clinician-scientist: report of the ANA long range planning committee. Ann Neurol. 2006;60:278–85.

55. O'Connor PG, Nyquist JG, McLellan AT. Integrating addiction medicine into graduate medical education in primary care: the time has come. Ann Intern Med. 2011;154:56–9.

56. Childers JW, Broyles LM, Hanusa BH, Kraemer KL, Conigliaro J, Spagnoletti C, McNeil M, Gordon AJ. Teaching the teachers: faculty preparedness and evaluation of a retreat in screening, brief intervention, and referral to treatment. Subst Abuse. 2012;33:272–7.

57. Polydorou S, Gunderson EW, Levin FR. Training physicians to treat substance use disorders. Curr Psychiatry Rep. 2008;10:399–404.

58. Christison GW, Haviland MG. Requiring a one-week addiction treatment experience in a six-week psychiatry clerkship: effects on attitudes toward substance-abusing patients. Teach Learn Med. 2003;15:93–7.

59. Edwards K. "Short stops": peer support of scholarly activity. Acad Med. 2002;77:939.

60. Alford D, Bridden C, Jackson A, Saitz R, Amodeo M, Barnes H, Samet J. Promoting substance use education among generalist physicians: an evaluation of the chief resident immersion training (CRIT) program. J Gen Intern Med. 2009;24:40–7.

61. Guest G, Bunce A, Johnson L. How many interviews are enough? an experiment with data saturation and variability. Field Methods. 2006;18:59–82.

62. Strang J, Hunt C, Gerada C, Marsden J. What difference does training make? A randomized trial with waiting-list control of general practitioners seeking advanced training in drug misuse. Addiction. 2007;102:1637–47.

21

Associations of criminal justice and substance use treatment involvement with HIV/HCV testing and the HIV treatment cascade among people who use drugs in Oakland, California

Barrot H. Lambdin[1,2,3]*, Alex H. Kral[1], Megan Comfort[1,2], Andrea M. Lopez[1] and Jennifer Lorvick[1]

Abstract

Background: People who smoke crack cocaine and people who inject drugs are at-risk for criminal justice involvement as well as HIV and HCV infection. Compared to criminal justice involvement, substance use treatment (SUT) can be cost-effective in reducing drug use and its associated health and social costs. We conducted a cross-sectional study of people who smoke crack cocaine and people who inject drugs to examine the association between incarceration, community supervision and substance use treatment with HIV/HCV testing, components of the HIV treatment cascade, social and physical vulnerability and risk behavior.

Methods: Targeted sampling methods were used to recruit people who smoke crack cocaine and people who inject drugs (N = 2072) in Oakland, California from 2011 to 2013. Poisson regression models were used to estimate adjusted prevalence ratios between study exposures and outcomes.

Results: The overall HIV prevalence was 3.3% (95% CI 2.6–4.1). People previously experiencing incarceration were 21% (p < 0.001) and 32% (p = 0.001), respectively, more likely to report HIV and HCV testing; and were not more likely to report receiving HIV care or initiating ART. People previously experiencing community supervision were 17% (p = 0.001) and 15% (p = 0.009), respectively, more likely to report HIV and HCV testing; and were not more likely to report receiving HIV care or initiating ART. People with a history of SUT were 15% (p < 0.001) and 23% (p < 0.001), respectively, more likely to report receiving HIV and HCV testing, 67% (p = 0.016) more likely to report HIV care, and 92% (p = 0.012) more likely to report HIV treatment initiation. People previously experiencing incarceration or community supervision were also more likely to report homelessness, trouble meeting basic needs and risk behavior.

Conclusions: People with a history of substance use treatment reported higher levels of HCV and HIV testing and greater access to HIV care and treatment among HIV-positive individuals. People with a history of incarceration or community supervision reported higher levels of HCV and HIV testing, but not greater access to HIV care or treatment among HIV-positive individuals., Substance use treatment programs that are integrated with other services for HIV and HCV will be critical to simultaneously address the underlying reasons drug-involved people engage in drug-related offenses and improve access to essential medical services.

Keywords: Criminal justice, Substance use treatment, HIV, Hepatitis C, People who use drugs, Implementation science

*Correspondence: blambdin@rti.org
[1] RTI International, 351 California St, Suite 500, San Francisco, CA 94104, USA
Full list of author information is available at the end of the article

Background

Since the 1980s, the "War on Drugs" has contributed to drastic increases in incarceration in the United States, including a threefold increase in drug-related arrests and an eightfold increase in the prison population [1–3]. Consequently, the US has the highest documented incarceration rate in the world at 716 inmates per 100,000 residents [4], and an astonishing 4,751,400 people on probation or parole [5]. Because law enforcement policies target people who use drugs, 64.5% of people who are incarcerated experience a substance use disorder; however, only 11% receive any type of substance use treatment while incarcerated [6].

People who smoke crack cocaine (PWSC) and people who inject drugs (PWID) are not only at high risk for incarceration, but they are also at high risk for HIV and hepatitis C virus (HCV) infection. Thus, the estimated HIV prevalence is nearly three times higher among incarcerated populations than the general population (1.5 vs. 0.6%) and HCV prevalence is 9–27 times higher (12–35% compared to 1.3%) [7–9].

Access to care and adherence to treatment are key to reducing morbidity and mortality from HIV and HCV. For HIV, antiretroviral therapy (ART) is associated with improved clinical outcomes, longer survival and secondary prevention of infection, including reduced HIV transmission risk at the community level [10–12]. For HCV, the advent of direct acting antiretroviral (DAA) medications, with a relatively short course of treatment and minimal side effects, has led to cure rates of 90%, and the possibility of virtually eliminating HCV transmission. Benefitting from these therapies, however, requires participation in a series of sequential steps, often referred to as the HIV or HCV treatment cascade [13, 14]. These include diagnosis of HIV/HCV, linkage to care, clinical evaluation, treatment initiation, retention in care, and treatment adherence, with the ultimate goal of making viral load undetectable [13–15].

The lives of people using illicit drugs can be chaotic due to stigma, severe poverty, probation/parole requirements, comorbidities, serious mental illness, and the psychological and clinical effects of the substances they ingest, making it difficult to access and adhere to treatment for HIV or HCV in community settings. Incarceration can provide a point of access for HIV/HCV services [16–20], but this does not always translate to successful navigation of the care continuum [21–25]. Community supervision can provide another opportunity to facilitate access to HIV/HCV services, but this opportunity is often not realized [26, 27].

Research has suggested that substance use treatment (SUT) can effectively address the underlying reasons why many people who use drugs become engaged in drug-related offenses [28]. Further evidence suggests that SUT is cost-effective in reducing drug use and its associated health and social costs, as compared to incarceration [29]. SUT has been shown to help people lower their risk of HIV acquisition and transmission, improve their access and adherence to HIV treatment and reduce their viral load [30–33].

In this cross-sectional study of PWSC and PWID, we examine the association of a history of incarceration, community supervision and substance use treatment with access to HIV/HCV testing, components of the HIV treatment cascade, social and physical vulnerability and risk behavior. We additionally assess for predictors of HIV and HCV status.

Methods

Study setting

Our study includes a community-based sample of PWSC and PWID in Oakland, California. Oakland is a racially diverse, mid-sized city in Alameda County with a population of 400,000 people. Alameda County was the first county in the United States to declare a state of emergency in 1998 due to a disproportionally high HIV prevalence among the African American population, an emergency that continues to this day [34]. In 2013, the HIV prevalence was 113 per 100,000 people with 80 new diagnoses per 100,000 among African American men [35, 36]. In addition, the adult incarceration prevalence in Alameda County was 1471 per 100,000 men (nearly double the national average) and 86 per 100,000 women in 2010, and the prevalence of community supervision (probation or parole) was 1580 per 100,000 people, with most people clustered in 6 contiguous zip codes of Oakland [37, 38]. Residents in these areas also carry a disproportionate burden of poor health, low income and unstable housing [39].

Study population

Using targeted sampling methods [40, 41], an outreach worker recruited participants from July 2011 to July 2013 in street settings within the cluster of zip codes having high community supervision levels [42], and collected data at three easily accessible field sites. From July 2011 to July 2013, an outreach worker recruited a total of 2323 participants in neighborhoods surrounding the three field sites. Inclusion criteria for the study included crack cocaine or injection drug use in the 6 months prior to interview and age ≥18. Drug use was verified by use of a screening instrument that obscured eligibility requirements. Approximately 10% of recruited participants did not meet eligibility criteria, leading to 2072 participants for this study.

Participants engaged in an informed consent process, a quantitative interview and HIV testing, as well as pre- and post-test counseling. The quantitative interview was conducted face-to-face, with interviewers posing items verbally and recording responses in a computer-based personal interviewing system (Blaise®, Westat). Rapid testing for HIV infection was conducted using the OraQuick ADVANCE® rapid HIV antibody test. Reactive results on the OraQuick test were confirmed with a second point-of-care test, the Clearview STAT-PAK®. Interview staff were trained in HIV testing and counseling as well as data collection techniques. Participants who were HIV antibody positive were eligible for a separate intervention study, complete with a new informed consent process [43].

All study procedures were reviewed and approved by a federally accredited Institutional Review Board at RTI International. Participants received $20 remuneration for their contribution to the research, as well as referrals to medical and social services as appropriate.

Measures

Outcome variables included measures for HIV/HCV testing, the HIV treatment cascade, social and physical vulnerability, risky injection or sexual behavior, and HIV/HCV status. HCV testing was defined as having ever had an HCV antibody test. Variables for steps of HIV treatment cascade included HIV testing, defined as receiving an HIV antibody testing ever; received HIV care, defined as ever receiving HIV care among those who are HIV positive; and initiated ART, defined as ever starting ART among those who are HIV positive. HIV status was determined through rapid testing (see above) and HCV status was self-reported. Indicators for social and physical vulnerability included homelessness, defined as currently homeless; trouble meeting basic needs (derived from research by Gelbert et al. [44]), defined as trouble finding a place to sleep, wash, use the bathroom or trouble having enough clothes or food to eat in the past 6 months; and income, categorized as income of <$900 or ≥$900 in the past month. Derived from the National Institute on Drug Abuse's validated Risk Behavior Assessment [45], risky injection or sexual behavior was defined as receptive syringe sharing or unprotected sex with more than 1 partner in the past 6 months.

Our primary exposure variable for criminal justice involvement included two variables: (a) incarceration, defined as spending time in city jail, county jail or federal prison since the age of 18, and (b) community supervision, defined as having ever been on probation or parole. The primary exposure variable for substance use treatment involvement was defined as having ever received methadone detoxification, methadone maintenance, buprenorphine or suboxone, residential treatment (containing counseling, group therapy or cognitive behavioral

therapy) or other outpatient treatment (containing counseling, group therapy or cognitive behavioral therapy).

Derived from the Urban Health Study questionnaire [46–49]—a community-based study with people who use drugs in Oakland for 15 years—other covariates of interest as potential confounders included current age; sexual risk group: categorized as men who have sex with women, men who have sex with men or men and women, women non-sex workers, women sex workers and transgender people; race/ethnicity: defined as African American, Caucasian, Latino/a, or Mixed Race/Other; high school education: defined as having received a high school diploma or GED; steady partnership: current relationship with a steady partner; having children and a history of injection drug use. The measures for social and physical vulnerability, criminal justice involvement, substance use treatment involvement were included as explanatory variables in assessing associations with HCV and HIV status.

Statistical analysis

Descriptive statistics, including frequencies, median and interquartile range, were calculated to describe the distribution of variables in the study population. We calculated the prevalence and accompanying 95% confidence intervals for HIV and HCV status. Poisson regression models with robust variances were built to estimate adjusted prevalence ratios [42]. Our primary analysis of interest included assessing the impact of criminal justice and substance use treatment involvement with metrics for HCV testing and the steps of the HIV treatment cascade, risky behavior and social and physical vulnerability. Socio-demographic covariates considered for the multivariable model were determined based on their theoretical ability to confound the relationship of our exposures and outcomes. Backward stepwise regression with a criterion p value of 0.2 identified potential covariates for inclusion in the final multivariable model. Additionally, we examined the associations of socio-demographic, criminal justice and substance use treatment involvement and vulnerability with HIV and HCV status. Variables having a p value <0.2 with HIV or HCV status in bivariate analyses were considered for inclusion in the multivariable models, using backward stepwise regression with a criterion p value of 0.2. Statistical significance was set at p = 0.05. All statistical analyses were conducted in Stata v14 [50].

Results
Study population

A total of 2072 people who smoked crack cocaine or injected drugs were included in this analysis. Table 1 outlines characteristics of our study population. The median age of respondents was 49 years [interquartile range

Table 1 Characteristics of people who inject drugs or smoke crack cocaine, 2011–2013 (N = 2072)

	HIV-negative (n = 2004)	HIV-positive (n = 68)	Total (n = 2072)
Age			
18–29	139 (7)	0 (0)	139 (7)
30–39	274 (14)	7 (10)	281 (13)
40–49	644 (32)	28 (41)	672 (32)
50–59	726 (36)	27 (40)	753 (36)
≥60	222 (11)	6 (9)	228 (11)
Male	1177 (59)	39 (57)	1216 (59)
Men who have sex with men	46 (2)	16 (23)	62 (3)
Men who have sex with women	1129 (56)	23 (34)	1152 (56)
Female	827 (41)	25 (37)	852 (41)
Non-sex worker	485 (24)	21 (31)	506 (24)
Sex worker	342 (17)	4 (6)	346 (17)
Transgender	1 (<1)	4 (6)	5 (<1)
Racial/ethnic group			
African American	1721 (86)	63 (93)	1784 (86)
Caucasian	100 (5)	3 (4)	103 (5)
Latino	76 (4)	0 (0)	76 (4)
Black Latino	10 (<1)	0 (0)	10 (<1)
Asian/Pacific Islander	8 (<1)	0 (0)	8 (<1)
Native American	13 (<1)	0 (0)	13 (<1)
Mixed	47 (2)	2 (3)	49 (2)
Other	30 (1)	0 (0)	30 (1)
High school education	1260 (63)	43 (63)	1303 (63)
Steady partnership	967 (48)	36 (53)	1003 (48)
Have children	1597 (80)	50 (73)	1647 (79)
Drug use history			
Injected drugs (only)	42 (2)	1 (<1)	43 (2)
Injected opioids (only)	31 (1)	0 (0)	31 (1)
Injected stimulants (only)	4 (<1)	1 (<1)	5 (<1)
Injected opioids and stimulants	7 (<1)	0 (0)	7 (<1)
Smoked crack/cocaine (only)	1476 (74)	50 (73)	1526 (74)
Injected drugs and smoked crack/cocaine	486 (24)	17 (<1)	510 (25)
Injected opioids and smoked crack/cocaine	245 (12)	5 (<1)	254 (12)
Injected stimulants and smoked crack/cocaine	26 (1)	6 (<1)	33 (2)
Injected opioids and stimulants and smoked crack/cocaine	215 (11)	6 (<1)	223 (11)
Homeless	1011 (50)	36 (53)	1047 (50)
Trouble meeting needs	1420 (71)	55 (81)	1475 (71)
Income <$900	1513 (76)	55 (82)	1568 (76)
Risky injection or sexual behavior	785 (40)	19 (28)	804 (39)
Incarcerated	1844 (92)	62 (91)	1906 (92)
Community supervision	1613 (86)	57 (89)	1670 (86)
Substance use treatment	1330 (67)	46 (68)	1376 (66)

(IQR) 41–55], and nearly 60% were male. Regarding our exposures of interest, 92, 86 and 66% had been incarcerated since the age of 18, ever been in community supervision and ever involved in substance use treatment, respectively.

In terms of engagement in HIV care, 85% had ever been tested for HIV prior to study participation, and the HIV prevalence was 3.3% (95% confidence interval (CI) 2.6–4.1). Among people living with HIV (n = 68), 71% reported having ever received HIV care, and 64%

reported having ever initiated antiretroviral therapy (ART) (Fig. 1). With regards to HCV testing, 65% had ever been tested for HCV, and the self-reported HCV prevalence was 31% (95% CI 29–34%).

Criminal justice involvement

Criminal justice involvement was statistically associated with several HIV/HCV service access, vulnerability and risk behavior variables. Of note, people who reported a history of incarceration since the age of 18 were more likely to report testing for HIV ever (adjusted prevalence ratio (aPR) = 1.21; 95% CI 1.10–1.34; p < 0.001) and testing for HCV ever (aPR = 1.32; 95% CI 1.12–1.56; p = 0.001). Among people living with HIV, no statistically significant associations were observed between reported history of incarceration and receipt of HIV care

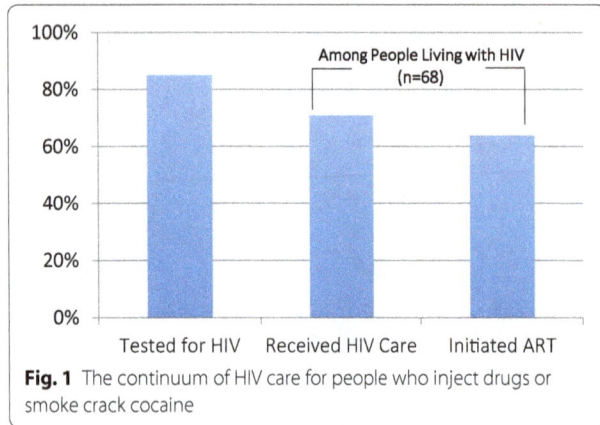

Fig. 1 The continuum of HIV care for people who inject drugs or smoke crack cocaine

or initiation of ART (Table 2). In addition, people who reported a history of incarceration were significantly more likely to report homelessness (1.22; 95% CI 1.00–1.48; p = 0.049), having trouble meeting basic needs (aPR = 1.14; 95% CI 1.01–1.28; p = 0.031) and risky injection or sexual behavior (aPR = 1.31; 95% CI 1.04–1.66; p = 0.024) (Table 3).

Like people who have a history of incarceration, people who reported a history of community supervision were more likely to report testing for HIV ever (aPR = 1.17; 95% CI 1.09–1.25; p = 0.001) and testing for HCV ever (aPR = 1.15; 95% CI 1.04–1.29; p = 0.009). No statistically significant associations were observed between reported history of community supervision and receipt of HIV care or initiation of ART (Table 2). In addition, people who reported a history of community supervision were significantly more likely to report homelessness (aPR = 1.33; 95% CI 1.14–1.55; p < 0.001), having trouble meeting basic needs (aPR = 1.12; 95% CI 1.02–1.23; p = 0.014) and risky injection or sexual behavior (aPR = 1.18; 95% CI 1.00–1.40; p = 0.048) (Table 3).

Substance use treatment

With regards to SUT, people who reported a history of substance use treatment were more likely to report receiving HIV testing ever (aPR = 1.15; 95% CI 1.10–1.20; p < 0.001) and HCV testing ever (aPR = 1.23; 95% CI 1.14–1.33; p < 0.001). Among people living with HIV, those who reported a history of SUT were more likely to report receiving HIV care (aPR = 1.67; 95% CI 1.10–1.25; p = 0.016) and initiating HIV treatment (aPR = 1.92; 95%

Table 2 Associations of criminal justice involvement and substance use treatment on HCV testing and steps of engagement in HIV care

	HCV testing		HIV testing		HIV care		Initiated ART	
	aPR (95% CI)	p value	aPR (95% CI)	p value	aPR (95% CI)	p value	aPR (95% CI)	p value
Incarceration	1.32 (1.12–1.56)	p = 0.001	1.21 (1.10–1.34)	p < 0.001	0.82 (0.52–1.29)	p = 0.394	0.79 (0.48–1.28)	p = 0.336
Community supervision	1.15 (1.04–1.29)	p = 0.009	1.17 (1.09–1.25)	p = 0.001	1.35 (0.59–3.07)	p = 0.470	2.04 (0.64–6.49)	p = 0.227
Substance use treatment	1.23 (1.14–1.33)	p < 0.001	1.15 (1.10–1.20)	p < 0.001	1.67 (1.10–2.55)	p = 0.016	1.92 (1.15–3.21)	p = 0.012

Age, gender, race, education, steady partnership, having children and injection drug use history assessed as potential confounders in all analyses

Table 3 Associations of criminal justice involvement and substance use treatment on vulnerability and risk behavior

	Homelessness		Trouble meeting needs		Income ≥ $900		Risky injection or sexual behavior	
	aPR (95% CI)	p value	aPR (95% CI)	p value	aPR (95% CI)	p value	aPR (95% CI)	p value
Incarceration	1.22 (1.00–1.48)	0.049	1.14 (1.01–1.28)	0.031	1.14 (0.84–1.55)	0.391	1.31 (1.04–1.66)	0.024
Community supervision	1.33 (1.14–1.55)	<0.001	1.12 (1.02–1.23)	0.014	1.22 (0.96–1.56)	0.104	1.18 (1.00–1.40)	0.048
Substance use treatment	1.05 (0.96–1.15)	0.245	1.00 (0.94–1.06)	0.952	1.19 (1.00–1.41)	0.045	1.10 (0.98–1.23)	0.119

Age, gender, race, education, steady partnership, having children and injection drug use history assessed as potential confounders in all analyses

CI 1.15–3.21; p = 0.012), as compared to people who had no history of SUT (Table 2). People who reported a history of SUT were more likely to report a current income ≥$900 (aPR = 1.19; 95% CI 1.00–1.41; p = 0.045); however, no statistically significant associations were observed between reported history of SUT and homelessness, trouble meeting needs or risky behavior (Table 3).

Predictors of HIV and HCV status

In multivariable analysis of HIV seropositive status, men who reported having sex with men (aPR = 12.49; 95% CI 6.95–22.44; p < 0.001) and people who reported being transgender (aPR = 38.32; 95% CI 20.10–73.03; p < 0.001) had a higher likelihood of being HIV-positive. With regards to HCV, people who reported being older in age (aPR = 1.47 per 10 years; 95% CI 1.35–1.59; p < 0.001), men who have sex with men (aPR = 1.74; 95% CI 1.32–2.31; p < 0.001), transgender (aPR = 1.70; 95% CI 1.12–2.57; p = 0.010), Caucasian (aPR = 1.41; 95% CI 1.16–1.72); p < 0.001), drug injectors (aPR = 7.06; 95% CI 5.17–9.64; p < 0.001) and homeless [aPR = 1.30; 95% CI 1.14–1.48; p = 0.001) had a higher likelihood of self-reporting being HCV-positive (Table 4).

Discussion

With data from 2072 PWSC and PWID, people who reported a history of SUT were more likely to report higher levels of HIV and HCV screening, HIV care and ART initiation and were not more likely to report increased vulnerability or risky behavior. Other research has also suggested that people with a history of SUT have improved access to HIV care and treatment [30–33]. Researchers have also suggested that SUT can attend to the root causes of drug-related offenses among drug-involved offenders [28]. Yet as of 2011, 21.6 million people aged 12 or older had a substance use disorder, but only 2.3 (11%) million people received SUT [51]. There remains a great opportunity to invest and expand the use of SUT for drug-involved people with criminal justice histories in order to attend to their substance use disorder [28] and facilitate access to other essential health care such as HIV care and treatment.

In addition, our results suggested that people with a history of criminal justice involvement reported greater access to HIV and HCV testing, but did not report greater access to HIV care or treatment. Researchers and practitioners have urged medical and public health

Table 4 Associations with HIV and HCV positivity among PWID and PWSC in Oakland, 2011–2013 (N = 2072)

	HIV-positive				HCV-positive			
	PR (95% CI)	p value	aPR (95% CI)	p value	PR (95% CI)	p value	aPR (95% CI)	p value
Age (per 10 years)	1.11 (0.99–1.03)	0.208			1.65 (1.52–1.80)	<0.001	1.47 (1.35–1.59)	<0.001
Sexual risk group								
Men who have sex with women	1.00 (ref)		1.00 (ref)		1.00 (ref)		1.00 (ref)	
Men who have sex with men	12.93 (7.20–23.20)	<0.001	12.49 (6.95–22.44)	<0.001	1.57 (1.15–2.14)	0.002	1.74 (1.32–2.31)	<0.001
Female non-sex workers	2.08 (1.16–3.72)	0.014	1.71 (0.98–2.99)	0.058	0.84 (0.68–1.04)	0.107	1.06 (0.89–1.25)	0.513
Female sex worker	0.58 (0.20–1.66)	0.310	0.56 (0.19–1.60)	0.277	0.86 (0.68–1.08)	0.197	1.21 (0.98–1.48)	0.069
Transgender	40.07 (22.07–72.76)	<0.001	38.32 (20.10–73.03)	<0.001	0.99 (0.20–4.96)	0.997	1.70 (1.12–2.57)	0.010
Racial/ethnic group								
African American	1.00 (ref)				1.00 (ref)		1.00 (ref)	
Caucasian	0.83 (0.26–2.60)	0.748			2.06 (1.67–2.54)	<0.001	1.41 (1.16–1.72)	<0.001
Latino	NC				1.88 (1.46–2.42)	<0.001	1.25 (0.99–1.59)	0.060
Mixed race/other	0.57 (0.14–2.29)	0.429			1.22 (0.88–1.70)	0.232	1.00 (0.73–1.37)	0.997
High school education	1.01 (0.62–1.65)	0.810			0.94 (0.80–1.10)	0.452		
Steady partnership	1.20 (0.75–1.91)	0.448			0.81 (0.69–0.96)	0.012		
Have children	0.72 (0.42–1.22)	0.217			1.01 (0.83–1.24)	0.896		
Ever injected drugs	1.19 (0.74–1.90)	0.470			8.98 (6.63–12.16)	<0.001	7.06 (5.17–9.64)	<0.001
Homeless	1.10 (0.69–1.76)	0.686			1.21 (1.03–1.42)	0.017	1.30 (1.14–1.48)	<0.001
Trouble meeting needs	1.71 (0.94–3.12)	0.077	1.61 (0.91–2.85)	0.101	1.27 (1.05–1.54)	0.012		
Income ≥ $900	0.69 (0.37–1.27)	0.230			1.16 (0.98–1.38)	0.088		
Incarcerated	0.87 (0.38–1.99)	0.746			2.45 (1.37–4.39)	0.002		
Community supervision	1.34 (0.62–2.90)	0.464			1.41 (1.05–1.88)	0.022		
Substance use treatment	1.06 (0.64–1.74)	0.826			1.91 (1.53–2.39)	<0.001	1.20 (0.99–1.45)	0.060

NC: model did not converge for this category

professionals to take advantage of the opportunities provided by the criminal justice system in providing care for a highly underserved population [16, 52, 53]. Both the California state prison and Alameda county jail systems have an opt-out model for HIV testing, and the community supervision system provides testing referrals as indicated by the court or probation/parole officer. While our study did not evaluate these specific policies, it is encouraging that a history of criminal justice involvement was associated with higher reported levels of testing.

Accessing HIV services can quickly become complicated and disjointed for people with a history of criminal justice involvement. People incarcerated for longer sentences might be able to reap the benefits of HIV care and treatment during incarceration, but lose them once released [54]. Further, people who are going in and out of jail for low-level drug use or 'quality of life' violations are likely to miss any stabilizing benefit as they are caught in a criminal justice cycle that continually changes their environment. Our findings suggest that people with a history of criminal justice system involvement do not have greater access to HIV care or treatment.

Our findings are also consistent with previous research suggesting that involvement with the criminal justice system is associated with increased social and physical vulnerability [55, 56]. Prior studies have found an increased likelihood of homelessness [57], unemployment [58], lack of educational opportunities [55] and lack of health insurance [59] among people who have been involved in the criminal justice system. Furthermore, our findings showed increased injection- and sexual-related risk behavior among people with a history of criminal justice involvement is consistent with previous research that suggests this dynamic can be driven by factors such as poverty, mental health disorders and concurrent sexual partnerships, that are a by-product of involvement with the criminal justice system [55, 60].

The principal limitation of the study is the observational nature of the research design. Although we adjusted for measured participant characteristics to address concerns of confounding, the potential for unmeasured or mismeasured factors to bias our results existed. In addition, concerns regarding the temporality between exposures and outcomes given the cross-sectional nature of our study exist. We attempted to ameliorate this concern by defining exposure periods prior to outcomes when possible, but this does not convey the same level of rigor as a longitudinal study. Our study had the largest sample and most power for the earlier stage of the HIV care continuum (testing), and included a small number of people living with HIV, which may have impacted the study's power to detect associations for the following stages of the continuum (receiving HIV care and initiating ART). Furthermore, this study was not designed to look for relationships between different types of substance use treatment for different substance use disorders on study outcomes.

Another limitation is the self-report of behaviors and HCV status for the survey, and as a result, recall and social desirability are potential biases impacting the metrics collected as part for this analysis. Specifically, metrics for vulnerability (e.g., homelessness), sexual risk factors (e.g., multiple partners), injection risk factors (e.g., sharing needles) may be prone to social desirability bias. Due to stigmatization of behaviors and conditions, these types of biases are common when studying people who use drugs [61]. However, the resulting misclassification would be non-differential with regards to our primary exposures of interest and would generally bias our results toward the null [62]. On the other hand, prior research has illustrated that self-reported behaviors from drug users are both reliable and valid for epidemiological purposes [63].

Strengths of the study included the community-recruited sample of study participants. Most studies of HIV care engagement typically use service utilization data, while our sample provides a snapshot of access to services among people recruited from a community setting. Interviewing participants in community settings that are independent of any criminal justice or substance abuse treatment institution may increase participants' comfort with disclosing stigmatizing behavior compared to participants who are interviewed within institutional settings. In addition, our study included a large sample of criminal justice involved individuals who would not be captured in prison or jail populations, including people who were on probation or parole, who had absconded, or who had warrants out for their arrest. Furthermore, we had data of high quality that were collected specifically for the purposes of research.

Conclusion

Challenges remain in improving access to components of the HIV continuum and reducing vulnerabilities and risk among PWSC and PWID who have a history of the criminal justice system involvement. Innovative models that improve access to the HIV care continuum for these populations is vital. In addition, utilizing SUT programs, as appropriate, that are integrated with other services for HIV, HCV and mental health disorders will be critical to simultaneously address poor access to HIV and HCV services and the underlying reasons people who use drugs engage in drug-related offenses.

Authors' contributions
BHL analyzed and interpreted the data and led the drafting of the manuscript. AHK, AL, MC and JL interpreted the data and were major contributors in drafting the manuscript. All authors read and approved the final manuscript

Author details
[1] RTI International, 351 California St, Suite 500, San Francisco, CA 94104, USA.
[2] University of California, San Francisco, San Francisco, CA, USA. [3] University of Washington, Seattle, WA, USA.

Acknowledgements
We would like to thank the research staff and study participants for sharing their time and expertise. The article processing charge for this article was funded by the National Institute on Drug Abuse (NIDA), the National Drug Abuse Treatment Clinical Trials Network and the NIDA/SAMHSA Blending Initiative.

Competing interests
The authors declare that they have no competing interests.

Conference presentations
A portion of these data have been presented previously at the International AIDS Society Conference in July 2015 at Vancouver, Canada.

Ethics approval
All study procedures were reviewed and approved by a federally accredited Institutional Review Board at RTI International.

Funding
This research was conducted with funding from the National Institute of Mental Health (R01MH094090), the National Institute of Minority Health and Health Disparities (R01MD007679), and the National Institute of Drug Abuse (R34DA037787).

References
1. Moore LD. Who's using and who's doing time: incarceration, the war on drugs, and public health. Am J Public Health. 2008;98(5):782–6.
2. Bonczar TP. Prevalence of imprisonment in the U.S. population, 1974–2001. Washington: Bureau of Justice Statistics, US Department of Justice; 2003.
3. Glaze LE, Danielle K. Correctional populations in the United States, 2013. Washington: US Department of Justice, Office of Justice Programs, Bureau of Justice Statistics; 2014.
4. Wagner P, Sakala L, Begley J. States of incarceration: the global context. 2015. Accessed 10 June 2015.
5. Bonczar T, Herberman E. Probation and parole in the United States, 2013. 2013. Accessed 10 June 2015.
6. University TNCoAaSAaC. Behind bars II: substance abuse and America's prison population. 2010. Accessed 6 June 2015.
7. CDC. Monitoring selected national HIV prevention and care objectives by using HIV surveillance data—United States and 6 dependent areas. HIV surveillance report, vol 8, no 5 2011. Accessed 10 June 2015.
8. Wenbaum C, Lyerla R, Margolis HS. Prevention and control of infections with hepatitis viruses in correctional settings. MMWR. 2003;52(RR01):1–33.
9. CDC. HIV in correctional settings. 2014. Accessed 10 June 2015.
10. Kitahata MM, Gange SJ, Abraham AG, et al. Effect of early versus deferred antiretroviral therapy for HIV on survival. N Engl J Med. 2009;360(18):1815–26.
11. Sterne J, May M, Costagliola D, et al. Timing of initiation of antiretroviral therapy in AIDS-free HIV-1-infected patients: a collaborative analysis of 18 HIV cohort studies. Lancet. 2009;373(9672):1352–63.
12. Cohen MS, Chen YQ, McCauley M, et al. Prevention of HIV-1 infection with early antiretroviral therapy. N Engl J Med. 2011;365(6):493–505.
13. Gardner EM, McLees MP, Steiner JF, Del Rio C, Burman WJ. The spectrum of engagement in HIV care and its relevance to test-and-treat strategies for prevention of HIV infection. Clin Infect Dis. 2011;52(6):793–800.
14. Linas BP, Barter DM, Leff JA, et al. The hepatitis C cascade of care: identifying priorities to improve clinical outcomes. PLoS ONE. 2014;9(5):e97317.
15. Ogbuagu O, Bruce RD. Reaching the unreached: treatment as prevention as a workable strategy to mitigate HIV and its consequences in high-risk groups. Curr HIV/AIDS Rep. 2014;11(4):505–12.
16. Glaser JB, Greifinger RB. Correctional health care: a public health opportunity. Ann Intern Med. 1993;118(2):139–45.
17. Baillargeon J, Giordano TP, Harzke AJ, et al. Predictors of reincarceration and disease progression among released HIV-infected inmates. AIDS Patient Care STDS. 2010;24(6):389–94.
18. Beckwith CG, Zaller ND, Fu JJ, Montague BT, Rich JD. Opportunities to diagnose, treat, and prevent HIV in the criminal justice system. J Acquir Immune Defic Syndr. 2010;55(Suppl 1):S49–55.
19. Allen SA, Spaulding AC, Osei AM, Taylor LE, Cabral AM, Rich JD. Treatment of chronic hepatitis C in a state correctional facility. Ann Intern Med. 2003;138(3):187–90.
20. Strock P, Mossong J, Hawotte K, Arendt V. Access to treatment of hepatitis C in prison inmates. Dig Dis Sci. 2009;54(6):1325–30.
21. Basu S, Smith-Rohrberg D, Hanck S, Altice FL. HIV testing in correctional institutions: evaluating existing strategies, setting new standards. AIDS Public Policy J. 2005;20(1–2):3–24.
22. Sylla, M. HIV treatment in U.S. jails and prisons. San Francisco AIDS Foundation Online Newsletter. http://www.sfaf.org/beta/2008_win/jails_Prisons (2008). Accessed 24 Aug 2015.
23. Haley DF, Golin CE, Farel CE, et al. Multilevel challenges to engagement in HIV care after prison release: a theory-informed qualitative study comparing prisoners' perspectives before and after community reentry. BMC Public Health. 2014;14:1253.
24. Pope LG, Smith TE, Wisdom JP, Easter A, Pollock M. Transitioning between systems of care: missed opportunities for engaging adults with serious mental illness and criminal justice involvement. Behav Sci Law. 2013;31(4):444–56.
25. Baillargeon J, Giordano TP, Rich JD, et al. Accessing antiretroviral therapy following release from prison. JAMA. 2009;301(8):848–57.
26. Belenko S, Langley S, Crimmins S, Chaple M. HIV risk behaviors, knowledge, and prevention education among offenders under community supervision: a hidden risk group. AIDS Educ Prev. 2004;16(4):367–85.
27. Gordon MS, Kinlock TW, McKenzie M, Wilson ME, Rich JD. Rapid HIV testing for individuals on probation/parole: outcomes of an intervention trial. AIDS Behav. 2013;17(6):2022–30.
28. McVay D, Schiraldi V, Ziedenberg J. Treatment or incarceration? National and state findings on the efficacy and cost savings of drug treatment versus imprisonment. 2014. Accessed 10 June 2015.
29. Zarkin GA, Cowell AJ, Hicks KA, et al. Benefits and costs of substance abuse treatment programs for state prison inmates: results from a lifetime simulation model. Health Econ. 2012;21(6):633–52.
30. Palepu A, Tyndall MW, Joy R, et al. Antiretroviral adherence and HIV treatment outcomes among HIV/HCV co-infected injection drug users: the role of methadone maintenance therapy. Drug Alcohol Depend. 2006;84(2):188–94.
31. Reddon H, Milloy MJ, Simo A, Montaner J, Wood E, Kerr T. Methadone maintenance therapy decreases the rate of antiretroviral therapy discontinuation among HIV-positive illicit drug users. AIDS Behav. 2014;18(4):740–6.
32. Roux P, Carrieri MP, Villes V, et al. The impact of methadone or buprenorphine treatment and ongoing injection on highly active antiretroviral therapy (HAART) adherence: evidence from the MANIF2000 cohort study. Addiction. 2008;103(11):1828–36.
33. Uhlmann S, Milloy MJ, Kerr T, et al. Methadone maintenance therapy promotes initiation of antiretroviral therapy among injection drug users. Addiction. 2010;105(5):907–13.
34. Briscoe A. Report on continuing exixstence of a local state of emergency in Alameda County relative to the transmission of HIV and hepatitis C through the use of contaminated needles. In: Agency ACHCS, editors. http://www.acgov.org/board/bos_calendar/documents/DocsAgendaReg_06_24_14/HEALTH%20CARE%20SERVICES/Consent%20Calendar/PUBHLTH_204473.pdf (2014). Accessed 24 August 2015.
35. Davis M. Alameda County African American HIV/AIDS state of emergency report. In: Uni ACPHDHEaS, editors. http://www.acgov.org/board/bos_calendar/documents/DocsAgendaReg_10_13_14/HEALTH%20CARE%20

SERVICES/Regular%20Calendar/HIV_African_American_State_of_Emergency_Update_Health_10_13_14.pdf (2014). Accessed 24 August 2015.

36. County A. Healthy Alameda County. In: Department PH, editors. http://www.healthyalamedacounty.org/ (2015). Accessed 15 May 2015.

37. Institute CS. Sentencing practices in california by county, calendar year 2010. In: (CJCJ) CoJaCJ, editors. http://casi.cjcj.org/2011.

38. Council US. Alameda County probationer as of July 2010 and Parolee as of Oct 2010. 2010. Accessed 24 Aug 2015.

39. Department ACPH. How place, racism and poverty matter for health in Alameda County. 2013. Accessed 15 May 2015.

40. Kral AH, Malekinejad M, Vaudrey J, et al. Comparing respondent-driven sampling and targeted sampling methods of recruiting injection drug users in San Francisco. J Urban Health. 2010;87(5):839–50.

41. Watters J, Biernack P. Targeted sampling: options for the study of hidden populations. Soc Probl. 1989;36:416–30.

42. Zou G. A modified poisson regression approach to prospective studies with binary data. Am J Epidemiol. 2004;159(7):702–6.

43. Comfort M, Lopez A, Powers C, Kral AH, Lorvick J. How institutions deprive: ethnography, social work, and interventionist ethics among the hypermarginalized. Russell Sage J Soc Sci. 2015;1(1):100–19.

44. Gelberg L, Gallagher T, Andersen R, Koegel P. Competing priorities as a barrier to medical care among homeless adults in Los Angeles. Am J Public Health. 1997;87(2):217–20.

45. Dowling-Guyer S, Johnson ME, Fisher DG, et al. Reliability of drug users' self-reported HIV risk behaviors and validity of self-reported recent drug use. Assessment. 1994;1(4):383–92.

46. Seal KH, Kral AH, Gee L, et al. Predictors and prevention of nonfatal overdose among street-recruited injection heroin users in the San Francisco Bay Area, 1998–1999. Am J Public Health. 2001;91(11):1842–6.

47. Lorvick J, Kral AH, Seal K, Gee L, Edlin BR. Prevalence and duration of hepatitis C among injection drug users in San Francisco, Calif. Am J Public Health. 2001;91(1):46–7.

48. Kral AH, Bluthenthal RN, Lorvick J, Gee L, Bacchetti P, Edlin BR. Sexual transmission of HIV-1 among injection drug users in San Francisco, USA: risk-factor analysis. Lancet. 2001;357(9266):1397–401.

49. Kral AH, Lorvick J, Gee L, et al. Trends in human immunodeficiency virus seroincidence among street-recruited injection drug users in San Francisco, 1987–1998. Am J Epidemiol. 2003;157(10):915–22.

50. Stata Statistical Software. Release 14 [computer program]. College Station: StataCorp LP; 2015.

51. (NIDA) NIoDA. Principles of drug addiction treatment: a research-based guide. 3rd ed. http://www.drugabuse.gov/publications/principles-drug-addiction-treatment-research-based-guide-third-edition/acknowledgments2012.

52. Pathela P. Incarceration: a prime opportunity for sexually transmitted infection control. Sex Transm Dis. 2014;41(3):166–7.

53. Spaulding AC, Seals RM, Page MJ, Brzozowski AK, Rhodes W, Hammett TM. HIV/AIDS among inmates of and releasees from US correctional facilities, 2006: declining share of epidemic but persistent public health opportunity. PLoS ONE. 2009;4(11):e7558.

54. Iroh PA, Mayo H, Nijhawan AE. The HIV care cascade before, during and after incarceration: a systematic review and data synthesis. Am J Public Health. 2015;105(7):e5–16.

55. Dumont DM, Allen SA, Brockmann BW, Alexander NE, Rich JD. Incarceration, community health, and racial disparities. J Health Care Poor Underserved. 2013;24(1):78–88.

56. Lorvick J, Comfort M, Krebs CP, Kral AH. Health service use and social vulnerability in a community-based sample of women on probation and parole, 2011-2013. Health Justice. 2015;3(13):1–6.

57. Drucker E. A plague of prisons: the epidemiology of mass incarceration in America. New York: The New Press; 2011.

58. Pager D, Western B, Sugie N. Sequencing disadvantage: barriers to employment facing young black and white men with criminal records. Ann Am Acad Polit Soc Sci. 2009;623:195–213.

59. Mallik-Kane K, Cisher C. Health and priosner reentry: how physical, mental and substance abuse conditions shape the process of reintegration. Washington: Urban Institute; 2008.

60. Khan MR, Golin CE, Friedman SR, et al. STI/hiv sexual risk behavior and prevalent STI among incarcerated African American men in committed partnerships: the significance of poverty, mood disorders, and substance use. AIDS Behav. 2015;19(8):1478–90.

61. Perlis TE, Des Jarlais DC, Friedman SR, Arasteh K, Turner CF. Audio-computerized self-interviewing versus face-to-face interviewing for research data collection at drug abuse treatment programs. Addiction. 2004;99(7):885–96.

62. Koepsell TD, Weiss NS. Epidemiologic methods: studying the occurence of illness. New York: Oxford University Press; 2003.

63. Darke S. Self-report among injecting drug users: a review. Drug Alcohol Depend. 1998;51(3):253–63.

22

Prevalence and personal attitudes towards tobacco smoking among Palestinian healthcare professionals

Isra Y. Mizher[1], Shahd I. Fawaqa[1] and Waleed M. Sweileh[2*]

Abstract

Background: Little is known about tobacco smoking behaviors of healthcare professionals in the Middle East where stress conditions are high and tobacco smoking regulations are either absent or loose. The objective of this study was to identify the prevalence of and attitudes toward tobacco smoking among healthcare professionals.

Methods: Trained senior medical students conducted a cross–sectional survey study in all governmental and non-governmental hospitals in Nablus city (Palestine) using a self-administered questionnaire containing both open-and closed-ended questions.

Results: In total, 708 healthcare professionals participated in the study. The mean age of the participants was 31.4 ± 9.6 years. Forty-five (6.4%) participants were ex-smokers, 419 (59.2%) were never smokers, and 244 (34.5%) were current tobacco smokers. One hundred and forty-two (58.2%) tobacco smokers reported that they smoke inside the hospital and 119 (48.8%) reported that they think of quitting smoking. Univariate analysis indicated that age, gender, marital status, family history of tobacco smoking, country of graduation, and night shifts were significantly associated with tobacco smoking status. No significant difference ($p = 0.156$) in prevalence of tobacco smoking was found between physicians and other healthcare professionals. Binary logistic regression indicated that older age, male gender, and having a positive family history of smoking were significant predictors of being a current tobacco smoker. Non-smokers had significantly higher frequency of patient counseling than current smokers.

Conclusion: Palestinian healthcare professionals have relatively higher prevalence of tobacco smoking compared to the general population. Urgent national intervention and strict implementation of "No Smoking Law" in health institutions and in public places are needed to root out this negative behavior.

Background

Tobacco smoking is responsible for the death of nearly 7 million people yearly, 6 million of them are killed by direct tobacco use, while 890,000 are killed by second-hand smoking [1]. In addition, tobacco smoking is the second leading cause of cardiovascular diseases (CVD), contributing to approximately 12% of all cardiovascular disease deaths [2]. Tobacco smoking is also the single greatest avoidable risk factor for cancer mortality, as it has a relationship with many types of cancer [3, 4]. Furthermore, tobacco smoking plays a major role in physical fitness and survival [5].

The 2010 report by the *Palestinian Central Bureau of Statistics* (PCBS) revealed that 22.5% of adults (≥ 18 years old) were current tobacco smokers [6]. The report indicated that the percentage of male smokers reached 37.6 against 2.6% of female smokers. The report also stated that tobacco smoking plays a key role in the escalating numbers of lung cancers and childhood respiratory problems [7]. International reports also indicated that water tobacco smoking (hookah), which is a method of tobacco smoking, is gaining popularity where the highest prevalence of waterpipe smoking was in Lebanon (36.9%)

*Correspondence: waleedsweileh@yahoo.com
[2] Department of Physiology, Pharmacology, and Toxicology, College of Medicine and Health Sciences, An-Najah National University, Nablus 44839, Palestine
Full list of author information is available at the end of the article

followed by that in West Bank in the occupied Palestinian territory (32.7%) and Latvia (22.7%) [8]. Waterpipe smoking is common in the Middle East [9]. It is present in different flavors and is served in restaurants and coffee shops. The Council of Arab Ministers of Health called for banning smoking in all its forms in public and closed places, and prohibiting advertising and promotion of tobacco, its products and derivatives [10].

Physicians and other healthcare professionals should play a positive role in the prevention and treatment of tobacco smoking. Healthcare professionals who have direct contact with patients, should increase patients' awareness about harms of smoking and should provide medical consultation for patients who want to quit smoking [11, 12]. Tobacco smoking among healthcare professionals negatively affects the attitude and impression of patients about healthcare professionals and negatively affects their willingness to quit smoking. Furthermore, it was found that physicians who smoke are less likely to advise their patients about smoking [13, 14] and their smoking status influence their patients' response to quit smoking [15, 16]. Therefore, reducing the prevalence of tobacco smoking among healthcare professionals will effectively reduce its prevalence among the general population [17].

Combating tobacco smoking among healthcare professionals requires availability of data on the prevalence of this habit among this leading group of people. However, data on the prevalence of and attitudes toward tobacco smoking among healthcare professionals are lacking which negatively affects the ability of policy makers to develop national plans to ban tobacco smoking. Therefore, the general aim of the current study was to determine the prevalence of and attitudes toward tobacco smoking among healthcare professionals. The aim of this study is in accordance with World Health Organization (WHO) which recommends strengthening tobacco smoking surveillance and monitoring among various population categories and age groups [18, 19]. The findings of the current study helps the Palestinian legislative bodies to develop interventional strategies to minimize the health effects of tobacco smoking.

Methods
Study design and study population
This was a cross-sectional study that targeted healthcare professionals in two governmental and five non-governmental hospitals in the city of Nablus. The number of healthcare professionals in Nablus city is estimated to be less than 2000 while the estimated number of healthcare professionals in the selected seven hospitals is estimated to be 800. None of the hospitals included in the study had a clear, written, and implemented no-smoking policy.

However, verbal recommendations and wall signs of "no smoking" are loosely adopted in these hospitals.

Sample size
Sample size was calculated using the Raosoft sample size calculator [20]. The sample size was calculated by anticipating at least 20% prevalence of tobacco smoking with $z = 1.96$ for a 95% confidence level, margin of error of 5%, and a response rate of 50%. The minimum sample size required to estimate a population parameters was estimated as 323. The study was conducted from September 01, 2017 to November 01, 2017.

Recruitment of participants
Two senior medical students visited the target hospitals three times weekly (Sunday, Tuesday, and Thursday) during the study period. The study questionnaire was distributed to healthcare professionals in all hospital departments on Sundays and Tuesdays and the filled questionnaire were collected back on Thursdays. Healthcare professionals were asked to fill in the questionnaire during working hours in their workplace. Completing the questionnaire took an average of 10 min. The participants were assured of the confidentiality of the information that they provided.

The study tool
A self-administered questionnaire was developed for the purpose of this study. The questionnaire was developed based on previously published studies [21, 22]. The questionnaire consisted of three parts. The first part was about demographic characteristics of the participants, night shifts, family history of smoking, and their attitudes in dealing with patients who smoke. The first part included several questions about the role of the healthcare provider in advising patients about smoking and explaining its health hazards. The second part included questions to current tobacco smokers while the third part included questions to ex-smokers. Current smokers were asked about forms of tobacco smoking they use (cigarettes, waterpipe, or both), at what age they started smoking, for how long, and the quantity they smoke by day or week. Current smokers were also asked if they smoke inside the hospital and weather stressful conditions (yes, no) inside the hospital increase their tendency to smoke. Current smokers were also asked if they think of quitting smoking and by which means. Ex-smokers were asked about the age and the reason (medical, financial, other) for quitting smoking. In the current study, definitions of current and former cigarette smokers were obtained the Centre for Disease Control and Prevention guidelines [23] while waterpipe smokers were defined as in the study of Bahrain [22].

Statistical analysis

Data collected were coded and entered into Statistical Package for Social Sciences (IBM SPSS statistics; version 21; Armonk, NY: IBM Corporation program. The main outcome variable was prevalence of current tobacco smoking expressed as a proportion (%). Most variables, such as gender, marital status, place of study, night shifts, place of living were entered as dichotomous variables (0; 1). Age variable was divided into four categories. Smoking status was divided into three categories: current smokers, never smokers, and ex-smokers. Descriptive categorical variables were expressed as proportion while descriptive continuous variables were expressed as mean ± standard deviation (SD) and/or medians and interquartile range (25th quartile–75th quartile). Statistical analysis for the association of various variables with smoking status was carried out using Chi square test using a significance level of less than 5%. Variables that showed significant association with smoking status in univariate analysis were entered into binary logistic regression to find significant predictors of smoking status. For the part pertaining to the attitudes of healthcare professionals towards smoking in clinical settings, the frequency of "yes" and "no" answers were calculated and statistically tested using Chi square test. Finally, for the ex-smokers, analysis was carried out separately because this category turned out to be small and because it is a unique category compared with current smokers and never smokers.

Ethical consideration

Ethical approval was obtained from NNU-IRB committee, the Palestinian Ministry of Health (MOH), and each hospital's medical director. A verbal consent was taken from each participant before filling in the questionnaire.

Results

Of the 800 questionnaires that were distributed, a total of 708 were completed and returned to the researchers. The response rate was 88.5%. The mean ± SD of the age of the participants was 31.4 ± 9.6 years while the median (25th quartile–75th quartile) age was 28 [Q1–Q3 = 25–35] years. The sample included 387 (54.7%) males and 321 (45.3%) females. Forty-five (6.4%) were ex-smokers and this category of participants was analyzed separately to avoid any bias in data analysis and interpretation. The remaining 663 participants were either never smokers (419; 59.2%) or current smokers (244; 34.5%). Data regarding current smokers were analyzed in terms of socio-demographic characteristics, predictors of being a current smoker, types of smoking, and attitudes toward smoking habits in clinical settings.

Smoking behaviors

When asked about how long they have been smoking, 50% reported that they have been smoking for at least 9 years. The mean ± SD of the starting age of smoking among current smokers was 21.1 ± 5.1 years. One hundred and forty-two (58.2%) current smokers reported that they smoke inside the hospital and 137 (56.1%) reported doing so because of the stressful conditions inside the hospital. When asked about where they smoke inside the hospital, the majority reported that they do so in hospital corridors or inside the medical staff rooms or food court. Sixty-eight (27.9%) of current smokers reported feeling embarrassed to smoke in the presence of patients and 170 (69.7%) reported that they wish they were not smokers. Only 5 (2.0%) reported that they would smoke in close distance to patients. Approximately half (119; 48.8%) of the current smokers reported that they think of quitting smoking using nicotine patches (30; 25.2%) or by strong will (89; 74.8%). When asked about why they think of quitting smoking, 87 (35.7%) cited economic reasons while the remaining stated health reasons. More than half (126; 51.9%) of current smokers reported smoking cigarettes only while the remaining (48.1%) reported smoking both cigarettes and waterpipe.

Current versus never-smokers

Never and current smokers included 192 (29.0%) physicians and 471 (71%) nurses and other healthcare professionals. The non-physician group include 325 (49.0%) nurses while the remaining were medical laboratory technologists, pharmacists, and medical technicians. One hundred and twenty-three (18.6%) physicians were specialists. Socio-demographic characteristics of current smokers and never-smokers are shown in Table 1. The majority (363; 54.8%) of participants were in the age category of 25–34.9 years. Younger age category (< 25 years) had significantly lower odds [OR = 0.231; 95% CI (0.124–0.427)] of being smokers compared to older age category (> 45 years). The participants included 349 males and 314 females. Male healthcare professionals had significantly higher odds of being smokers than female healthcare professionals [OR = 7.099, 95% CI (4.889–10.309)]. The majority of participants were unmarried (383; 57%). Married healthcare professionals had significantly lower odds of being smokers than unmarried health professionals [OR = 0.685; 95% CI (0.496–0.948)]. More than half of the participants (358; 54%) had a family history of at least one of their parents being smoker. Healthcare professionals with positive family history of smoking had significantly higher odds of being smokers [OR = 2.446, 95% CI (1.759–3.401)]. When asked about place of study, the majority of participants were graduates of local

Table 1 Sociodemographic characteristics of current and never smokers

Variable	Total $N=663$	Current smokers $N=244$	Never smokers $N=419$	p value
Age (years)				0.000
<25	141 (21.27%)	27 (19.15%)	114 (80.85%)	
25–34.9	363 (54.75%)	144 (39.69%)	219 (60.33%)	
35–44.9	84 (12.69%)	35 (41.69%)	49 (58.33%)	
≥45	75 (11.31%)	38 (50.67%)	37 (49.33%)	
Gender				0.000
Male	349 (52.64%)	196 (56.16%)	153 (43.84%)	
Female	314 (47.37%)	48 (15.29%)	266 (84.71%)	
Marital status				0.022
Married	280 (42.23%)	89 (31.79%)	191 (68.21%)	
Unmarried	383 (57.77%)	155 (40.47%)	228 (59.53%)	
Living address				0.770
Urban	332 (50.07%)	124 (37.34%)	208 (62.65%)	
Suburban	331 (49.92%)	120 (36.25%)	211 (63.74%)	
Family history of smoking				0.000
Positive	358 (54.00%)	165 (46.10%)	193 (53.91%)	
Negative	305 (46.00%)	79 (25.90%)	226 (74.10%)	
Occupation				0.156
Physicians	192 (29.00%)	79 (41.14%)	113 (58.9%)	
Paramedics	471 (71.04%)	165 (35.03%)	306 (65%)	
Place of study				0.000
Inside the country	522 (78.73%)	171 (32.76%)	351 (67.24%)	
Abroad	141 (21.27%)	73 (51.77%)	68 (48.22%)	
Place of work				0.651
Governmental hospitals	313 (47.21%)	118 (37.70%)	195 (62.30%)	
Non-governmental hospitals	350 (52.79%)	126 (36.00%)	224 (64.00%)	
Night or on-call shifts				0.014
Yes	411 (62.00%)	166 (40.39%)	245 (59.61%)	
No	252 (38.00%)	78 (30.95%)	174 (69.04%)	

Palestinian Universities (522, 78%). Healthcare professionals who studied in local universities had significantly lower odds of being smokers than health professionals who studied abroad [OR = 0.454, 95% CI (0.311–0.662)]. Approximately two-thirds of the participants reported having night shifts or having on-call shifts. Healthcare professional who had night or on-call shifts had significantly higher odds of being a smoker than those who do not [OR = 1.511, 95% CI (1.085–2.106)]. No significant difference in frequency of smoking was found between physicians and other healthcare professionals ($p = 0.156$). Similarly, both place of work and living address were not significantly associated with the status of smoking.

Significant variables in univariate analysis were entered in binary logistic regression using enter method to find the predictors of smoking status. The dependent variable was smoking status (current smoker vs. never smoker) while the independent variables were age category, gender, marital status, place of study, family history of

smoking, and having night/on-call shifts. The results of binary logistic regression indicated that older age categories, male gender, and positive family history of smoking were significant predictors of a healthcare professional being a smoker (Table 2).

The attitude of current smokers and never-smokers toward smoking was investigated. Approximately 92% of non-smokers were convinced that health professionals should advise patients to quit smoking while 81% of current smokers reported that they were convinced that they should advise patients to quit smoking ($p < 0.001$). Approximately 45% of non-smoker healthcare professionals reported that they always advise their patients to quit smoking while only 32% of current smokers reported doing so ($p < 0.005$). Furthermore, 116 (27.7%) of non-smokers reported that they follow up with their patients in smoking cessation while only 45 (18.4%) of current smokers said that they do so with their patients ($p < 0.007$).

Table 2 Binary logistic regression for significant predictors of smoking status

Variable	B	p value	OR	95% CI for OR	
				Lower	Upper
Age category (< 25): reference					
Age category (25–34.9)	0.890	0.002	2.436	1.382	4.294
Age category (35–44.9)	0.938	0.019	2.556	1.164	5.612
Age category (>45)	1.227	0.002	3.413	1.542	7.551
Gender (male) Gender (female): reference	2.000	0.000	7.390	4.867	11.223
Marital status (single) Marital status (married): reference	− 0.058	0.798	0.944	0.607	1.468
Place of graduation (local universities) Place of graduation (Abroad): reference	0.172	0.455	1.188	0.756	1.867
Night or on-call shifts No Yes (reference)	− 0.041	0.843	0.960	0.642	1.437
Family history of smoking Positive Negative (reference)	1.005	0.000	2.732	1.881	3.968
Constant	− 3.164	0.000	0.042		

OR odds ratio, *CI* confidence limit

Approximately 89% of non-smokers reported that they endorse regulations to ban smoking of healthcare professionals in hospitals and clinical settings while 73% of smokers reported to agree on regulations that ban smoking of healthcare professionals in hospitals and clinical settings ($p < 0.000$). No significant difference was found between current smokers and non-smokers with regard to efforts and time spent with patients to explain negative health effects of smoking ($p = 0.112$) (Table 3).

Characteristics of ex-smokers

Of the 708 participants, there were 45 healthcare professionals who identified themselves as ex-smokers. The majority of ex-smokers (26; 55.6%) stated that they were regular smokers for at least 5 years. Ex-smokers were 38 (84.4%) males and 7 (15.6%) females. Mean ± SD age of ex-smokers was 37 ± 12.1 years. Approximately half (51.1%) of ex-smokers had a positive family history of smoking. The majority of ex-smokers were married (77.8%). Ex-smokers included 19 (42.2%) physicians. When asked about the cause of quitting smoking, the majority (31; 68.9%) stated that they were concerned about the health consequences of smoking while the remaining stated economic reasons for quitting smoking. When asked about the method they used to quit smoking, only 6 (13.3%) stated using nicotine replacement therapy while the remaining stated strong will and sports as methods of quitting smoking.

Discussion

In the current study, we investigated the prevalence of tobacco smoking among healthcare professionals working in governmental and non-governmental hospitals in Nablus district, north of Palestine. The current study showed that the prevalence of tobacco smoking among healthcare professionals was relatively higher than that reported in the general population as well as among the youth population in West Bank [6, 24]. Unfortunately, there is no previously published data about the prevalence of tobacco smoking among healthcare professionals in Palestine for comparative purposes. Therefore, the current study serves as a baseline data for future comparisons and for future interventional programs to combat tobacco smoking at the national level.

No doubt that occupational stress is one potential reason for the high prevalence of tobacco smoking among healthcare professionals compared to that of the general population [25, 26]. A second potential reason is the loose implementation of the Palestinian "No Smoking law" [27]. A third reason is the wrong belief that waterpipe smoking is less harmful than cigarette smoking [28]. A fourth potential reasons is the lack of well-trained experts in the treatment of nicotine addiction and in the delivery of smoking cessation therapy. The Palestinian Ministry of Health should invest in building capacities and starting specialized clinics for tobacco smoking cessation therapy to help in combating tobacco smoking. These factors should be

Table 3 Counseling behaviors of current and never smokers

Question	Total	Never smokers	Current smokers	p value
Are you convinced that a healthcare worker should advise the patient to stop smoking?				
Yes	581 (87.63%)	384 (91.64%)	197 (80.73%)	0.000
No	82 (12.36%)	35 (8.35%)	47 (19.26%)	
Do you advise your patient to stop smoking?				
Always	266 (40.12%)	188 (44.87%)	78 (31.96%)	0.005
Sometimes	329 (49.62%)	192 (45.82%)	137 (56.15%)	
Never	68 (10.25%)	39 (9.30%)	29 (11.88%)	
Do you explain the negative health effects of smoking to your patient?				
Yes	550 (82.95%)	355 (84.73%)	195 (79.91%)	0.112
No	113 (17.04%)	64 (15.27%)	49 (20.08%)	
Do you follow up with your smoking patients if they reduce or quite smoking?				
Yes	161 (24.28%)	116 (27.68%)	45 (18.44%)	0.007
No	502 (75.71%)	303 (72.31%)	199 (81.56%)	
Have you recorded any cases that quitted smoking?				
High numbers	9 (1.35%)	8 (1.90%)	1 (0.40%)	0.193
Low numbers	184 (27.75%)	111 (26.49%)	73 (29.91%)	
Zero	470 (70.89%)	300 (71.59%)	170 (69.67%)	
Do you know if there are any policies that ban smoking of healthcare workers inside hospitals?				
Yes	263 (39.67%)	166 (39.62%)	97 (39.75%)	0.972
No	400 (60.33%)	253 (60.38%)	147 (60.24%)	
In your opinion, Is it a necessity to have policies that ban smoking and punish who smokes inside hospitals?				
Yes	550 (83.00%)	372 (88.87%)	178 (73.00%)	0.000
No	113 (17.04%)	47 (11.21%)	66 (27.04%)	
Total	663 (100%)	419 (100%)	244 (100%)	

considered in any tailored national intervention program to decrease the prevalence of tobacco smoking.

There are several studies about prevalence of tobacco smoking among healthcare professionals in the Middle East region. The findings of the current study was higher than that reported from Bahrain [22], Saudi Arabia [29, 30], and Oman [31], but lower than that reported from Jordan [32]. At the international level, the findings of the current study was closer to that reported from Central/Eastern Europe (37%) and higher than that in Africa (29%), Central and South America (25%), and Asia (17.5%) [33]. It was fortunate that only five of current smokers reported smoking in close distance to patients. This is in agreement with a study published from Croatia [26] but not in agreement with other studies [34]. Healthcare professionals who participated in our study are familiar with the harmful effects of smoking and passive smoking on patients, children, and pregnant women and tend to avoid smoking in front of patients.

The current study showed that the significant predictors of current tobacco smoking were older age, male gender, and positive family history of smoking. The findings of the current study regarding predictors of smoking status were in agreement with those published in other studies [35–37]. Gender differences in the prevalence of smoking are due to the conservative culture in the Middle East. Women who smoke are subjected to social stigma. Therefore, the data regarding prevalence of tobacco smoking among females might be inaccurate due to fear of females of social stigma. Despite this, interventional programs to combat smoking should focus on males and give women a participatory role in education and increasing awareness among males. The strong association between tobacco use and parental history of tobacco use indicates that smokers might have inherited this bad habit from their parents which make them victims of their living environment.

The current study showed that almost half of the current tobacco smokers use both cigarette smoking and waterpipe. The relationship between waterpipe tobacco smoking and cigarettes had been discussed is complex and showed cultural variations [38]. The availability of various flavors of waterpipe and the social acceptability of waterpipe are considered a precursor for future cigarette smoking [39]. A longitudinal smoking study carried out in Irbid (Jordan) suggested that waterpipe tobacco smoking may be an initial trigger to future cigarette smoking among never users [40]. A Canadian study argued that waterpipe smokers have higher prevalence of substance use than non-smokers [41]. A recent study from Palestine concluded that there is a high prevalence of waterpipe smoking that surpassed the prevalence of cigarette smoking [24]. The authors of the Palestinian study concluded that interventions to curb the practice of tobacco smoking among Palestinian youth should be tailored differently to waterpipe smoking and cigarette smoking. The common use of waterpipe smoking among healthcare professionals could be attributed to the increasing trend of waterpipe smoking among youth and university students [42]. It should be emphasized here that cigarette smoking is usually an individual and might be a hidden behavior. However, the waterpipe smoking is usually practiced within social groups and in public places which negatively affects the public image of healthcare professionals and negatively affects their abilities to provide clinical intervention in smoking cessation therapy.

The current study has few limitations. First, the study was not a national study. Only healthcare professionals in Nablus city participated in the study. It should be emphasized here that different regions in Palestine might have different patterns and prevalence of smoking [24]. Second, the recruitment of the participants and the study setting might have created certain bias or underestimation of the prevalence of tobacco smoking among female healthcare professionals. Third, the tool used in this study was developed by the authors and not an internationally validated one. Fourth, the prevalence of tobacco smoking was not correlated with any laboratory or psychological measure of nicotine addiction. Future studies should include measures of nicotine addiction and correlate it with prevalence and attitude toward smoking. Fifth, the cross-sectional design of the study which limits the ability of the investigators to generalize the findings of the study or claim any causal relationship between demographic variables and smoking status.

Conclusion

Our study indicated that the prevalence of tobacco smoking among healthcare professionals in hospitals is relatively higher than that reported elsewhere including the general population in Palestine. This finding could create a negative image about healthcare professionals who should behave as a model for disease prevention. We have also shown that male gender, parental history of tobacco smoking, and older age are significant predictors that need to be targeted in future plans to decrease prevalence of smoking. In Palestine, there is weak implementation of the "No Smoking Law" issued in 2005 [27] and it is hoped that the current findings signal a warning to health policy makers and legislative bodies to strengthen the implementation of the law and impose penalties for those who violate the law in health institutions. The ultimate goal is to formulate a national plan in which healthcare professionals can take the lead in both increasing awareness and in delivering appropriate smoking cessation therapy.

Abbreviation
IRB: Institutional Review Board.

Authors' contributions
IM, and SF collected data, performed the analyses and literature search, and drafted the manuscript. WS conceptualized and designed the study, coordinated the study and data analysis, interpreted the data, and assisted in final write-up of the manuscript. All authors read and approved the final manuscript.

Author details
[1] College of Medicine and Health Sciences, An-Najah National University, Nablus 44839, Palestine. [2] Department of Physiology, Pharmacology, and Toxicology, College of Medicine and Health Sciences, An-Najah National University, Nablus 44839, Palestine.

Acknowledgements
The authors would like to thank An-Najah National University for giving the opportunities to this study.

Competing interests
The authors declare that they have no competing interests.

Consent for publication
Not applicable.

Funding
No funding was available for this study.

References
1. World Health Organization (WHO); Tobacco (Fact sheet). http://www.who.int/mediacentre/factsheets/fs339/en/. 28 Jan 2018.
2. World Health Organization (WHO); World No Tobacco Day, Tobacco and heart disease. http://www.who.int/mediacentre/events/2018/world-no-tobacco-day/en/. 28 Jan 2018.
3. Motorykin O, Matzke MM, Waters KM, Massey Simonich SL. Association of carcinogenic polycyclic aromatic hydrocarbon emissions and smoking with lung cancer mortality rates on a global scale. Environ Sci Technol. 2013;47(7):3410–6.
4. Islami F, Torre LA, Jemal A. Global trends of lung cancer mortality and smoking prevalence. Transl Lung Cancer Res. 2015;4(4):327–38.
5. West R. Tobacco smoking: health impact, prevalence, correlates and interventions. Psychol Health. 2017;32(8):1018–36.
6. Palestinian Central Bureau of Statistics (PCBS): Palestinian Family Survey, 2010 (Final Report). In: Ramallah—State of Palestine; 2013.
7. Palestinian Central Bureau of Statistics (PCBS) and the Ministry of Health (MoH): The Palestinian Central Bureau of Statistics (PCBS) and the Ministry of Health (MoH) are issuing a Press Release on the occasion of International Day of Giving up Smoking (Word No Tobacco Day) In: Rmallah—State of Palestine; 2012.
8. Jawad M, Lee JT, Millett C. Waterpipe tobacco smoking prevalence and correlates in 25 Eastern Mediterranean and Eastern European countries: cross-sectional analysis of the Global Youth Tobacco Survey. Nicotine Tob Res. 2015;18(4):395–402.
9. Jaghbir M, Shreif S, Ahram M. Pattern of cigarette and waterpipe smoking in the adult population of Jordan. East Mediterr Health J. 2014;20(9):529–37.
10. Asharq Al-Awsat; Arab Countries Considering broad ban on smoking. https://aawsat.com/english/home/article/1191901/arab-countries-considering-broad-ban-smoking. 02 July 2018.
11. Joshi V, Suchin V, Lim J. Smoking cessation: barriers, motivators and the role of physicians—a survey of physicians and patients. Proc Singap Healthc. 2010;19(2):145–53.
12. Sreedharan J, Muttappallymyalil J, Venkatramana M. Nurses' attitude and practice in providing tobacco cessation care to patients. J Prev Med Hyg. 2010;51(2):57–61.
13. Abdullah AS, Guangmin N, Kaiyong H, Jing L, Yang L, Zhang Z, Winickoff JP. Implementing tobacco control assistance in pediatric departments of chinese hospitals: a feasibility study. Pediatrics. 2018;141(Supplement 1):S51–62.
14. Parna K, Rahu K, Rahu M. Smoking habits and attitudes towards smoking among Estonian physicians. Public Health. 2005;119(5):390–9.
15. Stead LF, Buitrago D, Preciado N, Sanchez G, Hartmann-Boyce J, Lancaster T. Physician advice for smoking cessation. Cochrane Database Syst Rev. 2013;2017(12):165.
16. Meshefedjian GA, Gervais A, Tremblay M, Villeneuve D, O'Loughlin J. Physician smoking status may influence cessation counseling practices. Can J Public Health. 2010;101(4):290–3.
17. Shkedy YOFR, Mizrachi A. Smoking habits among Israeli hospital doctors: a survey and historical review. Israel Med Assoc J IMAJ. 2013;15(7):339–43.
18. World Health Organization (WHO): WHO Study Group on Tobacco Product Regulation (TobReg), Waterpipe tobacco smoking: health effects, research needs and recommended actions for regulators. In: Edited by ed. n; 2015.
19. World Health Organization (WHO). Global action plan for the prevention and control of NCDs 2013–2020. Geneva: World Health Organization; 2013.
20. Raosoft; Sample size calculator. http://www.raosoft.com/samplesize.html. 02 July 2018.
21. Zinonos S, Zachariadou T, Zannetos S, Panayiotou AG, Georgiou A. Smoking prevalence and associated risk factors among healthcare professionals in Nicosia general hospital, Cyprus: a cross-sectional study. Tob Induc Dis. 2016;14(1):14.

22. Borgan SM, Jassim G, Marhoon ZA, Almuqamam MA, Ebrahim MA, Soliman PA. Prevalence of tobacco smoking among health-care physicians in Bahrain. BMC Public Health. 2014;14(1):931.

23. CDC. State-specific secondhand smoke exposure and current cigarette smoking among adults—United States, 2008. MMUR?. 2009;58(44):1232–5.

24. Tucktuck M, Ghandour R, Abu-Rmeileh NME. Waterpipe and cigarette tobacco smoking among Palestinian university students: a cross-sectional study. BMC Public Health. 2017;18(1):1.

25. Ficarra MG, Gualano MR, Capizzi S, Siliquini R, Liguori G, Manzoli L, Briziarelli L, Parlato A, Cuccurullo P, Bucci R, et al. Tobacco use prevalence, knowledge and attitudes among Italian hospital healthcare professionals. Eur J Public Health. 2011;21(1):29–34.

26. Juranić B, Rakošec Ž, Jakab J, Mikšić Š, Vuletić S, Ivandić M, Blažević I. Prevalence, habits and personal attitudes towards smoking among health care professionals. J Occup Med Toxicol. 2017;12(1):20.

27. Palestinian Legislative Council: Public Health Law. In: Ramallah—Palestine; 2005.

28. Akl EA, Jawad M, Lam WY, Co CN, Obeid R, Irani J. Motives, beliefs and attitudes towards waterpipe tobacco smoking: a systematic review. Harm Reduct J. 2013;10:12.

29. Al-Haddad NS, Al-Habeeb TA, Abdelgadir MH, Al-Ghamdy YS, Qureshi NA. Smoking patterns among primary health care attendees, Al-Qassim region, Saudi Arabia. East Mediterr Health J. 2003;9(5–6):911–22.

30. Mahfouz AA, Shatoor AS, Al-Ghamdi BR, Hassanein MA, Nahar S, Farheen A, Gaballah II, Mohamed A, Rabie FM. Tobacco use among health care workers in Southwestern Saudi Arabia. Biomed Res Int. 2013;2013:960292.

31. Al-Lawati JA, Nooyi SC, Al-Lawati AM. Knowledge, attitudes and prevalence of tobacco use among physicians and dentists in Oman. Ann Saudi Med. 2009;29(2):128–33.

32. Shishani K, Nawafleh H, Jarrah S, Froelicher ES. Smoking patterns among Jordanian health professionals: a study about the impediments to tobacco control in Jordan. Eur J Cardiovasc Nurs. 2011;10(4):221–7.

33. Abdullah AS, Stillman FA, Yang L, Luo H, Zhang Z, Samet JM. Tobacco use and smoking cessation practices among physicians in developing countries: a literature review (1987–2010). Int J Environ Res Public Health. 2013;11(1):429–55.

34. Duaso M, Duncan D. Health impact of smoking and smoking cessation strategies: current evidence. Br J Community Nurs. 2012;17(8):356–63.

35. Stamatopoulou E, Stamatiou K, Voulioti S, Christopoulos G, Pantza E, Stamatopoulou A, Giannopoulos D. Smoking behavior among nurses in rural greece. Workplace Health Saf. 2014;62(4):132–4.

36. Lam TH, Jiang C, Chan YF, Chan SSC. Smoking cessation intervention practices in Chinese physicians: do gender and smoking status matter? Health Soc Care Community. 2011;19(2):126–37.

37. Jiménez-Ruiz CA, Miranda JAR, Pinedo AR, Martinez EDH, Marquez FL, Cobos LP, Reina SS, Orive JIDG, Ramos PDL. Prevalence of and attitudes towards smoking among Spanish health professionals. Respiration. 2015;90(6):474–80.

38. Jawad M, Lee JT, Millett C. The relationship between waterpipe and cigarette smoking in low and middle income countries: cross-sectional analysis of the global adult tobacco survey. PLoS ONE. 2014;9(3):e93097.

39. Jensen PD, Cortes R, Engholm G, Kremers S, Gislum M. Waterpipe use predicts progression to regular cigarette smoking among Danish youth. Subst Use Misuse. 2010;45(7–8):1245–61.

40. Mzayek F, Khader Y, Eissenberg T, Al Ali R, Ward KD, Maziak W. Patterns of water-pipe and cigarette smoking initiation in schoolchildren: Irbid longitudinal smoking study. Nicotine Tob Res. 2012;14(4):448–54.

41. Dugas E, Tremblay M, Low NC, Cournoyer D, O'Loughlin J. Water-pipe smoking among North American youths. Pediatrics. 2010;125(6):1184–9.

42. Jawad M, McEwen A, McNeill A, Shahab L. To what extent should waterpipe tobacco smoking become a public health priority? Addiction. 2013;108(11):1873–84.

23

Barriers and facilitators of the HIV care continuum in Southern New England for people with drug or alcohol use and living with HIV/AIDS: perspectives of HIV surveillance experts and service providers

Lauretta E. Grau[1]*, Abbie Griffiths-Kundishora[1], Robert Heimer[1], Marguerite Hutcheson[2], Amy Nunn[3], Caitlin Towey[3] and Thomas J. Stopka[2]

Abstract

Background: Contemporary studies about HIV care continuum (HCC) outcomes within substance using populations primarily focus on individual risk factors rather than provider- or systems-level influences. Over 25% of people living with HIV (PLWH) have substance use disorders that can alter their path through the HCC. As part of a study of HCC outcomes in nine small cities in Southern New England (population 100,000–200,000 and relatively high HIV prevalence particularly among substance users), this qualitative analysis sought to understand public health staff and HIV service providers' perspectives on how substance use may influence HCC outcomes.

Methods: Interviews with 49 participants, collected between November 2015 and June 2016, were analyzed thematically using a modified social ecological model as the conceptual framework and codes for substance use, HCC barriers and facilitators, successes and failures of initiatives targeting the HCC, and criminal justice issues.

Results: Eight themes were identified concerning the impact of substance use on HCC outcomes. At the individual level, these included coping and satisfying basic needs and could influence all HCC steps (i.e., testing, treatment linkage, adherence, and retention, and viral load suppression). The interpersonal level themes included stigma issues and providers' cultural competence and treatment attitudes and primarily influenced treatment linkage, retention, and viral load suppression. These same HCC steps were influenced at the health care systems level by organizations' physical environment and resources as well as intra-/inter-agency communication. Testing and retention were the most likely steps to affect at the policy/society level, and the themes included opposition within an organization or community, and activities with unintended consequences.

Conclusions: The most substantial HCC challenges for PLWH with substance use problems included linking and retaining in treatment those with multiple co-morbidities and meeting their basic living needs. Recommendations to improve HCC outcomes for PLWH with substance use problems include increasing easy access to effective drug and mental health treatment, expanding case management and peer navigation services, training staff about harm reduction, de-stigmatizing, and culturally competent approaches to interacting with patients, and increasing information-sharing and service coordination among service providers and the social service and criminal justice systems.

Keywords: HIV/AIDS, Substance use, HIV care continuum

*Correspondence: Lauretta.Grau@yale.edu
[1] Yale School of Public Health, PO Box 208034, New Haven, CT
06520-8034, USA
Full list of author information is available at the end of the article

Background

The HIV care continuum (HCC) framework assesses patients at various steps of human immunodeficiency virus (HIV) diagnosis and care—from identification of cases, to linkage to care and antiretroviral treatment, to retention in care, and ultimately to viral suppression [1]. Each step builds upon the previous, and the proportion of PLWH within each step has important implications for achieving the ultimate goals of viral suppression and reduced HIV transmission [2]. Monitoring the outcome at each HCC step enables us to better identify where and how to intervene—be it a specific HCC step, geographic area, or at-risk population. The HCC is also a tool by which to monitor the UNAIDS 90-90-90 goal of identifying 90% of those infected, linking 90% of those identified to treatment, and achieving 90% viral suppression among those in treatment; it is believed that reaching this goal by 2020 would end the HIV epidemic by 2030 [3].

Despite reported overall improvements in HCC outcomes [4–6], negative associations between substance use and virtually every step on the continuum persist [7–10]. And although medical management of a patient's HIV infection and substance use problems can be complex [11], medication-assisted treatment improved HCC outcomes for PLWH with opioid use disorders [12] and decreased injection risk behavior [13]. Nonetheless, PLWH with substance use problems do not fare as well as other risk groups [4, 9, 14]. PLWH who used substances intermittently or continually were significantly more likely to develop opportunistic infections or experience disease progression or mortality when compared to PLWH with no reported substance use [15]. Substance use problems interfered with progression along the HCC for female PLWH; its treatment and that of related co-morbidities (e.g., depression) could help increase retention in care [16]. In addition to the potential instability that substance use can bring to the lives of PLWH, other sources of instability (i.e., financial, homelessness, housing insecurity, stigma, and food insecurity) also influence HCC retention rates for these individuals [17–19].

It is estimated that over one-quarter of PLWH have substance use disorders [20]. Recent studies have primarily focused on individual risk factors [21–24]. To our knowledge, there is scant information in the literature that examines HIV provider perspectives on the role of substance use in HCC outcomes, how structural or provider factors may influence progression on the continuum for those who use substances, or the role of substance use in continuum outcomes in smaller urban areas. Structural influences such as organizational, social, policy, or economic factors can include the convenience of access to and the array of HIV-related services offered, confidentiality issues, or the existence of laws that discriminate against marginalized populations such as people with substance use problems, commercial sex workers, or undocumented immigrants or seasonal workers. Provider influences can include provider attributes such as provider-initiated HIV testing and counseling as a strong motivator to be tested [25, 26], prescribers' opinions about when to initiate antiretroviral treatment [14], interpersonal skills, and cultural competence and can alter the path of PLWH at various steps of the HCC.

Several initiatives have helped to reduce the negative impact of substance use on HIV prevention, diagnosis, and treatment [27]. These include drug treatment programs that routinely test for HIV [28] and provide HIV prevention education [28]. Harm reduction programs such as syringe services programs (SSPs) that distribute condoms [29, 30] and provide access to testing and HIV and substance abuse treatment have also been demonstrated to be effective [31–38]. Evidence-based interventions that promote linkage and retention, such as case management, improved screening for substance used disorders and mental health, and peer navigators can be effective in improving retention rates [19].

Most HCC research has occurred in large urban and metropolitan areas [39, 40], with less known about HCC outcomes in smaller urban areas where a large share of new HIV infections occur. Structural and sociodemographic factors and geographic access to local resources differ between these larger urban areas and smaller cities and can also vary across smaller cities [41]. In Southern New England, thousands remain undiagnosed, and known cases have been lost to follow-up, thereby jeopardizing their own health and the health of the larger community. Within Connecticut, 8239 of 10,636 PLWH (77%) were engaged in care through 2014. Of those engaged, 81% were retained in care, and 86% were virally suppressed [42]. Among the nearly 20,000 PLWH in Massachusetts as of 2015, 75% were engaged in care, 59% were retained in care, and 28% did not have a viral load test through 2014. Among those who had a viral load test, 65% were virally suppressed, with even lower rates of viral suppression in Western Massachusetts [43]. The number of new HIV diagnoses in Rhode Island increased 33% from 2013 to 2014; 67% of PLWH were engaged in care, 48% were retained in care, and 57% were virally suppressed [44].

This qualitative study was part of a larger pilot project that explored the geographic differences in HCC outcomes in nine small cities in Southern New England (Lowell, Springfield, Worcester, New Bedford, Providence, Hartford, Waterbury, New Haven, and Bridgeport) and addressed the funders' interest in conducting HCC research in small cities across Southern New England. The current analysis used key informant (KI) interviews with HIV service providers and public health staff to understand how substance use problems shape HCC outcomes and to identify potential recommendations to promote receipt of HIV diagnosis, linkage to and retention in care, and viral suppression among PLWH with drug or alcohol problems. Given the time and resource limits of the pilot study, however, we sought to assess HCC outcomes from the multiple perspectives of these individuals (cf., interviews with PLWH) based on our assumption that their knowledge about the existing structural and organizational factors that may influence HCC outcomes would inform a less commonly studied research area and have important implications for future interventions to improve HCC outcomes.

Methods

City selection

We included cities with populations of 100,000–200,000 and relatively high HIV prevalence, particularly among people who use drugs and men who have sex with men (MSM). In addition, the cities differed in terms of how they have responded to the HIV epidemic, with only some implementing SSPs.

Study sample

Using a purposive sampling strategy that targeted staff with HCC-associated responsibilities (e.g., service provision, surveillance, monitoring), potential participants were initially identified through recommendations by state public health officials, an internet search of HIV service organizations in the nine cities, and purposive and snowball sampling of the authors' colleagues working in the HIV field who satisfied the inclusion criteria. Given the extent of the authors' (LG, RH, AN, TS) previous HIV and harm reduction research, many participants had established relationships with these individuals. Enrolled subjects subsequently referred us to other potential subjects.

Potential subjects were contacted by telephone or email and, if eligible, were scheduled for an interview. Inclusion criteria were: (1) individuals working in or responsible for HCC-related work in one of the nine cities (e.g., HIV surveillance staff at state or local health departments, Ryan White policy makers or administrators, HIV-associated service providers such as health care providers, early intervention specialists, disease intervention specialists, case managers, social workers, peer navigators); (2) at least five years of experience in the HIV field; and (3) English speaking. There were no refusals to participate among those who were eligible for the study.

We interviewed 49 participants between November 2015 and June 2016; there were no follow-up interviews. All were scheduled as individual, face-to-face interviews

with trained interviewers (LG, MH, AK, CT, TS). One interviewer was male; all held advanced degrees in the fields of public health or social science or had previous qualitative research experience. Seven KIs had invited other staff members to join based upon the belief that those other people could offer additional information about one of the interview domains. We honored the original KI's decision and confirmed that these additional KIs satisfied inclusion criteria. The interviews lasted approximately 60 min, were digitally recorded, and subsequently transcribed verbatim (transcripts were not reviewed by participants). The study was deemed exempt from human subjects research by the IRBs at Yale, Tufts, and Brown University. The interviews began after an informed consent discussion, and participants received a $25 gift card as reimbursement for the interview.

Data collection and analysis

The entire research team developed and reviewed a draft interview guide that included the five HCC steps as interview domains and assessed participants' perceptions about the specific successes and challenges encountered for each step (i.e., HIV testing, treatment linkage, initiation of antiretroviral therapy, treatment retention, and viral suppression). Probes for each HCC step included asking about the perceived *availability* and *accessibility* of HIV-associated services, treatment *acceptability* by PLWH, and *affordability* of such care [45].

While the five HCC steps served to structure and organize the flow and topics covered during the interviews, we used a modified social ecological model as the conceptual framework by which to organize the salient themes about the relationship between substance use and HCC outcomes [2, 46, 47]. The modified social ecological model is a multilevel model that situates the individual within the social and structural context when examining health outcomes [46]. The individual level includes demographic, biologic, and behavioral factors and intrapsychic factors such as self-efficacy and motivation. The individual level is contained within the social or interpersonal level which, in turn, is contained within the community level (which focused exclusively on the health and social service systems in the current analysis), and all are contained within the society or policy level. The latter two levels focus on structural factors.

Once transcripts were available, the coding team (LG, AK, MH) independently coded six transcripts and met weekly to discuss coding decisions and develop the codebook. Any coding discrepancies were resolved by consensus. Additional codes and further refinement of the codebook also occurred during these sessions. When no new codes were identified (i.e., thematic saturation was achieved) and acceptable inter-coder reliability had been achieved, the remaining transcripts were independently coded (by AK or MH) and reviewed by the first author when entering the data into ATLAS.ti (Version 7.1.7). Codes pertaining to substance use, HCC barriers and facilitators, successes and failures of initiatives targeting the HCC, and criminal justice issues were analyzed thematically [48, 49] in an iterative fashion, using an inductive approach wherein themes were grounded in the data. The coding team identified common patterns across the dataset, grouped them into themes, and sought negative instances where the data did not fit the existing themes as part of the confirmability process [50]. To improve readability without compromising content, all colloquialisms, hesitations, and non-verbal utterances were removed from the quotes. Participants did not review the analytic findings.

Themes were grouped by level within the modified social ecological model and specifically focused on the impact of substance use on HCC outcomes. Hence, the interpersonal level themes were restricted to those that shaped the client-provider relationship or motivation to seek testing or treatment and community level themes to those involving care for PLWH. A total of nine themes were identified across the four levels of the modified social ecological (Fig. 1). It should be noted that the influence of each theme on the HCC could be positive or negative, depending upon the degree to which each is present or absent.

Results

Description of the study sample

The majority of participants held supervisory or administrative positions within AIDS service organizations (ASOs) and had detailed knowledge about the types and quality of local services available (Table 1). Interviews with regional Ryan White administrators and state-level epidemiologists and program managers provided

Table 1 Description of study sample and interview types

Interview characteristics	Participants no. (%)
State (N = 44 interviews)	
Connecticut	18 (41)
Massachusetts	21 (48)
Rhode Island	5 (11)
Interviews per city (N = 38)	
Bridgeport, CT	4 (10.5)
Hartford, CT	4 (10.5)
New Haven, CT	4 (10.5)
Waterbury, CT	4 (10.5)
Lowell, MA	5 (13)
New Bedford, MA	4 (10.5)
Springfield, MA	6 (16)
Worcester, MA	4 (10.5)
Providence, RI	3 (8)
Organization type (N = 44 interviews)[a]	
State Health Department	5 (11)
Local Health Department	3 (7)
Ryan White (local and regional)	4 (1)
AIDS Service Organization	36 (82)
Staff type (N = 49 participants)[a]	
Regional/state program administration	6 (12)
Local administrative/supervisory	31 (63)
Medical providers (MD/APRN)	8 (16)
Case management/EIS/DIS	6 (12)
Sex (N = 49 participants)	
Female	23 (47)
Male	26 (53)

A total of 49 individuals participated in the interviews

[a] Some interviews involved participants with multiple job responsibilities

a broader, "bird's eye view" of the HCC and local services. Interviews with local medical providers (16%) and caseworkers (12%) provided examples of HCC successes

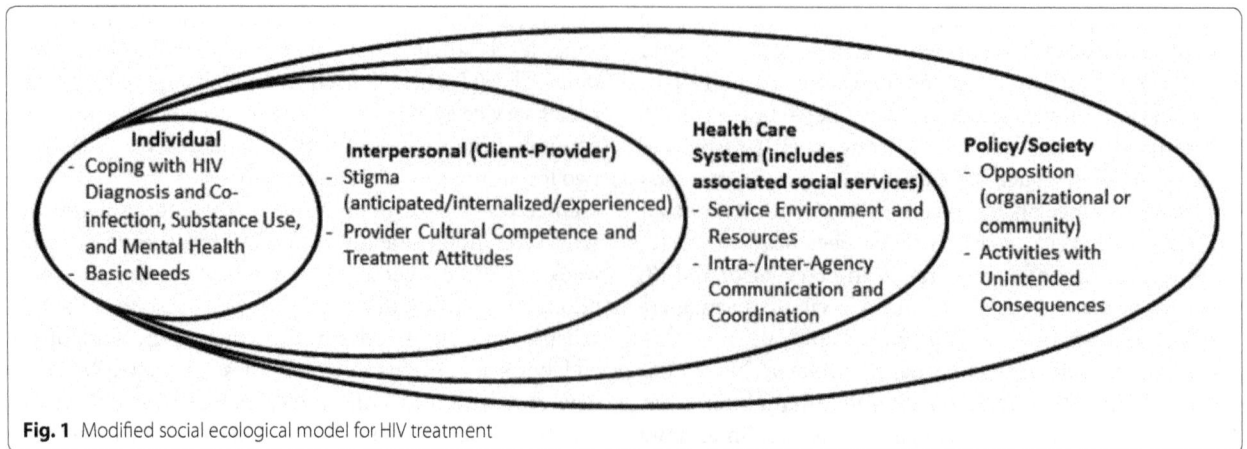

Fig. 1 Modified social ecological model for HIV treatment

and failures from participants' experiences working with PLWH with substance use problems.

Successful initiatives to improve the HCC

Before identifying the themes about how substance use problems shape HCC outcomes, it is important to acknowledge the improvements that have already been achieved in reducing the negative impact of drug and alcohol use on HCC outcomes. These included reductions in HIV incidence in conjunction with HIV testing and prevention efforts at SSPs, community expansion of medication-assisted treatment, and efforts within the Department of Corrections. A medical provider acknowledged that expanded syringe access through SSPs and pharmacy sales has *"kind of done it already [fewer HIV cases among entering inmates within the Department of Corrections] with injection drug use."* Others noted the community's belief in the public health benefits of SSPs, in one case assuming operation of the SSP when city officials wanted to discontinue it.

> *We don't see as many intravenous drug users getting infected as we did, obviously, because they have access to syringes. (Participant 13, Male, ASO administrator)*

> *And [the community has] come together to do the [SSP] van and to expand services going—that's the heart that exists here. There was no turf. It's like we need, for our folks, we're going to do what it takes. (Participant 11, Male, Ryan White administrator)*

Efforts within the criminal justice system have also improved HCC outcomes by identifying new infections or resuming treatment among entering inmates who had been lost to treatment. These advances were acknowledged by virtually all participants with knowledge about Department of Corrections activities or data.

> *We are not testing nearly as much as we used to at the DoC, and that's mostly because the number of positives dropped dramatically when the epidemic shifted away from injection drug use. (Participant 39, Male, Medical Provider)*

Individual level themes

The advances noted above, notwithstanding, PLWH who use drugs or alcohol continue to face challenges that can affect HCC outcomes. These include the individual's coping style, comorbid conditions (e.g., hepatitis C virus co-infection, substance abuse, mental health), and resources to meet basic needs (e.g., housing, food security, transportation, clothing, childcare).

Coping with HIV diagnosis and comorbidities

Receiving an HIV diagnosis, being co-infected, or having mental health problems (whether associated with or independent of the HIV diagnosis) can be a source of stress that some PLWH may attempt to cope with by self-medicating with alcohol or drugs. Ongoing substance use problems can, in turn, pose significant barriers to the HCC steps of treatment linkage, adherence, and viral suppression. Many identified the need for mental health services to address either the co-morbid condition or maladaptive coping style.

> *Mental health is a big one. "I'm depressed; therefore, I'm not taking it [HIV medications]." (Participant 1, Female, ASO administrator)*

> *A lot of times what we've found is it's people with mental health issues trying to make themselves feel better by using substance. (Participant 9, Male, ASO administrator)*

How problems with substance use and co-morbidities manifest can be highly idiosyncratic. Many participants reported that clients with ongoing substance use or who had experienced relapse—particularly with opioids—often stopped receiving their regular HIV care. By contrast, a few participants observed that some PLWH remained highly engaged in their treatment despite using drugs or alcohol. The possible reasons for these observed differences remained unclear, however.

> *[HIV infection is] a tremendous psychological stress that people carry with them day in, day out, and some people respond well to it and some don't. (Participant 39, Male, Medical Provider) Some people end up, when they're actively using drugs, [they] are out there and not taking meds and not keeping their appointments, and just disappear and have a whole other mode of circling and who they're seeing. And on the other hand we have folks that are actively using heroin and have a pretty stable pattern of life and [are] coming in for their visits and taking all their meds and, and the heroin is not destabilizing. (Participant 31, Male, Medical Provider)*

> *And I think that even those individuals who are in care who are using...I think they do not want to do harm to their families or the women and/or men in their lives. I think they want to make sure that they are protecting them and their selves, and so I think that has all to do with the retention rate. (Participant 15, Female, City Health Department)*

Inherent in attempts to cope with a given health problem is the level of motivation to seek help.

Although less frequently mentioned, motivation to enter mental health or substance abuse treatment was viewed as critical to successful HIV treatment linkage, retention, and adherence. Participants noted that for substance abuse problems in particular, bureaucratic hassles and ineffective treatments can seriously reduce the chances of entry into treatment that could mitigate substance use problems that interfere with HIV treatment adherence.

> With substance abuse, there has to be a desire to actually want to get help. I would let them know where those resources are, but I can't like physically force them to go. (Participant 5, Female, Case worker)

> You want to get in the detox because you're finally sick of drinking and using drugs, and it's such a dehumanizing process. You go through this long intake and then they say, "Oh, we don't take your insurance, try this other place," or "Okay, we're going to put you on the waiting list. You'll have to call us three times a day to find out if we get a bed open." And it's days and usually by the time a bed does open, so many people have lost their motivation and just said, "Screw it, I'm going to go out and get another bag of dope." (Participant 12, Female, ASO administrator)

> [Detox is] a band-aid. It doesn't—it has yet to work once since I've been at [this clinic]. (Participant 48, Female, Medical Provider)

Fulfilling basic living needs

Basic needs such as housing, food, and transportation, if unmet, can also pose significant challenges to PLWH. Participants reported that these unmet needs can be stressful, leading to substance use or relapse and are often higher priorities than is treatment linkage or adherence. Housing opportunities were a *"major, major issue"* according to participants, and the possibility of stable housing was especially limited for those with substance use problems.

> Everything just piggybacks each other, housing, transportation, food, income, medication, doctors' appointments, everything just piggybacks each other. (Participant 47, Female, Case worker)

> But it's very hard to place somebody in housing that doesn't have a job or somebody who is multiple evictions. Those things are still factors in placing folks in housing. Somebody with significant or severe mental

health and substance abuse challenges, those things still are challenges for people accessing stable housing. (Participant 18, Female, Ryan White administrator)

> I mean, the care of HIV itself is not the problem. It's just all of the other social situations surrounding it that make it challenging. So we have one patient that I think I saw last who came in here today who is living in her car. (Participant 24, Female, ASO administrator)

> Somebody might let the medicines go while they're working on the housing. (Participant 31, Male, Medical Provider)

Interpersonal level themes
Stigma

PLWH are susceptible to three types of stigma: (1) enacted stigma or individuals' belief that they had a stigmatizing experience associated with their having HIV infection, mental health problems, or drug or alcohol use, (2) anticipated stigma or individuals' expectation of experiencing stigma in some future situation or context, and (3) internalized stigma or the degree to which individuals endorse the negative attributes associated with one or all of these health problems [51]. Although many acknowledged that HIV stigma has decreased over time, participants primarily discussed stigma in terms of anticipated HIV stigma within the clients' communities (most notably immigrant or minority communities) and far less frequently from service providers. The anticipated stigma which could impact HCC outcomes was most frequently based on concerns about being stigmatized because of potential confidentiality breaches within these small cities.

> There's stigma about HIV. There's stigma about mental illness. There's stigma about addiction. There's stigma about a number of things. So it seems sort of multi-layered issues. (Participant 39, Male, Medical provider)

> Stigma. They don't want people to see—in a small city, people know each other...That is big. People will see them going into a clinic. People will see them going into an HIV anything, and they don't want to be seen doing that. (Participant 29, Female, ASO administrator and clinician)

> So I think one of the challenges to testing is stigma, and what happens, and who has access to your information, and what... what if my partner finds out? What if my family finds out? (Participant 30, Female, ASO administrator)

I tell my clients right off the bat, because I live in [this city] and I'm in the area and I see a lot of you, when I'm with my family to keep your information confidential and so that your information isn't breached. When I'm with my family I don't speak to my clients. (Participant 45, Female, Case worker)

Participants occasionally noted how PLWH may have experienced stigma from their HIV service providers and organizations. It could involve actual experiences with specific providers or how the physical layout of services within the organization could shape stigma perceptions. Of note is that no one mentioned staff training on stigma issues.

I have patients here who say they feel stigmatized every time they're interacting with their medical provider, their ID specialists. They're being treated like an addict. (Participant 6, Male, ASO administrator)

Our offices are separate from the adult medicine offices, so even some members of the community, when they come up here, they know if you look to the left, this is where people living with HIV go, and [to the right] is where people who are not living with HIV go. One of our goals is to change that, because, I mean I personally think that it drives stigma. Just the idea that you're living with HIV, you can't receive your medical care where everybody else is receiving their medical care. (Participant 42, Male, ASO administrator)

More frequently, participants identified organizational strategies to reduce the potential for stigma. These included giving clinics names that did not identify them as uniquely HIV clinics or incorporating HIV services into non-HIV clinics.

Instead of calling it the HIV department or the infectious disease department, Cardenio (sic) means caring and loving in Spanish...and the thought behind it was the caring, and loving, and compassion that somebody can receive. When we moved to this building, we really had a hard time identifying how do we designate our area, how do people know that they can come to this floor without feeling stigmatized and so it's our attempt for somebody to be able to come in and say, "I'm here to see the Cardenio (sic) department" versus "I'm here for HIV services." (Participant 37, Female, ASO administrator)

And in that same vein, to reduce the stigma, we don't want to be just an HIV testing van, hep C testing van. Our signs are we do blood pressure, glucose

screening, so you can all come in. You can get a vaccination. (Participant 28, Female, Medical Provider)

Staff cultural competence and treatment attitudes

Positive client-provider relationships were thought to be critical to the success of HIV treatment linkage, adherence, and retention. Although the merits of a harm reduction approach (i.e., "meeting people where they are at") and staff assuming a respectful, non-judgmental, and supportive stance with their clients are key to positive relationships for any health problem and client population, participants noted that these can be particularly important when interacting with PLWH with drug or alcohol problems. They recognized that shame and guilt issues—about substance use in addition to HIV—can be incapacitating at times. Sensitive and culturally competent interactions, both in the workplace and when staff encounter clients out in the community, are critical to ensuring that clients remain engaged or re-engage in care. However, it should also be noted that discussion about cultural competence most often focused on the number of languages spoken by staff and far less frequently on the attitudes or behaviors that demonstrate cultural competence.

We're culturally competent here and when we hire staff, we try to get a good array of people that come from different cultures and speak the languages [spoken in this region]. (Participant 2, Female, ASO administrator)

For me, the surface of culturally competent care is care delivered in the language that the person feels most comfortable speaking and understanding. And maybe even the person speaking that language coming from a similar background to the person that's receiving the education or [care]...So it's our effort to make sure that we can, at the very least, provide language services...My philosophy, and when I talk to our staff is [that] it's more about just withholding judgment. I mean, part of being culturally competent is knowing that you can't be completely culturally competent because if you were, then you're just basing that competency on norms which don't apply to everybody. So when people are coming in and talking about certain attitudes and certain beliefs and understandings about the care that they're coming into access, for me, it's more about just greeting that understanding with an open mind and trying to understand where it's coming from and trying to do what you can to address those issues without being, I guess, condescending or without the appearance of being rude or without making the person feel like they are stupid. Which can be complicated because if somebody holds a belief really firmly, and you're trying to have a discussion with them that sort of is contradicting that belief, then that can be a difficult conversation. (Participant 42, Male, ASO administrator)

Attitudes concerning initiation of antiretroviral therapy varied, particularly for PLWH with drug or alcohol problems, with most stating that it should be initiated as soon as possible. By contrast, providers in one city stated their reluctance to initiate treatment until the patients' housing, substance use, mental health, or other medical or social service problems were stabilized—some estimating this process could take as long as 6 months.

It just doesn't make sense to prescribe somebody antiretrovirals and they don't have a place to live, ya know, or they...they're actively using drugs and they have uncontrolled schizophrenia, really? It doesn't make sense, so I really feel strongly you got to address those things first. (Participant 3, Male, Medical Provider)

I have people using crack who have non-detectable viral loads, so it makes me think that they [ART and crack use] can happen at the same time. (Participant 48, Female, Medical Provider)

I've known this for years, you got to give them access and availability to a pill, no matter what. (Participant 32, Male, State Health Department)

Health care systems level themes

Themes at the health care systems level occurred internally within a given organization as well as across organizations and agencies. They were thought to influence HIV treatment, linkage, and retention for people who use drugs or alcohol and included two themes: (1) the organization's environment such as the services that were available, its physical location and layout, and hours of operation and (2) intra- and inter-agency communications and coordination of services.

Service organization environment and resources

Virtually all participants noted the complexity of service needs for PLWH with drug or alcohol problems and agreed that increased availability of and easy accessibility to these needed services was key to improving HCC outcomes. Beyond providing for the basics such as housing, clothing, and food, participants reported that clients often required transportation or daycare services so they could attend their various HIV-related appointments.

Clients often needed case management services or other specialty services (e.g., treatment for substance use or mental health problems, hepatitis C virus treatment, physical therapy for motor problems, support and group therapy meetings) or help in managing their finances. The extent to which "one-stop shopping" was possible increased the potential for successful HCC outcomes. Co-locating multiple medical and social services, having flexible office hours, the opportunity for walk-in visits, and being able to address multiple health and social service problems in a single visit facilitated HIV treatment retention and adherence. ASOs that offered on-site services with substance abuse counselors, psychiatric nurses, and/or infectious disease specialists (to treat both HIV and hepatitis C infections) were believed to greatly enhance client care and consequently HCC outcomes. Although medication-assisted treatment services were not co-located at any of the ASOs in this study, referrals to local providers were offered in an attempt to facilitate access to and availability of these services.

[Directly observed therapy] can get done at either place [van or storefront], but usually we like to see them on the van and then we can address any other issues, medical or social, and then we link them either back up to [their case worker] or back up to their primary doctor. And I also can do some primary care with them as well, so they don't have to try to get an appointment to see their primary medical doctor if I can see them in five minutes—the van is like an urgent care center and it's kind of, it's very quick, very fast. (Participant 28, Female, Medical Provider)

And even if I see somebody who might want to have me as a source of their HIV care, I will refer them to the health center, because they've got a whole other bucket of needs that I can't really fulfill, so sort of one-stop shopping. (Participant 43, Male, Medical Provider)

The importance of case management and peer-to-peer programs was repeatedly linked to successful HCC outcomes. It was clear in interviews with medical providers that they respected and viewed case managers, peer navigators, early intervention specialist, and disease intervention specialists as highly knowledgeable about their patients' current life situations. Providers relied upon these staff for re-engaging clients who use drugs or alcohol—often among the most difficult to retain in care—after missed appointments. Hence, co-location of medical and case management services afforded opportunities for frequent staff interactions and quicker response when patients missed appointments.

It all depends when the doctor calls you and said, "I haven't seen this patient in a while," and then I go look for them and then go try to find them. Usually I can find them maybe in a couple hours. Maybe it'll take me a day—because I already have [an] idea. See, there's a lot of clients that we see on the van that we already know their routines, so it's like I walk down the street, like I'll go from here to downtown, might see ten people living with HIV that I know, so the first thing I ask them, "When was the last time you seen your doctor?" So they said, "Well, I haven't seen the doctor in six months, I'm having a drinking problem." I grab the phone, make an appointment... we link them right there. (Participant 33, Male, Case worker)

I was able to hire a nurse and a peer specifically to carry about twenty cases of the most difficult patients to retain in care. And that money is running out [at] the end of July on [that] project, but the state just decided to pick it up because here it's been extremely—extremely successful. (Participant 13, Male, ASO administrator)

Intra- and inter-agency communications and coordination

Most cities attempted to facilitate information-sharing and open communications among HIV service providers in order to best serve their clients. Some accomplished this by having new clients sign consents permitting the organizations to share information between organizations such as medical laboratories, hospitals, social service and medical providers, drug treatment programs, and the Department of Corrections. City-wide meetings also took place to address HCC issues. The local PLWH community participated in some of these meetings in order to empower and engage them in local efforts to improve HCC outcomes and inform service providers about the types of successes, challenges, and recommendations that could guide client-centered and community-engaged prevention and care. Regional Ryan White meetings were another way that providers evaluated and discussed strategies to improve the HCC at the local or regional level. Yet although formal meetings were helpful, it appeared that informal communications were more frequently used to solve problems for individual clients.

The patients already signed a consent to let us work with any of their providers and [access their electronic medical record]. (Participant 28, Female, Medical Provider)

[The ASOs in the region] meet once a month. They will look at quality data. They will look at expendi-tures. They will look at service utilization data. They will talk about barriers. They will talk every single month about what's going on in this community and what they can do and even down to expenditures where I can say "You know what, I have emergency financial assistance money in my organization and you know what, we're going to run out. Does anybody have—?" "Oh, we have plenty. Why don't you refer your clients over to us and we'll take care of it for them." (Participant 11, Male, Ryan White Administrator)

Coordination with the Department of Corrections was also crucial to HCC outcomes when PLWH transitioned back to the community, particularly for those with histories of substance use as is the case for many—if not the majority—of those incarcerated.

What gets you in jail, it's—I mean there are some folks with violence charges and things like that, domestic and, but it's mainly addiction that's behind it, (Participant 31, Male, Medical Provider)

Participants noted that, prior to incarceration, many PLWH may have discontinued their HIV treatment. Incarceration represented an opportunity to resume HIV treatment that would be important to continue after release. Recognizing the high risk of relapse and potential need for post-incarceration substance abuse treatment, participants considered coordination of the responsibilities of parole/probation officers and case managers to be particularly critical to ensuring that the person remained in HIV treatment and did not return to prison due to probation/parole violation (which often involves illicit drug use).

We start working with them at least three months before they are released and then we assess what would be those challenges for them to stay in care once they are out of the jail. (Participant 36, Male, Case Worker)

When they come out of jail, I'll go to probation and meet with them. I'll talk to the probation. I have a drug counselor. I have a psychiatrist. I have primary care that we could help them. We maintain the medicines and once I tell them the plans that we got, the probation office is happy with us because we got a good relation with the probation officer because we'll do their work [perform weekly urine screens, find the person]. (Participant 33, Male, Case worker)

Less frequently, participants reported that transfer of care was less than ideal in terms of notifying the ASO in a timely way of a prisoner's release.

[The case worker] sometimes get notice that morning that so-and-so inmate is being released today, and they have to find a place for this person to go, and sometimes there's no place for them to go. (Participant 1, Female, ASO administrator)

So we tested him at the jail. He got connected with some kind of service. I don't believe he got connected with medical care there because he was going to leave and once he was out, he just disappeared until we found him months later. (Participant 40, Female, ASO administrator)

Policy/society level themes

We identified two themes at the policy/society level: opposition and activities with unintended consequences.

Organizational and community opposition

The first addresses opposition in the form of policies or actions that could pose challenges to improving the HCC for at-risk populations such as those who use drugs or alcohol. The opposition could occur within an organization or within the larger community. The distinction is that organizations have unique internal procedures and contexts, and the larger community rarely has the opportunity to influence the organization's decisions or policies. By contrast, community residents often can influence decisions about the budgets, programs, and policies of the local government.

Substance use-related visits to emergency departments (e.g., overdose/poisoning, trauma/falls while intoxicated, end-stage liver disease from alcohol use or hepatitis C infection) are not uncommon. Yet organizational opposition resulted in discontinuing routine, opt-out HIV testing in one hospital's Emergency Department based on organizational doubt about the public health benefit of opt-out testing and desire to minimize potential bad publicity about legal problems during the pending sale of the hospital. This decision thereby decreased opportunities to identify cases among at-risk individuals who may have never been tested elsewhere.

The [new] director of the emergency room...just does not think this is the place for public health issues in [the] emergency room. That's his attitude and you shouldn't be doing [HIV testing] here...I literally just came from a meeting an hour and a half ago and they said "We're not interested at this hospital in pursuing that right now."...[the hospital is] in the middle of some legal stuff going on with that right now...the hospital is [also] being bought by another company and we're getting to the closing and [the hospital is] just not interested in any bad publicity

right now, so it's not a good time for me to be talking about [routine HIV testing] in our emergency room, but it's still something I'm very excited about. (Participant 3, Male, Medical Provider)

Despite the strong empirical evidence that SSPs can improve HCC outcomes [31, 32, 34–36, 38], programs faced challenges in operating in certain cities because of community opposition to the program, perceptions that SSPs are no longer needed, or inability to sustain regular hours when the SSP van required maintenance.

[The city council said,] "And so why would needle exchange help, because it's not helping that the [HIV] numbers are down. So because the hepatitis C numbers were up is what really got [the city council] to do something different. But otherwise they'd say, "Why do we need it? What do we need testing for? The numbers are down." (Participant 14, Female, City Health Department)

[The SSP clients] go, "You're not here," and we go, "Yeah, we're really sorry, but we couldn't get the van out," or sometimes the van, the van's a vehicle, like a car, so everyone's like, "I need another van," because we need one to [substitute just like] you need two cars in a house to take one to the mechanic, so this thing has to go in and get oil changes, mechanic, go get gasoline, it's not like it's a structure that stands. (Participant 33, Male, Case worker)

Activites with unintended consequences

Finally, anti-crime efforts and attempts to "clean up" high-risk neighborhoods resulted in the unintended consequence of increasing barriers to HIV testing and linkage efforts, particularly for people who inject drugs and men who have sex with men.

Well, a lot of abandoned buildings have been torn down. They redesigned the bus terminal and there's policing out there, so there's not a lot of people just hanging out anymore, same as the train station. So [activities of men who have sex with men have] gone more underground. Same as the drug use. It's gone more underground. (Participant 30, Female, ASO administrator)

Discussion and conclusions

The HCC strengths and successes noted by participants in the nine cities were many, although the 90-90-90 goal of the Joint United Nations Programme on HIV/AIDS [3] was not yet met by any of the ASOs participating in this study. ASO administrators were quick to note steady improvement in HCC outcomes over time, however. The most substantial HCC challenges noted were in linking and retaining HIV patients with multiple co-morbidities (substance use disorder, hepatitis C viral infection, mental health problems) and essential needs such as housing, food security, and transportation. These findings were consistent with previous studies and were thought to occur at all levels of the modified social ecological model [16, 19, 52–54].

At the individual level, per those interviewed, PLWH with ongoing or relapses in drug or alcohol use often had chaotic lives that frequently led to discontinuation of HIV treatment. These observations were consistent with the literature. Alcohol use was associated with poor HIV health outcomes [55–57]. Drug use often increased in response to tendencies to cope with receiving a diagnosis of HIV infection [58]. Expanding the availability of and easy access to effective drug and mental health treatments is recommended to reduce risk of delaying or discontinuing HIV treatment. The lives of PLWH with substance use problems could be further stabilized by ensuring secure living conditions (e.g., housing, food security, transportation) [59]. In addition, encouraging clients to actively engage in decisions about their care and to connect with other HIV consumers could increase opportunities for socioemotional support and promote a sense of community that may be particularly important for those whose social capital is largely confined to fellow substance users.

At the interpersonal level, it is well known that developing and maintaining positive client-staff relationships is essential to the successful provision of any healthcare or social service [60, 61] and was noted as essential to improving HCC outcomes in this and other studies [58]. Cultural competence and a non-judgmental, harm reduction approach were key to positive interactions, particularly for clients with internalized or anticipated stigma as a result of their substance use. It is, therefore, recommended that all staff receive periodic training on harm reduction, de-stigmatizing, and culturally competent approaches to interacting with PLWH with substance use problems in order to limit the potential for negative interactions that could ultimately compromise client-staff relationships and increase risk of discontinuing treatment.

We identified several themes at the health care system and policy/society levels—levels that are less frequently addressed in HCC research [14, 25]. At the health care system level, many of those incarcerated had histories of substance use, and although they qualified for housing benefits as PLWH, the availability of this entitlement was limited. In addition, incarceration provided an opportunity to return many to HIV treatment. This return to treatment is important to sustain post-release by not only linking these individuals to HIV treatment but also to substance abuse treatment services when indicated. Hence, permitting ASOs, other social and health service providers, and the Departments of Corrections to easily share individual patients' data (e.g., current HCC status, medical care, social service needs and benefits) would permit quicker identification of and a more coordinated effort to satisfying individuals' service needs as well as improving HIV treatment adherence and retention rates. By obtaining consent from everyone at the time of HIV diagnosis and linkage, such information could be shared with the relevant parties. It is suggested that consents be routinely updated when changes in care and services occur. The goal would be for all systems to remain as flexible and responsive as possible to the individual PLWH's personal needs and preferences while preserving confidentiality. Bureaucratic barriers made such efforts difficult at times, particularly with respect to housing and in cases where PLWH were about to be released from detoxification treatment, prison, or jail. These barriers can create challenges for the HCC steps of treatment retention and viral suppression.

Perhaps the most compelling structural issue noted at the health care system level was the importance of case workers and peer navigators in retaining clients in care or returning them to care [52, 58, 62], particularly for cases of relapse in substance use. Although funding concerns were noted more generally and went beyond the scope of the current analysis, ASO administrators and providers were acutely aware that fluctuations in funding negatively impacted staffing considerations and desires to expand peer-to-peer programs. Coupled with the evidence from modelling studies that treatment retention is critical to improving HCC outcomes [63, 64] and that PLWH who either have ongoing substance use or who relapse are often among the most difficult clients to retain [7, 9, 65], case workers and peers are central to maintaining or returning them to treatment [66, 67], and salaries for these individuals should be ensured at all times.

Another key issue for those interviewed was making a comprehensive array of services available under one roof (i.e., "one-stop shopping"). Consistent with other studies, these services should be convenient [25], acceptable to consumers, and effective in addressing their treatment needs [16, 68]. The data indicated that agencies worked, with little evidence of inter-agency competition, to optimize coordination of both health and social services as much as possible when "one-stop shopping" was impossible. For those with opioid and alcohol dependence, medication-assisted treatment has been demonstrated to be cost-effective [69] and improves HCC outcomes [11, 14, 70]. Although co-location of HIV and medication-assisted treatment services did not exist at any of the organizations included in this study, it may be particularly important and worth exploring, given participants' assertions of the tight-knit nature and close proximity of many local community collaborations and in the interest of better serving PLWH and improving HCC outcomes.

At the policy/society level, the community usually has little influence on organizational opposition to internal policies or decisions; this is in marked contrast to that of its potential influence at the community level. Hence, it is crucial to maximize communities' potential influence at this level by ensuring that local governments are transparent about policies and activities and are open to discussions about harm reduction and HIV and substance abuse treatment efforts that include not only the members of the general community but also those with substance use problems. In addition, attempts to "clean up" neighborhoods in at least one of the nine cities made public health outreach efforts to test, link, or return PLWH to treatment particularly difficult for hard-to-reach populations such as people who inject drugs and men who have sex with men. To mitigate the potential for negative collateral consequences resulting from such policy decisions, public health officials and consumers should be involved in the decision-making process.

All three states permit syringe purchase at pharmacies without a prescription [71] as part of efforts to reduce HIV incidence. Yet SSPs were not legally authorized in five of the nine cities at the time of this study, despite the proven effectiveness of SSPs in HIV prevention and as a resource for HIV testing [32, 34, 36, 38], access to social and health services [72–75], HIV treatment [31, 35], and referral to drug treatment for injectors and non-injectors alike [33, 37]. In addition, many SSPs offer opioid overdose prevention and response training and distribution of naloxone which can save lives of PLWH who use opioids. It is therefore recommended that SSPs be implemented or expanded as a means of continuing the low HIV incidence among people who use drugs. SSPs can play an integral role in improving HCC outcomes by facilitating access to HIV testing, diagnosis, and linkage to treatment. Expansion of SSPs is occurring at a relatively fast pace in Massachusetts, following new amendments to syringe access legislation. In 2016, new SSPs in Worcester, Brockton, Lawrence, Greenfield, and North Adams were authorized and have the potential to greatly improve HCC outcomes in these small cities and non-urban areas.

The study had several limitations. First, the qualitative data were collected only from experienced HIV providers and public health staff. Hence, it is unclear whether the experiences and perceptions of PLWH about what shapes HCC outcomes are consistent with those of the KIs interviewed in this pilot study. In a follow-up study, we will soon interview PLWH both in and out of treatment to clarify this issue. Second, it appeared that participants were more willing to discuss the strengths and successes of their programs rather than HCC barriers or challenges attributable to organizational limitations. However, thematic saturation was achieved, and we therefore assume that additional interviews would not have identified additional themes. It is hoped that such limitations and gaps in knowledge could be addressed in future interviews with PLWH. Finally, the qualitative findings and associated recommendations are based upon a limited number of interviews within each city and state. Future studies are necessary to determine if additional themes exist, whether any of these findings apply to other locations, and whether the suggested recommendations will improve HCC outcomes for PLWH with drug and alcohol problems.

In conclusion, HCC outcomes have improved over time, but challenges persist. For PLWH with substance use problems and reside in smaller cities, there is a critical need for increased availability of and access to medication-assisted treatment and mental health services. Ideally, these and other ancillary services should be co-located with HIV treatment services. Expansion of case management and peer navigation services is also recommended in order to improve HIV treatment retention and re-engagement for this population. Finally, the data suggest that improved communication and coordination of services are necessary to improve HCC outcomes for PLWH who use substances. These objectives may be more easily achieved in small cities.

Authors' contributions
LEG and TJS were the Co-Principal Investigators and were responsible for the overall design and execution of the study and overall monitoring of data collection at the three sites. RH and AN provided guidance on the study design and interpretation of the data. AK, MH, and CT assisted in data collection, codebook development, and coding. LEG, TS, RH, and AN agreed to ensuring that questions related to the accuracy or integrity of any part of the work are appropriately investigated and resolved. All authors read and approved the final manuscript.

Author details
[1] Yale School of Public Health, PO Box 208034, New Haven, CT 06520-8034, USA. [2] Tufts University School of Medicine, Boston, MA 02111, USA. [3] Brown University School of Public Health, Providence, RI 02912, USA.

Acknowledgements
The authors would especially like to thank the community of public health staff and HIV service providers in the three states for their thoughtful insights and enthusiasm about this project.

Competing interests
The authors declare that they have no competing interests.

Consent for publication
An informed written consent was obtained from the subjects who were interviewed as part of this study.

Funding
This work was funded by Grants from the National Institute of Mental Health (P30MH062294) and National Institute of Allergy and Infectious Diseases (P30AI042853).

References

1. Centers for Disease Control and Prevention. Selected national HIV prevention and care outcomes in the United States. 2016. https://www.cdc.gov/hiv/pdf/library/factsheets/cdc-hiv-national-hiv-care-outcomes.pdf. Accessed 1 Dec 2016.
2. Mugavero MJ, Amico KR, Horn T, Thompson MA. The state of engagement in HIV care in the United States: from cascade to continuum to control. Clin Infect Dis. 2013;57:1164–71.
3. UNAIDS. 90-90-90 An ambitious treatment target to help end the AIDS epidemic. 2014. http://www.unaids.org/sites/default/files/media_asset/90-90-90_en_0.pdf. Accessed 1 Dec 2016.
4. Chakraborty H, Iyer M, Duffus WA, Samantapudi AV, Albrecht H, Weissman S. Disparities in viral load and CD4 count trends among HIV-infected adults in South Carolina. AIDS Patient Care ST. 2015;29:26–32.
5. Rebeiro PF, Gange SJ, Horberg MA, Abraham AG, Napravnik S, Samji H, et al. Geographic variations in clinical retention in care among HIV-infected adults in the United States. PLoS ONE. 2016;11:e0146119.
6. Toren KG, Buskin SE, Dombrowski JC, Cassels SL, Golden MR. Time from HIV diagnosis to viral load suppression: 2007–2013. Sex Transm Dis. 2016;43:34–40.
7. Chitsaz E, Meyer JP, Krishnan A, Springer SA, Marcus R, Zaller N, et al. Contribution of substance use disorders on HIV treatment outcomes and antiretroviral medication adherence among HIV-infected persons entering jail. AIDS Behav. 2013;17:S118–27.
8. Cofrancesco J, Scherzer R, Tien PC, Gilbert CL, Southwell H, Sidney S, et al. Illicit drug use and HIV treatment outcomes in a US cohort. AIDS. 2008;28:357–65.
9. Lucas GM, Gebo KA, Chaisson RE, Moore RD. Longitudinal assessment of the effects of drug and alcohol abuse on HIV-1 treatment outcomes in an urban clinic. AIDS. 2002;16:767–74.
10. Rosen MI, Black AC, Arnsten JH, Goggin K, Remien RH, Simoni JN, et al. Association between use of specific drugs and antiretroviral adherence: findings from MACH 14. AIDS Behav. 2013;17:142–7.
11. Bruce RD, Kresina TF, McCance-Katz EF. Medication-assisted treatment and HIV/AIDS: aspects in treating HIV-infected drug users. AIDS. 2010;24:331–40.
12. Altice FL, Bruce RD, Lucas GM, Lum PJ, Korthius PT, Flanigan TP, et al. HIV treatment outcomes among HIV-infected, opioid-dependent patients receiving buprenorphine/naloxone treatment within HIV clinical care settings: results from a multisite study. J Acquir Immune Def Synd. 2011;56:S22–32.
13. Edelman EJ, Chantarat T, Caffrey S, Chaudhry A, O'Connor PG, Weiss L, et al. The impact of buprenorphine/naloxone treatment on HIV risk behaviors among HIV-infected, opioid-dependent patients. Drug Alcohol Depend. 2014;139:79–85.
14. Vagenas P, Azar MM, Copenhaver MM, Springer SA, Molina PE, Altice FL. The impact of alcohol use and related disorders on the HIV continuum of care: a systematic review. Curr HIV-AIDS Rep. 2015;12:421–36.
15. Lucas GM, Griswold M, Gebo KA, Keruly J, Chaisson RE, Moore RD. Illicit drug use and HIV-1 disease progression: a longitudinal study in the era of highly active antiretroviral therapy. Am J Epidemiol. 2006;163:412–20.
16. Messer LC, Quinlivan EB, Parnell H, Roytburd K, Adimora AA, Bowditch N, et al. Barriers and facilitators to testing, treatment entry, and engagement in care by HIV-positive women of color. AIDS Patient Care ST. 2013;27:398–407.
17. Colasanti J, Kelly J, Pennisi E, Hu YJ, Root C, Hughes D, et al. Continuous retention and viral suppression provide further insights into the HIV care continuum compared to the cross-sectional HIV care cascade. Clin Infect Dis. 2016;62:648–54.
18. Colasanti J, Stahl N, Farber EW, del Rio C, Armstrong WS. An exploratory study to assess individual and structural level barriers associated with poor retention and re-engagement in care among person living with HIV/AIDS. J Acquir Immune Defic Syndr. 2017;74:S113–20.
19. Del Rio C, Mayer K. A tale of 2 realities: What are the challenges and solutions to improving engagement in HIV care? Clin Infect Dis. 2013;57:1172–4.
20. Substance Abuse and Mental Health Services Administration. The NSDUH report: HIV/AIDS and substance use. 2010. http://www.samhsa.gov/data/2k10/HIV-AIDS/HIV-AIDs.htm. Accessed 7 Dec 2016.
21. Iralu J, Duran B, Pearson CR, Jiang Y, Foley K, Harrison M. Risk factors for HIV disease progression in a rural Soutwest American indian population. Public Health Rep. 2010;125:S43–50.
22. Kalichman SC, Grebler T, Amaral CM, McKerey M, White D, Kalichman MO, et al. Assumed infectiousness, treatment adherence and sexual behaviors: applying the Swiss statement on infectiousness to HIV positive alcohol drinkers. HIV Med. 2013;14:263–72.
23. Palepu A, Milloy MJ, Kerr T, Zhang R, Wood E. Homelessness and adherence to antiretroviral therapy among a cohort of HIV-infected injection drug users. J Urban Health. 2011;88:545–55.
24. Sullivan KA, Messer LC, Quinlivan EB. Substance abuse, violence, and HIV/AIDS (SAVA) syndemic effects on viral suppression among HIV positive women of color. AIDS Patient Care ST. 2015;29:S42–8.
25. Leblanc NM, Dalmacio DF, Barroso J. Facilitators and barriers to HIV screening: a qualitative meta-synthesis. Qual Health Res. 2016;26:294–306.
26. Robertson M, Wei SC, Beer L, Adedinsewo D, Stockwell S, Dombrowski JC, et al. Delayed entry into HIV medical care in a nationally representative sample of HIV-infected adults receiving medical care in the USA. AIDS Care. 2016;28:325–33.
27. Springer SA, Larney S, Alam-Mehrjerdi Z, Altice FL, Metzger D, Shoptaw S. Drug treatment as HIV prevention among women and girls who inject drugs from a global perspective: progress, gaps, and future directions. J Acquir Immune Def Synd. 2015;69:S155–61.
28. Aletraris L, Roman PM. Provision of onsite HIV services in substance use disorder treatment programs: a longitudinal analysis. J Subst Abuse Treat. 2015;57:1–8.
29. Centers for Disease Control and Prevention. Syringe services programs. 2016. http://www.cdc.gov/hiv/risk/ssps.html. Accessed 1 Dec 2016.
30. University of California—Berkeley, Univeristy of California—San Francisco. The public health impact of needle exchange programs in the United States and Abroad. Summary, conclusions, and recommendations. 1993. http://caps.ucsf.edu/uploads/pubs/reports/pdf/NEPReportSummary1993.pdf. Accessed 7 Dec 2016.
31. Altice FL, Springer S, Buitrago M, Hunt DP, Friedland GH. Pilot study to enhance HIV care using needle exchange-based health services for out-of-treatment injecting drug users. J Urban Health. 2003;80:416–27.
32. Drucker E, Lurie P, Wodak A, Alcabes P. Measuring harm reduction: the effects of needle and syringe exchange programs and methadone maintenance on the ecology of HIV. AIDS. 1998;12:S217–30.
33. Heimer R. Can syringe exchange serve as a conduit to substance abuse treatment? J Subst Abuse Treat. 1998;15:183–91.
34. Heimer R, Grau LE, Curtin E, Khoshnood K, Singer M. Should HIV testing programs for urban injection drug users be expanded? Am J Public Health. 2007;97:110–6.
35. Lambers FA, Stolte IG, van den Berg CH, Coutinho RA, Prins M. Harm reduction intensity: Its role in HAART adherence amongst drug users in Amsterdam. Int J Drug Policy. 2011;22:210–8.
36. Paone D, Des Jarlais DC, Clark J, Shi Q, Krim M, Purchase D. Update: syringe-exchange programs—United States, 1996. Morb Mortal Wkly Rep. 1997;26:565–8.
37. Strathdee SA, Ricketts EP, Huettner S, Cornelius L, Bishai D, Havens JR, et al. Facilitating entry into drug treatment among injection drug users referred from a needle exchange program: Results from a community-based behavioral intervention trial. Drug Alcohol Depen. 2006;83:225–32.
38. Wodak A, Cooney A. Effectiveness of sterile needle and syringe programming in reducing HIV/AIDS among injecting drug users. In *Evidence for Action Technical Papers*. 2004. http://www.who.int/hiv/pub/prev_care/en/effectivenesssterileneedle.pdf. Accessed 7 Dec 2016.
39. Axelrad JE, Mimiaga MJ, Grasso C, Mayer KH. Trends in the spectrum of engagement in HIV care and subsequent clinical outcomes among men who have sex with men (MSM) at a Boston community health center. AIDS Patient Care ST. 2013;27:287–96.
40. Okeke N, McFarland W, Raymond HF AB. Closing the gap? The HIV continuum in care for African-American men who have sex with men, San

Francisco, 2004–2014. AIDS Behav. 2016. http://link.springer.com/article/1 0.1007%2Fs10461-016-1472-0. Accessed 5 July 2016.

41. Cook CL, Lutz BJ, Young ME, Hall A, Stacciarini JM. Perspectives of linkage to care among people diagnosed with HIV. J Assoc Nurses AIDS Care. 2015;26:110–26.

42. Connecticut Department of Public Health. HIV Surveillance Report. Trend in HIV infection cases by year of diagnoses. 2015. http://www.ct.gov/dph/lib/dph/aids_and_chronic/surveillance/statewide/ct_table4_hivaids.pdf. Accessed Mar 1 2017.

43. Massachusetts Department of Public Health. Massachusetts HIV/AIDS Data Fact Sheet: The Massachusetts HIV/AIDS Epidemic at a Glance. 2015. http://www.mass.gov/eohhs/docs/dph/aids/2015-profiles/epidemic-glance.pdf. Accessed Mar 1 2017.

44. Rhode Island Department of Health. 2015 Rhode Island HIV/AIDS epidemiological profile with surrogate data. 2016. http://www.health.ri.gov/publications/epidemiologicalprofiles/2015HIVAndSurrogateData.pdf. Accessed Mar 1 2017.

45. Blankenship K, Bray S, Merson M. Structural interventions in public health. AIDS. 2000;14:S11–21.

46. Baral S, Logie CH, Grosso A, Wirtz AL, Beyrer C. Modified social ecological model: a tool to guide the assessment of the risks and risk contexts of HIV epidemics. BMC Public Health. 2013;13:482.

47. Bronfenbrenner U. The ecology of human development: experiments by nature and design. Cambridge: Harvard University Press; 1979.

48. Braun V, Clarke V. Using thematic analysis in psychology. Qual Res Psychol. 2006;3:77–101.

49. Braun V, Clarke V. Successful qualitative research: a practical guide for beginners. 1st ed. Thousand Oaks: SAGE Publications Ltd; 2013.

50. Henwood K, Pidgeon NF. Qualitative research and psychological theorizing. Br J Psychol. 1992;83:97–111.

51. Earnshaw VA, Chaudoir SR. From conceptualizing to measuring HIV stigma: a review of HIV stigma mechanism measures. AIDS Behav. 2009;13:1160–77.

52. Gardner LI, Giordano TP, Marks G, Wilson TE, Craw JA, Drainoni ML, et al. Enhanced personal contact with HIV patients improves retention in primary care: a randomized trial in 6 US HIV clinics. Clin Infect Dis. 2014;59:725–34.

53. Krentz HB, MacDonald J, Gill MJ. High mortality among human immunodeficiency virus (HIV)-infected individuals before accessing or linking to HIV care: a missing outcome in the cascade of care? Open Forum Infect Dis. 2014;1:ofu011.

54. Castel AD, Tang W, Peterson J, Mikre M, Parenti D, Elion R, et al. Sorting through the lost and found: Are patient perceptions of engagement in care consistent with standard continuum of care measures? J Acquir Immune Def Synd. 2015;69:S44–55.

55. Kalichman SC, Amaral CM, White D, Swetsze C, Pope H, Kalichman MO, et al. Prevalence and clinical implications of interactive toxicity beliefs regarding mixing alcohol and antiretroviral therapies among people living with HIV/AIDS. AIDS Patient Care ST. 2009;23:449–54.

56. Samet JH, Horton NJ, Traphagen ET, Lyon SM, Freedberg KA. Alcohol consumption and HIV disease progression: Are they related? Alcohol Clin Exp Res. 2003;27:862–7.

57. Sankar A, Wunderlich T, Neufeld S, Luborsky M. Seropositive African Americans' beliefs about alcohol and their impact on anti-retroviral adherence. AIDS Behav. 2007;11:195–203.

58. Kuchinad KE, Hutton HE, Monroe AK, Anderson G, Moore RD. A qualitative study of barriers to and facilitators of optimal engagement in care among PLWH and substance use/misuse. BMC Res Notes. 2016;9:229.

59. Dombrowski JC, Simoni JM, Katz DA, Golden MR. Barriers to HIV care and treatment among participants in a public health HIV care relinkage program. AIDS Patient Care ST. 2015;29:279–87.

60. Charlesworth JM, McManus E. Delivering patient-centred care in rural family practice: using the patient's concept of health to guide treatment. BMJ Case Rep. 2017. https://www.ncbi.nlm.nih.gov/pubmed/28069782. Accessed 5 April 2017.

61. Dang BN, Westbrook RA, Njue SM, Giordano TP. Building trust and rapport early in the new doctor-patient relationship: a longitudinal qualitative study. BMC Med Educ. 2017;17:32.

62. Gardner LI, Metsch LR, Anderson-Mahoney P, Loughlin AM, delRio C, Strathdee S, et al. Efficacy of a brief case managment intervention to link recently diagnosed HIV-infected persons to care. AIDS. 2005;19:423–31.

63. Shah M, Risher K, Berry SA, Dowdy DW. The epidemiologic and economic impact of improving HIV testing, linkage, and retention in care in the United States. Clin Infect Dis. 2016;62:220–9.

64. Skarbinski J, Rosenberg E, Paz-Bailey G, Hall HI, Rose CE, Viall AH, et al. Human immunodeficiency virus transmission at each step of the care continuum in the United States. JAMA Intern Med. 2015;175:588–96.

65. Kamarulzaman A, Altice FL. Challenges in managing HIV in people who use drugs. Curr Opin Infect Dis. 2015;28:10–6.

66. Hallum-Montes R, Manoloudis T, D'Souza R, Wrisby C, Cicatelli B, Cousins S, et al. Results of a peer navigation pilot program to link HIV positive clients of harm reduction services with Ryan White Clinical Service Providers. J Public Health Epidemiol. 2013;5:56–8.

67. Tobias C, Cunningham WE, Cunningham CO, Pounds MB. Making the connection: the importance of engagement and retention in HIV medical care. AIDS Patient Care ST. 2007;21:S3–8.

68. Meyer JP, Althoff AL, Altice FL. Optimizing care for HIV-infected people who use drugs: evidence-based approaches to overcoming healthcare disparities. Clin Infect Dis. 2013;57:1309–17.

69. Schackman BR, Leff JA, Botsko M, Fiellin DA, Altice FL, Korthuis PT, et al. The cost of integrated HIV care and buprenorphine/naloxone treatment: results of a cross-site evaluation. J Acquir Immune Def Synd. 2011;56:S76–82.

70. Risher K, Mayer KH, Beyrer C. HIV treatment cascade in MSM, people who inject drugs, and sex workers. Curr Opin HIV AIDS. 2015;10:420–9.

71. Temple University Beasley School of Law. Non-prescription access to sterile syringes. 2008. http://www.temple.edu/lawschool/phrhcs/otc.htm. Accessed 1 Dec 2016.

72. Bowman S, Grau LE, Singer M, Scott G, Heimer R. Factors associated with hepatitis B vaccine series completion in a randomized trial for injection drug users reached through syringe exchange programs in three US cities. BMC Public Health. 2014;14:820.

73. Grau LE, Arevalo S, Catchpool C, Heimer R. Expanding harm reduction services via wound and abscess clinic. Am J Public Health. 2002;12:1915–7.

74. Grenfell P, Baptista Leite R, Garfein R, de Lussigny S, Platt L, Rhodes T. Tuberculosis, injecting drug use and integrated HIV-TB care: a review of the literature. Drug Alcohol Depend. 2013;129:180–209.

75. Perlman DC, Perkins MP, Solomon N, Kochems L, Des Jarlais DC, Paone D. Tuberculosis screening at a syringe exchange program. Am J Public Health. 1997;87:862–3.

Permissions

List of Contributors

Ann Kern-Godal and Espen Walderhaug
Department of Addiction Treatment, Oslo University Hospital, Sognsvannsveien 21, Building 22, 0424 Oslo, Norway

Espen Ajo Arnevik
Department of Addiction Treatment, Oslo University Hospital, Sognsvannsveien 21, Building 22, 0424 Oslo, Norway.
Department of Psychology, University of Oslo, Oslo, Norway

Edle Ravndal
Norwegian Centre for Addiction Research (SERAF), University of Oslo, Oslo, Norway

Amelia Gulliver, Louise Farrer, Kylie Bennett, Alison L Calear and Kathleen M Griffiths
National Institute for Mental Health Research, The Australian National University, Canberra, Australia

Jade KY Chan
School of Psychology, University of New South Wales, Sydney, Australia

Robert J Tait
National Institute for Mental Health Research, The Australian National University, Canberra, Australia
National Drug Research Institute, Faculty of Health Sciences, Curtin University, Perth, Australia

John-Kåre Vederhus
Addiction Unit, Sørlandet Hospital HF, PO Box 4164, 604 Kristiansand, Norway

Sarah E. Zemore
Alcohol Research Group, Emeryville, CA, USA.

Jostein Rise
Norwegian Institute for Alcohol and Drug Research, Oslo, Norway

Thomas Clausen
Addiction Unit, Sørlandet Hospital HF, PO Box 4164, 604 Kristiansand, Norway
Norwegian Center for Addiction Research, University of Oslo, Oslo, Norway
Fulbright Scholar (2014–15), Alcohol Research Group, Emeryville, CA, USA

Magnhild Høie
University of Agder, Grimstad, Norway

Monica Bawor
MiNDS Neuroscience Program, McMaster University, Hamilton, ON, Canada
Population Genomics Program, Chanchlani Research Centre, McMaster University, Hamilton, ON, Canada
Peter Boris Centre for Addictions Research, St. Joseph's Healthcare Hamilton, Hamilton, ON, Canada

Brittany B. Dennis
Population Genomics Program, Chanchlani Research Centre, McMaster University, Hamilton, ON, Canada
Peter Boris Centre for Addictions Research, St. Joseph's Healthcare Hamilton, Hamilton, ON, Canada
Department of Clinical Epidemiology and Biostatistics, McMaster University, Hamilton, ON, Canada

Charlie Tan
Michael G. DeGroote School of Medicine, McMaster University, Hamilton, ON, Canada

Guillaume Pare
Population Genomics Program, Chanchlani Research Centre, McMaster University, Hamilton, ON, Canada
Department of Clinical Epidemiology and Biostatistics, McMaster University, Hamilton, ON, Canada
Department of Pathology and Molecular Medicine, McMaster University, Hamilton, ON, Canada

Michael Varenbut, Jeff Daiter and Carolyn Plater
Canadian Addiction Treatment Centres (CATC), Richmond Hill, ON, Canada

Andrew Worster
Department of Clinical Epidemiology and Biostatistics, McMaster University, Hamilton, ON, Canada
Canadian Addiction Treatment Centres (CATC), Richmond Hill, ON, Canada
Department of Medicine, McMaster University, Hamilton, ON, Canada

David C. Marsh
Canadian Addiction Treatment Centres (CATC), Richmond Hill, ON, Canada
Northern Ontario School of Medicine, Laurentian Campus, Sudbury, ON, Canada

Meir Steiner
Department of Psychiatry and Behavioural Neurosciences, McMaster University, Hamilton, ON, Canada
Women's Health Concerns Clinic, St. Joseph's Healthcare Hamilton, Hamilton, ON, Canada
Department of Obstetrics and Gynecology, McMaster University, Hamilton, ON, Canada

Rebecca Anglin
Department of Medicine, McMaster University, Hamilton, ON, Canada
Department of Psychiatry and Behavioural Neurosciences, McMaster University, Hamilton, ON, Canada

Dipika Desai
Population Genomics Program, Chanchlani Research Centre, McMaster University, Hamilton, ON, Canada

Lehana Thabane
Department of Clinical Epidemiology and Biostatistics, McMaster University, Hamilton, ON, Canada

Alex H. Kral, Andrea M. Lopez and Jennifer Lorvick
RTI International, 351 California St, Suite 500, San Francisco, CA 94104, USA

Megan Comfort
RTI International, 351 California St, Suite 500, San Francisco, CA 94104, USA
University of California, San Francisco, San Francisco, CA, USA

Isra Y. Mizher and Shahd I. Fawaqa
College of Medicine and Health Sciences, An-Najah National University, Nablus 44839, Palestine

Waleed M. Sweileh
Department of Physiology, Pharmacology, and Toxicology, College of Medicine and Health Sciences, An-Najah National University, Nablus 44839, Palestine

Biostatistics Unit, Centre for Evaluation of Medicine, Hamilton, ON, Canada
System Linked Research Unit, Hamilton, ON, Canada

Zainab Samaan
MiNDS Neuroscience Program, McMaster University, Hamilton, ON, Canada
Population Genomics Program, Chanchlani Research Centre, McMaster University, Hamilton, ON, Canada
Peter Boris Centre for Addictions Research, St. Joseph's Healthcare Hamilton, Hamilton, ON, Canada.
Department of Clinical Epidemiology and Biostatistics, McMaster University, Hamilton, ON, Canada
Department of Psychiatry and Behavioural Neurosciences, McMaster University, Hamilton, ON, Canada
Mood Disorders Program, St. Joseph's Healthcare Hamilton, 100 West 5th St., Hamilton, ON L8N 3K7, Canada

Sigmund J. Kharasch
Division of Pediatric Emergency Medicine, Massachusetts General Hospital, Harvard Medical School, Zero Emerson Place, Suite 3B, Boston, MA 02114, USA

David R. McBride
Division of Student Affairs, University of Maryland, College Park, Campus Drive, Building 140, College Park, MD 20742, USA

Richard Saitz
Department of Community Health Sciences, Boston University School of Public Health, 801 Massachusetts Ave, 4th Floor, Boston, MA 02118, USA

Ward P. Myers
Department of Emergency Medicine, Boston Medical Center, Boston University School of Medicine, One Boston Medical Center Place, Boston, MA 02118, USA

Zarnie Khadjesari
Department of Primary Care and Population Health, UCL Royal Free Campus, Upper Third Floor, Rowland Hill Street, London NW3 2PF, UK.
Health Service and Population Research Department, Centre for Implementation Science, Institute of Psychiatry, Psychology and Neuroscience, King's College London, De Crespigny Park, London SE5 8AF, UK

Ian R. White
MRC Biostatistics Unit, Cambridge Institute of Public Health, Forvie Site, Robinson Way, Cambridge Biomedical Campus, Cambridge CB2 0SR, UK

Jim McCambridge and Christine Godfrey
Department of Health Sciences, Seebohm Rowntree Building, University of York, Heslington, York YO10 5DD, UK

Louise Marston, Paul Wallace and Elizabeth Murray
Department of Primary Care and Population Health, UCL Royal Free Campus, Upper Third Floor, Rowland Hill Street, London NW3 2PF, UK

Karen Chan Osilla, Susan M. Paddock, Elizabeth J. D'Amico, Brett A. Ewing and Katherine E. Watkins
RAND Corporation, 1776 Main Street, Santa Monica, CA 90407-2138, USA

Thomas J. Leininger
Department of Statistical Science, Duke University, Box 90251, Durham, NC 27708-0251, USA

Mersha Chetty and Sue Langham
PHMR Ltd, London, UK

James J. Kenworthy and William C. N. Dunlop
Mundipharma International Ltd, Cambridge Science Park, Milton Road, Cambridge CB4 0GW, UK

Andrew Walker
University of Glasgow, Glasgow, UK

Anette Søgaard Nielsen and Bent Nielsen
Department of Psychiatry, Odense University Hospital, DK-5000 Odense C, Denmark
Unit of Clinical Alcohol Research, Clinical Institute, University of Southern
Denmark, DK-5000 Odense C, Denmark

Adrienne Cheung and Anita Palepu
Department of Medicine, Centre for Health Evaluation and Outcome Sciences, University of British Columbia, 588B-1081 Burrard Street, Vancouver, BC V6Z 1Y6, Canada

Julian M Somers Akm Moniruzzaman and Michelle Patterson
Faculty of Health Sciences, Simon Fraser University, Vancouver, Canada

Charles J Frankish
School of Population and Public Health, Vancouver, Canada

Michael Krausz
School of Population and Public Health, Vancouver, Canada
Department of Psychiatry, University of British Columbia, Vancouver, Canada

Laura S. Ellerbe, Luisa Manfredi, Shalini Gupta, Tyler E. Phelps, Thomas R. Bowe and Alex H. S. Harris
Center for Innovation to Implementation, Department of Veterans Affairs (VA) Palo Alto Health Care System, 795 Willow Road (MPD-152), Menlo Park, CA 94025, USA

Anna D. Rubinsky
Department of Medicine, University of California, San Francisco and the San Francisco VA Medical Center, San Francisco, CA, USA

Jennifer L. Burden
Salem VA Medical Center, Salem, VA, USA

Keith Ahamad
British Columbia Centre for Excellence in HIV/AIDS, St. Paul's Hospital, 1081 Burrard Street, Vancouver, BC V6Z 1Y6, Canada. 2Department of Family Practice, University of British Columbia, 5950 University Boulevard Street, Vancouver, BC V6T 1Z3, Canada

MJ Milloy, Paul Nguyen, Sasha Uhlmann, Cheyenne Johnson and Thomas Kerr
British Columbia Centre for Excellence in HIV/AIDS, St. Paul's Hospital, 1081 Burrard Street, Vancouver, BC V6Z 1Y6, Canada

Todd P Korthuis
Department of Medicine, Oregon Health and Science University, 3181 SW Sam Jackson Park Rd, Portland, OR 97239, USA
Department of Public Health-Preventive Medicine, Oregon Health and Science University, 3181 SW Sam Jackson Park Rd, Portland, OR 97239, USA

Evan Wood
British Columbia Centre for Excellence in HIV/AIDS, St. Paul's Hospital, 1081 Burrard Street, Vancouver, BC V6Z 1Y6, Canada

Department of Medicine, University of British Co-lumbia, 10th Floor 2775 Laurel Street, Vancouver, BC V5Z 1M9, Canada
Division of Epidemiology and Population Health, BC Centre for Excellence in HIV/AIDS, 608-1081 Burrard Street, Vancouver, BC V6Z 1Y6, Canada

Anna E. Ordóñez
Department of Psychiatry and UCSF Weill Institute for Neurosciences, University of California, 401 Parnassus Avenue, San Francisco, CA 94143, USA
Office of Clinical Research, National Institute of Mental Health, 6001 Executive Blvd. MSC 9669, Bethesda, MD 20892, USA

Rachel Ranney, Maxine Schwartz
Department of Psychiatry and UCSF Weill Institute for Neurosciences, University of California, 401 Parnassus Avenue, San Francisco, CA 94143, USA

Carol A. Mathews
Department of Psychiatry and UCSF Weill Institute for Neurosciences, University of California, 401 Parnassus Avenue, San Francisco, CA 94143, USA
Department of Psychiatry, University of Florida, 100 S Newell Drive, Gainesville, FL 32610, USA

Derek D. Satre
Department of Psychiatry and UCSF Weill Institute for Neurosciences, University of California, 401 Parnassus Avenue, San Francisco, CA 94143, USA
Division of Research, Kaiser Permanente Northern California Region, 2000 Broadway, 3rd Floor, Oakland, CA 94612, USA

Anthony J. Accurso, Darius A. Rastegar, Sharon R. Ghazarian and Michael I. Fingerhood
Johns Hopkins Bayview Medical Center, 5200 Eastern Ave, Mason F. Lord Bldg, West Tower 5th floor, Baltimore, MD 21224, USA

Aaron D Fox, Joanna L Starrels and Chinazo O Cunningham
Albert Einstein College of Medicine, Bronx, NY 10461, USA
Montefiore Medical Center, Bronx, NY 10467, USA

Jeronimo Maradiaga
Albert Einstein College of Medicine, Bronx, NY 10461, USA

Linda Weiss
New York Academy of Medicine, New York, NY 10029, USA

Jennifer Sanchez
Montefiore Medical Center, Bronx, NY 10467, USA

Ryan P. Westergaard
Department of Medicine, University of Wisconsin School of Medicine and Public Health, Madison, WI, USA
University of Wisconsin-Madison, 1685 Highland Ave, MFCB 5223, Madison, WI 53705-2281, USA

Andrew Genz
Department of Epidemiology, Johns Hopkins Bloomberg School of Public Health, Baltimore, MD, USA

Kristen Panico
Department of Population, Family and Reproductive Health, Johns Hopkins Bloomberg School of Public Health, Baltimore, MD, USA

Pamela J. Surkan
Department of International Health, Johns Hopkins Bloomberg School of Public Health, Baltimore, MD, USA

Jeanne Keruly and Larry W. Chang
Department of Medicine, Johns Hopkins School of Medicine, Baltimore, MD, USA

Heidi E. Hutton
Department of Psychiatry and Behavioral Sciences, Johns Hopkins School of Medicine, Baltimore, MD, USA

Gregory D. Kirk
Department of Epidemiology, Johns Hopkins Bloomberg School of Public Health, Baltimore, MD, USA
Department of Medicine, Johns Hopkins School of Medicine, Baltimore, MD, USA

Jan Klimas
British Columbia Centres on Substance Use and Excellence in HIV/AIDS, St. Paul's Hospital, 608-1081 Burrard Street, Vancouver, BC V6Z 1Y6, Canada
Department of Medicine, University of British Co-lumbia, St. Paul's Hospital, 608-1081 Burrard Street, Vancouver, BC V6Z 1Y6, Canada
School of Medicine, University College Dublin, Health Sciences Centre, Belfield, Dublin 4, Ireland

Huiru Dong and Rolando Barrios
British Columbia Centres on Substance Use and Excellence in HIV/AIDS, St. Paul's Hospital, 608-1081 Burrard Street, Vancouver, BC V6Z 1Y6, Canada

Nadia Fairbairn and Eugenia Socías
British Columbia Centres on Substance Use and Excellence in HIV/AIDS, St. Paul's Hospital, 608-1081 Burrard Street, Vancouver, BC V6Z 1Y6, Canada
School of Medicine, University College Dublin, Health Sciences Centre, Belfield, Dublin 4, Ireland

Evan Wood, Thomas Kerr, Julio Montaner and M.-J. Milloy
British Columbia Centres on Substance Use and Excellence in HIV/AIDS, St. Paul's Hospital, 608-1081 Burrard Street, Vancouver, BC V6Z 1Y6, Canada
Department of Medicine, University of British Columbia, St. Paul's Hospital, 608-1081 Burrard Street, Vancouver, BC V6Z 1Y6, Canada

Claire Simeone
Opiate Treatment Outpatient Program, Division of Substance Abuse and Addiction Medicine, Zuckerberg San Francisco General Hospital and Trauma Center, University of California San Francisco School of Nursing, 995 Potrero Ave, Building 90, Ward 93, San Francisco, CA 94110, USA

Brad Shapiro
Opiate Treatment Outpatient Program, Division of Substance Abuse and Addiction Medicine, Departments of Psychiatry and Family and Community Medicine, Zuckerberg San Francisco General Hospital and Trauma Center, University of California San Francisco, San Francisco, CA, USA

Paula J. Lum
Division of HIV, Infectious Diseases, and Global Medicine, Department of Medicine, Zuckerberg San Francisco General Hospital and Trauma Center, University of California San Francisco, San Francisco, CA, USA

Scott P. Stumbo and Carla A. Green
Kaiser Permanente Northwest, Center for Health Research, 3800 N. Interstate Avenue, Portland, OR 97227-1110, USA

James H. Ford II
Center for Health Systems Research and Analysis, University of Wisconsin – Madison, 610 Walnut Street, Madison, WI 53726, USA

Carol Dawson-Rose, Yvette Cuca, Roland Zepf, Emily Huang and Bruce A. Cooper
UCSF School of Nursing, 2 Koret Way, San Francisco, CA 94143-0608, USA

Jessica E. Draughon
UCSF School of Nursing, 2 Koret Way, Box 0608, San Francisco, CA 94143-0608, USA.
Present Address: UC Davis Betty Irene Moore School of Nursing, 2450 48th Street, Suite 2600, Sacramento, CA 95817, USA

Paula J. Lum
Division of HIV, Infectious Diseases, and Global Medicine, UCSF Department of Medicine, San Francisco General Hospital, 1001 Potrero Ave, 307, Box 0874, San Francisco, CA 94110, USA

Maxine Stitzer, Colin Cunningham, Alexis S. Hammond and Heather Fitzsimons
Department of Psychiatry and Behavioral Sciences, Hopkins Bayview Medical Center, Johns Hopkins University School of Medicine, 5510 Nathan Shock Drive, Baltimore, MD 21224, USA

Tim Matheson
San Francisco Department of Public Health, 25 Van Ness Avenue Suite 500, San Francisco, CA 94102, USA

James L. Sorensen
UCSF Department of Psychiatry, Zuckerberg San Francisco General Hospital and Trauma Center, 1001 Potrero Avenue SFGH Building 20, Rm. 2117, San Francisco, CA 94110, USA

Daniel J. Feaster
Department of Public Health Sciences, University of Miami Miller School of Medicine, 1120 Northwest 14th Street, CRB 1059, Miami, FL 33136, USA

Lauren Gooden and Lisa R. Metsch
Department of Sociomedical Sciences, Mailman School of Public Health, Columbia University, 722 West 168th Street, Room 918, New York, NY 10032, USA

Stephanie M. Ruest
Section of Pediatric Emergency Medicine, Hasbro Children's Hospital, Alpert Medical School of Brown University, 593 Eddy St, Claverick 2, Providence, RI 02903, USA

Alexander M. Stephan
Department of Pediatrics, Massachusetts General Hospital for Children, Harvard Medical School, 55 Fruit St, Boston, MA 02114, USA

Peter T. Masiakos
Division of Pediatric Surgery, Massachusetts General Hospital for Children, Harvard Medical School, 55 Fruit St, Boston, MA 02114, USA

Paul D. Biddinger, Carlos A. Camargo and Sigmund Kharasch
Department of Emergency Medicine, Massachusetts General Hospital, Harvard Medical School, 55 Fruit St, Boston, MA 02114, USA

Bulat Idrisov
Clinical Addiction Research and Education Unit, Section of General Internal Medicine, Department of Medicine, Boston University School of Medicine/ Boston Medical Center, 801 Massachusetts Avenue, 2nd Floor, Boston, MA 02118, USA
Department of Infectious Diseases, Bashkir State Medical University, 3 Lenina St., Ufa, Bashkortostan Republic, Russian Federation 450000

Karsten Lunze
Clinical Addiction Research and Education Unit, Section of General Internal Medicine, Department of Medicine, Boston University School of Medicine/ Boston Medical Center, 801 Massachusetts Avenue, 2nd Floor, Boston, MA 02118, USA
Clinical Addiction Research and Education Unit, Section of General Internal Medicine, Department of Medicine, Boston Medical Center, 801 Massachusetts Avenue, 2nd Floor, Boston, MA 02118, USA

Debbie M. Cheng
Department of Biostatistics, Boston University School of Public Health, 801 Massachusetts Avenue, 3rd Floor, Boston, MA 02118, USA

Elena Blokhina
First St. Petersburg Pavlov State Medical University, Lev Tolstoy St. 6/8, St. Petersburg, Russian Federation 197022

Natalia Gnatienko and Carly Bridden
Clinical Addiction Research and Education Unit, Section of General Internal Medicine, Department of Medicine, Boston Medical Center, 801 Massachusetts Avenue, 2nd Floor, Boston, MA 02118, USA

Emily Quinn
Data Coordinating Center, Boston University School of Public Health, 85 E Newton St M921, Boston, MA 02118, USA

Alexander Y. Walley
Clinical Addiction Research and Education Unit, Section of General Internal Medicine, Department of Medicine, Boston University School of Medicine/ Boston Medical Center, 801 Massachusetts Avenue, 2nd Floor, Boston, MA 02118, USA

Kendall J. Bryant
HIV/AIDS Research, National Institute on Alcohol Abuse and Alcoholism, National Institute of Health, 5365 Fishers Lane, Bethesda, MD 20892, USA

Dmitry Lioznov
First St. Petersburg Pavlov State Medical University, Lev Tolstoy St. 6/8, St. Petersburg, Russian Federation 197022
Pasteur Research Institute of Epidemiology and Microbiology, Mira St. 14, St. Petersburg, Russian Federation 197101

Evgeny Krupitsky
First St. Petersburg Pavlov State Medical University, Lev Tolstoy St. 6/8, St. Petersburg, Russian Federation 197022
St. Petersburg Bekhterev Research Psychoneurological Institute, Bekhtereva St., 3, St. Petersburg, Russian Federation 192019

Jeffrey H. Sa met
Clinical Addiction Research and Education Unit, Section of General Internal Medicine, Department of Medicine, Boston University School of Medicine/ Boston Medical Center, 801 Massachusetts Avenue, 2nd Floor, Boston, MA 02118, USA
Department of Community Health Sciences, Boston University School of Public Health, 801 Massachusetts Avenue, Boston, MA 02118, USA

Michael M. Neeki, Arnold Sin and Rodney Borger
Department of Emergency Medicine, Arrowhead Regional Medical Center, Medical Office Building, Suite 7, 400 N Pepper Ave, Colton, CA 92324, USA

California University of Sciences and Medicine, 1405 W Valley Boulevard, Suite 101, Colton, CA 92321, USA

Fanglong Dong, Lidia Liang and Jake Toy
Western University of Health Sciences, College of Osteopathic Medicine of the Pacific, 309 E 2nd St., Pomona, CA 91766, USA

Sharon Brown, Braeden Carrico and Nina Jabourian
Department of Emergency Medicine, Arrowhead Regional Medical Center, Medical Office Building, Suite 7, 400 N Pepper Ave, Colton, CA 92324, USA

Farabi Hussain and David Wong
Department of General Surgery, Arrowhead Regional Medical Center, 400 N Pepper Ave, Colton, CA 92324, USA
California University of Sciences and Medicine, 1405 W Valley Boulevard, Suite 101, Colton, CA 92321, USA

Keyvan Safdari
Department of Anesthesiology, Arrowhead Regional Medical Center, 400 N Pepper Ave, Colton, CA 92324, USA
California University of Sciences and Medicine, 1405 W Valley Boulevard, Suite 101, Colton, CA 92321, USA

R. McNeil
Department of Medicine, B.C. Centre on Substance Use, St. Paul's Hospital, University of British Columbia, 608-1081 Burrard Street, Vancouver, BC V6Z 1Y6, Canada

W. Cullen
School of Medicine, Coombe Healthcare Centre, University College Dublin, Dolphins Barn, Dublin 8, Ireland

K. Ahamad, A. Mead and L. Rieb
Department of Medicine, B.C. Centre on Substance Use, St. Paul's Hospital, University of British Columbia, 608-1081 Burrard Street, Vancouver, BC V6Z 1Y6, Canada
Department of Family Practice, University of British Columbia, 1081 Burrard St., Vancouver, BC V6Z 1Y6, Canada

Department of Family and Community Medicine, St. Paul's Hospital, 1081 Burrard St., Vancouver, BC V6Z 1Y6, Canada

J. Klimas and E. Wood
Department of Medicine, B.C. Centre on Substance Use, St. Paul's Hospital, University of British Columbia, 608-1081 Burrard Street, Vancouver, BC V6Z 1Y6, Canada
School of Medicine, Coombe Healthcare Centre, University College Dublin, Dolphins Barn, Dublin 8, Ireland

W. Small
Department of Medicine, B.C. Centre on Substance Use, St. Paul's Hospital, University of British Columbia, 608-1081 Burrard Street, Vancouver, BC V6Z 1Y6, Canada
Faculty of Health Sciences, Simon Fraser University, Blusson Hall, 8888 University Drive, Burnaby, BC V5A 1S6, Canada

Barrot H. Lambdin
RTI International, 351 California St, Suite 500, San Francisco, CA 94104, USA
University of California, San Francisco, San Francisco, CA, USA
University of Washington, Seattle, WA, USA

Lauretta E. Grau, Abbie Griffiths-Kundishora and Robert Heimer
Yale School of Public Health, New Haven, CT 06520-8034, USA

Marguerite Hutcheson and Thomas J. Stopka
Tufts University School of Medicine, Boston, MA 02111, USA

Amy Nunn and Caitlin Towey
Brown University School of Public Health, Providence, RI 02912, USA

Index